Toxicology Emergencies

Editors

CHRISTOPHER P. HOLSTEGE
JOSHUA D. KING

EMERGENCY MEDICINE CLINICS OF NORTH AMERICA

www.emed.theclinics.com

Consulting Editor
AMAL MATTU

May 2022 • Volume 40 • Number 2

ELSEVIER

1600 John F. Kennedy Boulevard • Suite 1800 • Philadelphia, Pennsylvania, 19103-2899

http://www.theclinics.com

EMERGENCY MEDICINE CLINICS OF NORTH AMERICA Volume 40, Number 2
May 2022 ISSN 0733-8627, ISBN-13: 978-0-323-84886-2

Editor: Joanna Collett

Developmental Editor: Axell Ivan Jade Purificacion

Emergency Medicine Clinics of North America (ISSN 0733-8627) is published quarterly by Elsevier Inc., 360 Park Avenue South, New York, NY, 10010-1710. Months of issue are February, May, August, and November. Business and Editorial Offices: 1600 John F. Kennedy Boulevard, Suite 1800, Philadelphia, PA 19103-2899. Customer Service Office: 6277 Sea Harbor Drive, Orlando, FL 32887-4800. Periodicals postage paid at New York, NY, and additional mailing offices. Subscription prices are $100.00 per year (US students), $370.00 per year (US individuals), $963.00 per year (US institutions), $220.00 per year (international students), $476.00 per year (international individuals), $1002.00 per year (international institutions), $100.00 per year (Canadian students), $436.00 per year (Canadian individuals), and $1002.00 per year (Canadian institutions). International air speed delivery is included in all *Clinics'* subscription prices. All prices are subject to change without notice. **POSTMASTER:** Send address changes to *Emergency Medicine Clinics of North America*, Elsevier Periodicals Customer Service, 11830 Westline Industrial Drive, St. Louis, MO 63146. Customer Service (orders, claims, online, change of address): Elsevier Periodicals **Customer Service, 11830 Westline Industrial Drive, St. Louis, MO 63146. Tel: 1-800-654-2452 (U.S. and Canada); 314-453-7041 (outside U.S. and Canada). Fax: 314-453-5170. E-mail: journalscustomerservice-usa@elsevier.com (for print support); journalsonlinesupport-usa@elsevier.com (for online support).**

Reprints. For copies of 100 or more of articles in this publication, please contact the Commercial Reprints Department, Elsevier Inc., 360 Park Avenue South, New York, NY 10010-1710. Tel.: 212-633-3874; Fax: 212-633-3820; E-mail: reprints@elsevier.com.

Emergency Medicine Clinics of North America is covered in *MEDLINE/PubMed (Index Medicus), Current Contents/Clinical Medicine, EMBASE/Excerpta Medica, BIOSIS, SciSearch, CINAHL, ISI/BIOMED,* and *Research Alert.*

Contributors

CONSULTING EDITOR

AMAL MATTU, MD, FAAEM, FACEP
Professor and Vice Chair of Academic Affairs, Department of Emergency Medicine, University of Maryland School of Medicine, Baltimore, Maryland, USA

EDITORS

CHRISTOPHER P. HOLSTEGE, MD
Chief, Division of Medical Toxicology, Director, UVA Health's Blue Ridge Poison Center, Professor, Departments of Emergency Medicine and Pediatrics, University of Virginia School of Medicine, Charlottesville, Virginia, USA

JOSHUA D. KING, MD
Medical Director, Maryland Poison Center, Assistant Professor, Departments of Medicine and Pharmacy, Program Director, Nephrology Fellowship, University of Maryland, Baltimore, Maryland, USA

AUTHORS

ANN M. ARENS, MD
Department of Emergency Medicine, Hennepin Healthcare, Associate Professor, Department of Emergency Medicine, University of Minnesota, Minneapolis, Minnesota, USA

LAURA BECHTEL, PhD, DABCC
Director, Chemistry and Toxicology, Kaiser Permanente Colorado Health System, Denver, Colorado, USA

HEATHER A. BOREK, MD
Assistant Professor, Department of Emergency Medicine, Division of Medical Toxicology, University of Virginia School of Medicine, University of Virginia, Charlottesville, USA

DIANE P. CALELLO, MD, FACMT, FAAP, FAACT
Professor, Department of Emergency Medicine, Division of Medical Toxicology, Rutgers New Jersey School of Medicine, Newark, New Jersey, USA

RICHARD J. CHEN, MD
Attending Physician, Division of Medical Toxicology, Department of Emergency Medicine, Albert Einstein Medical Center, Philadelphia, Pennsylvania, USA

JON B. COLE, MD
Department of Emergency Medicine, Hennepin Healthcare, Professor, Department of Emergency Medicine, University of Minnesota, Minneapolis, Minnesota, USA

RICHARD C. DART, MD
PhD, Director, Rocky Mountain Poison and Drug Safety, Denver Health and Hospital Authority, Denver, Colorado, USA

DAVID L. ELDRIDGE, MD
Associate Professor, Department of Pediatrics, Brody School of Medicine at East Carolina University, Greenville, North Carolina, USA

AARON S. FREY, DO
Medical Toxicology Fellow, Division of Medical Toxicology, Instructor, Department of Emergency Medicine, University of Virginia School of Medicine, Charlottesville, Virginia, USA

SOPHIE GOSSELIN, MD, FRCPC, CSPQ, FAACT, FACMT
Centre Intégré de Santé et de Services Sociaux (CISSS), Montérégie-Centre Emergency Department, Hôpital Charles-Lemoyne, Greenfield Park, Centre Antipoison du Quebec, Department of Emergency Medicine, McGill University, Montreal, Québec, Canada

ROBERT S. HOFFMAN, MD, FAACT, FRCP Edin, FEAPCCT
Division of Medical Toxicology, Ronald O. Perelman Department of Emergency Medicine, NYU Grossman School of Medicine, New York, New York, USA

CHRISTOPHER P. HOLSTEGE, MD
Chief, Division of Medical Toxicology, Director, UVA Health's Blue Ridge Poison Center, Professor, Departments of Emergency Medicine and Pediatrics, University of Virginia School of Medicine, Charlottesville, Virginia, USA

BRYAN S. JUDGE, MD
Professor, Department of Emergency Medicine, Division of Medical Toxicology, Michigan State University College of Human Medicine, Spectrum Health Butterworth Emergency Department, Grand Rapids, Michigan, USA

SASHA K. KAISER, MD
Rocky Mountain Poison and Drug Safety, Denver Health and Hospital Authority, Denver, Colorado, USA

LOUISE W. KAO, MD
Professor of Clinical Emergency Medicine, Fellowship Director, Department of Emergency Medicine, Medical Toxicology, Indiana University School of Medicine, Indiana Poison Center, Indianapolis, Indiana, USA

JOSHUA D. KING, MD
Medical Director, Maryland Poison Center, Assistant Professor, Departments of Medicine and Pharmacy, Program Director, Nephrology Fellowship, University of Maryland, Baltimore, Maryland, USA

PAUL M. MANISCALCO, PhD(c), MPA, MS, EMT/P
President Emeritus, International Association EMS Chiefs, Potomac Falls, Virginia, USA

AVERY E. MICHIENZI, DO
Medical Toxicology Fellow and Clinical Instructor, Department of Emergency Medicine, Division of Medical Toxicology, University of Virginia, Charlottesville, Virginia, USA

KRISTINE A. NAÑAGAS, MD
Associate Professor of Clinical Emergency Medicine, Division Chief of Medical Toxicology, Department of Emergency Medicine, Indiana University School of Medicine, Indiana Poison Center, Indianapolis, Indiana, USA

RIKA N. O'MALLEY, MD
McLeod Health Seacoast, Little River, South Carolina, USA

MEHRUBA ANWAR PARRIS, MD, FAAEM
Assistant Professor, Department of Emergency Medicine, Division of Medical Toxicology, Rutgers New Jersey School of Medicine, Newark, New Jersey, USA

SHANNON J. PENFOUND, MPH
Indiana Poison Center Epidemiologist, Indianapolis, Indiana, USA

HALEY N. PHILLIPS, MD
Assistant Professor of Hospital Neurology, Department of Neurology, Emory University, Atlanta, Georgia, USA

JENNIFER A. ROSS, MD, MPH
Pediatric Addiction Medicine Fellow, Adolescent Substance Use and Addiction Program (ASAP), Boston Children's Hospital, Boston, Massachusetts, USA

ANNE-MICHELLE RUHA, MD
Chair, Department of Medical Toxicology, Banner University Medical Center Phoenix, Professor, University of Arizona College of Medicine, Phoenix, Arizona, USA

MATTHEW SALZMAN, MD
Assistant Professor, Division of Medical Toxicology and Addiction Medicine, Department of Emergency Medicine, Cooper Medical School of Rowan University, Camden, New Jersey, USA

LAURA TORMOEHLEN, MD
Associate Professor of Clinical Neurology and Emergency Medicine, Departments of Neurology and Emergency Medicine, Indiana University, Indiana University Neuroscience Center, Indianapolis, Indiana, USA

GEORGE P. WARPINSKI, MD
Medical Toxicology Fellow, Department of Medical Toxicology, Banner University Medical Center Phoenix, University of Arizona College of Medicine, Phoenix, Arizona, USA

Contents

EMERGENCY MEDICINE CLINICS OF NORTH AMERICA

FORTHCOMING ISSUES

August 2022
Respiratory and Airway Emergencies
Haney Mallemat and Terren Trott, *Editors*

November 2022
Cardiovascular Emergencies
Jeremy G. Berberian and Leen Albkaihed, *Editors*

February 2023
Trauma Emergencies
Kimberly A. Boswell and Christopher M. Hicks, *Editors*

RECENT ISSUES

February 2022
Allergy, Inflammatory, and Autoimmune Disorders in Emergency Medicine
Gentry Wilkerson and Salvador Suau, *Editors*

November 2021
Abdominal/GI Emergencies
Sara Manning and Nicole McCoin, *Editors*

August 2021
Pediatric Emergency Medicine
Le (Mimi) Lu, Ilene Claudius, and Christopher S. Amato, *Editors*

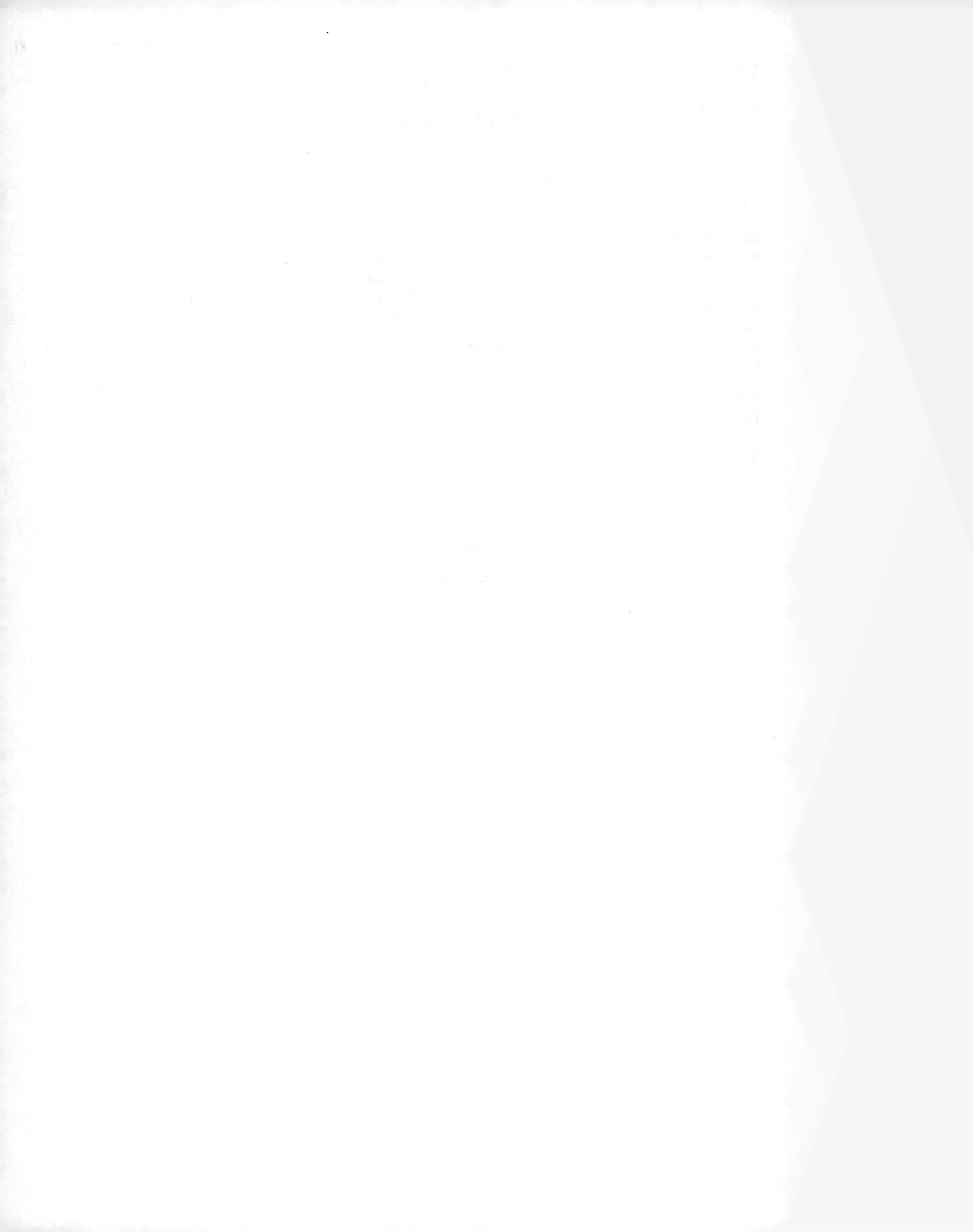

Foreword

Toxicology Emergencies

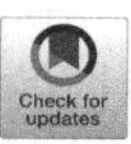

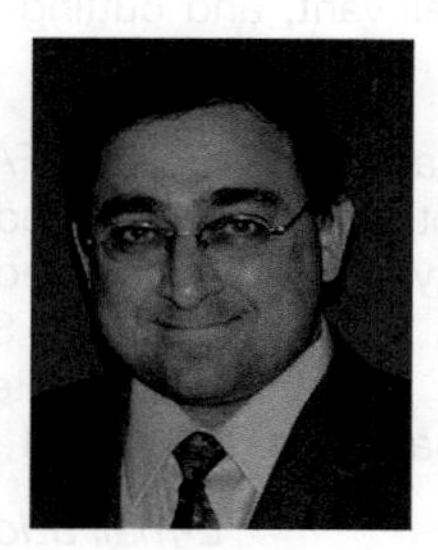

Amal Mattu, MD, FAAEM, FACEP
Consulting Editor

I recently cared for an elderly patient who presented to the emergency department for weakness and lightheadedness. During my evaluation, I asked the patient about her medications, and she pulled out a large bag. The bag contained 26 bottles of her medications...and unbelievably she was compliant with each one! Unfortunately, as I looked through the bottles, I discovered that she was taking two separate dosages of the same calcium-channel blocker and two separate dosages of the same beta-blocker, each prescribed by different providers. She was also taking multiple medications with anticholinergic effects, an over-the-counter antihistamine, and a couple of herbal supplements I had never heard of. There was little doubt that her symptoms were at least partly, if not completely, due to medication toxicity and drug interactions.

The elderly are certainly not the only patients in whom we encounter prescription medication-related toxicities. And on the other hand, toxicities do not occur purely from prescribed medications. An increasing number of patients in our emergency departments have medical issues partly or entirely due to prescribed drugs or illicit drugs. Toxicities can also occur from environmental sources of envenomations. This is certainly not new information to anyone who practices emergency medicine, and I think we all would agree that we are seeing more "toxic presentations" than ever before as the number and potency of prescription drugs and also abused drugs increase. The need for a sound knowledge of toxicology in emergency medicine is greater than ever before.

In this issue of *Emergency Medicine Clinics of North America*, Guest Editors Drs Holstege and King have assembled an outstanding group of authors to educate us on this increasing challenge in our specialty. Initial articles discuss the basic approach to the poisoned patient as well as emerging agents of abuse. An article then discusses the all-important topic of metabolic acidosis, simplifying a perennially confusing topic. Subsequent articles then discuss specific sources of toxicity and poisoning, including alcohols, caustics, carbon monoxide, snake envenomations, and cardiotoxins. Special

Emerg Med Clin N Am 40 (2022) xiii–xiv
https://doi.org/10.1016/j.emc.2022.03.001
0733-8627/22/© 2022 Published by Elsevier Inc.

articles focus on pediatric toxicology, antidotes, agitated toxidromes, toxin-induced seizures, and the use of the toxicology laboratory.

This issue of *Emergency Medicine Clinics of North America* represents a critically important addition to the emergency medicine literature. The Guest Editors and authors are to be commended for providing a single resource that covers a broad spectrum of toxicologic emergencies in a succinct, clinically relevant, and cutting-edge manner.

Amal Mattu, MD, FAAEM, FACEP
Department of Emergency Medicine
University of Maryland School of Medicine
110 South Paca Street
6th Floor, Suite 200
Baltimore, MD 21201, USA

E-mail address:
amattu@som.umaryland.edu

Preface
The Expanding Complexity of Poisonings Encountered in Emergency Medicine

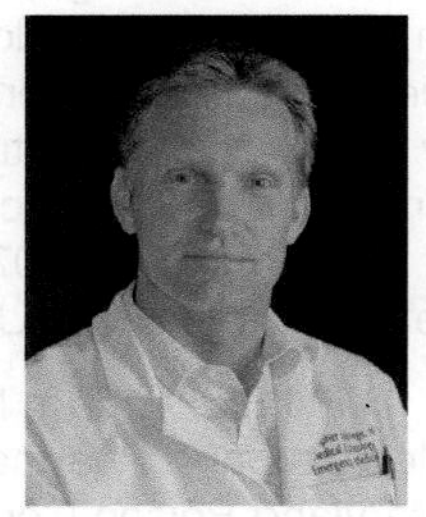

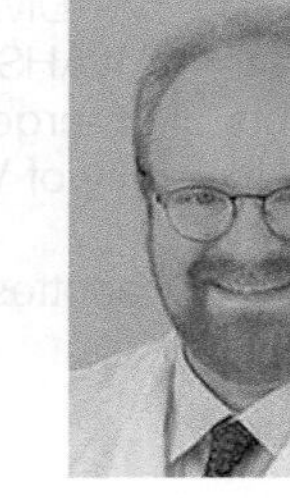

Christopher P. Holstege, MD Joshua D. King, MD
Editors

Innumerable potential toxins can inflict harm on humans, including pharmaceuticals, herbals, household products, environmental agents, occupational chemicals, substance use/misuse, and chemical terrorism threats. From the beginnings of written history, poisons and their effects have been well described. Paracelsus (1493–1541) correctly noted that "[a]ll substances are poisons; there is none which is not a poison. The right dose differentiates a poison…." As life in the modern era has become more complex, so has the study of poisons and the treatment of the patient inflicted with toxicity. Each year millions of human exposure cases are reported to poison centers across the globe, with many of those calls arising from emergency departments within their coverage area.

This issue of *Emergency Medicine Clinics of North America* is dedicated to the topic of Medical Toxicology. Medical Toxicology is a subspecialty recognized by the American Board of Medical Specialties. Physicians who have trained in this area focus their practice on the prevention, diagnosis, and management of poisoning. The field of Medical Toxicology has grown in conjunction with the emergence of new pharmaceuticals, substance use/misuse, chemicals within the workplace, and agents of terrorism. Medical Toxicology is one of very few fields where training and practice are open to those of any background; you will find that the authors for this issue share their toxicology training with Emergency Medicine, Pediatrics, Neurology, Internal Medicine, and other fields. This notwithstanding, a significant majority of medical toxicologists have primary boarding in Emergency Medicine, and nearly all medical toxicologists have a significant portion of their practice devoted to the care of patients in emergency medicine settings; the two fields are inextricably intertwined.

Emerg Med Clin N Am 40 (2022) xv–xvi
https://doi.org/10.1016/j.emc.2022.03.002
0733-8627/22/© 2022 Published by Elsevier Inc.

As the editors, we considered numerous topics for inclusion in this issue. We decided upon those topics we thought represented some of the more common, controversial, or emerging areas in our field. Within this issue, you will find a survey of topics that span the breadth of toxicology practice, ranging from toxins of recreational use to agents of malicious poisoning, management of poisonings across all age ranges, and toxins known since antiquity to those in existence for a scant few years. It is our hope that this issue will provide insight to emergency medicine personnel caring for potentially poisoned patients.

Christopher P. Holstege, MD
Division of Medical Toxicology
UVAHS Blue Ridge Poison Center
Departments of Emergency Medicine & Pediatrics
University of Virginia School of Medicine
P.O. Box 800774
Charlottesville, VA 22908-0774, USA

Joshua D. King, MD
Medicine and Pharmacy
Maryland Poison Center
University of Maryland Nephrology Fellowship
University of Maryland
220 Arch Street
Baltimore, MD 21201, USA

E-mail addresses:
ch2xf@virginia.edu (C.P. Holstege)
jdking@som.umaryland.edu (J.D. King)

Found Down: Approach to the Patient with an Unknown Poisoning

Mehruba Anwar Parris, MD, FAAEM[a,*,1],
Diane P. Calello, MD, FACMT, FAAP, FAACT[a,1]

KEYWORDS

• Toxicology • Poisonings • Decontamination • Toxidrome • Antidote

KEY POINTS

- The principles of emergency medicine (ABCs) should be applied to the initial management of the unknown toxicologic patient. Careful attention to history, vital signs, and physical examination may reveal a recognizable toxidrome or pattern of illness.
- Keeping nontoxicological and toxicologic mimics on the list of differential diagnoses will avoid misses in an unknown toxicologic patient's management.
- Urine drug immunoassays are often misleading. Focused quantitative testing for specific exposures is advised when possible but may not always be practical in the ED.
- High-quality supportive care guides the management of most patients with an unknown toxic exposure, but specific knowledge of potential decontamination methods, available antidotes, enhanced elimination techniques, and advanced supportive measures may improve patient prognosis and outcome.
- The involvement of a regional poison center and/or bedside medical toxicology service improves patient outcomes and cost of care.

INTRODUCTION

The patient in whom an unknown poisoning is suspected requires the clinician to simultaneously determine the cause of illness and to treat it. The undifferentiated poisoned patient is among the most challenging cases faced in the emergency department (ED), spurred in large part by its unknown nature and potential for life-threatening compromise. A systematic yet synchronized approach to assessment and management can increase the likelihood of the best outcome.

[a] Department of Emergency Medicine, Division of Medical Toxicology, Rutgers New Jersey School of Medicine, Newark, NJ, USA
[1] 140 Bergen St. Suite G1600, Newark, NJ 07103, USA.
* Corresponding author.
E-mail address: Mehruba.parris@rutgers.edu
Twitter: @EMToxNJ (M.A.P.)

Emerg Med Clin N Am 40 (2022) 193–222
https://doi.org/10.1016/j.emc.2022.01.011

CASE ILLUSTRATION

A 26-year-old woman is brought in by a family member. She was last seen normal the night before but is now somnolent and vomiting. Past medical history is notable for a prior suicide attempt but medications are not known. On physical examination, her vital signs demonstrate a temperature of 97.9°F, HR 110 bpm, BP 96/54 mm Hg, RR of 16/min, and SaO_2 93% on room air. She is arousable to loud verbal stimuli, tachycardic, has clammy skin and prolonged capillary refill. She has several episodes of bloody emesis in the ED.

EPIDEMIOLOGY

According to the American Association of Poison Control Centers (AAPCC) National Poison Data System (NPDS), there were 2.1 million human exposure cases reported to centers in 2019. Patients under 20 years of age comprised 57.5% of cases, and younger adults were the second most common age category with patients 20 to 39 accounting for 17.1%. Most exposures were unintentional. Death and/or major outcomes were rare (2%). However, for intentional exposures, death or major outcome was more likely (8.3%).[1]

The most common substances implicated are listed in **Table 1**, as are the most common substances in fatal exposures to multiple and single substances. Most cases involved a single substance (88%). Fatalities were more likely to be due to multiple substances (only 46% single substance exposures).

While most of the poison exposures reported to centers each year are managed at home, approximately 30% are either referred to or initiated within a health care facility. This includes unknown poisonings such as the case illustration provided above.

INITIAL CLINICAL APPROACH

Initial Stabilization

The emergency medicine mantra of airway, breathing, circulation (ABCs) is as central to the management of the patient with an unknown poisoning as it is in every patient that presents to the ED.

During the assessment of airway and breathing, paying attention to mucous membranes, secretions, lung sounds, and airway compliance may provide clues. If the patient requires airway support, rapid sequence intubation (RSI) is generally a good approach. However, other techniques may also be used:[2]

- Delayed sequence intubation (DSI)
- Awake intubation (caustic injury)
- Apneic oxygenation

Noninvasive ventilation methods may be considered for certain scenarios, such as bronchospasm from a pulmonary irritant, aspiration pneumonitis from hydrocarbons, or other moderate pulmonary effects. There is some emerging evidence to support its use in carbon monoxide poisoning as well.[3]

- High-velocity nasal cannula (HVNC)
- Bi-level or continuous positive pressure ventilation (Bi-PAP/CPAP)

Once intubated, ventilator settings will have to be optimized if there is a concern for direct pulmonary toxicity, pulmonary edema, or acute respiratory distress syndrome (ARDS). Ventilator settings should attempt to match a patient's intrinsic minute

Table 1
Most common substances implicated in overall poison exposures, fatal exposures, and single-substance fatalities (NPDS annual report 2019)

All Exposures	Fatal Exposures	Fatal Exposures- Single Substance
Analgesics[a]	Sedative/Hypnotic/Antipsychotic	Acetaminophen Alone
Household Cleaning Products	Opioids (prescription or illicit)	Opioids (prescription or illicit)
Cosmetics/Personal Care	Alcohols	Stimulants/Street Drugs
Antidepressants	Stimulants/Street Drugs	Fumes/Gases/Vapors
Sedative/Hypnotic/ Antipsychotic	Acetaminophen Alone	Alcohols
Cardiovascular Drugs	Calcium Channel Antagonists	Calcium Channel Antagonists
Antihistamines	Beta Blockers	Hypoglycemics
Foreign Bodies	Antidepressants	
Pesticides	SSRI Antidepressants	
Alcohols	Acetaminophen Combinations	

[a] Includes acetaminophen, salicylates, nonsteroidal anti-inflammatories, and opioid analgesics.

ventilation if a respiratory alkalosis is protective, such as in the case of oxidative phosphorylation inhibitors or uncouplers (eg, salicylates).

While assessing a patient's circulation, clinical evidence of perfusion, cardiac activity, and blood pressure should be assessed. If the patient has symptomatic hypertension due to poisoning:

- Benzodiazepines are first-line therapy.[4]
- Following that, the choice of antihypertensive therapy must be individualized for the likely agent causing hypertension (eg, avoidance of beta-blockers in acute cocaine intoxication).[5]

On the other hand, if a patient is found to be hypotensive:

- Fluid resuscitation and an inotrope or vasopressor is first-line therapy.
- Norepinephrine is an ideal initial agent for the undifferentiated toxicologic patient.[6]
- Determination of depressed cardiac function and/or vasoplegia via ultrasonography may help guide further pharmacotherapeutic interventions (see treatment section).
- A trial of atropine or glucagon while further stabilizing the patient is appropriate in the setting of bradycardia.

We can expand the ABCs for toxicologic patients to include disability and exposure (D&E). Disability assessment involves an initial neurologic examination to determine the level of CNS depression or excitability such as in excited delirium which may interfere with the patient's medical treatment. For agitation that is affecting patient/staff safety or severely limiting patient assessment:

- Escalating doses of benzodiazepines are preferred as they have predictable kinetics and are less likely to interact negatively with other agents or toxic exposures.

- Antipsychotics are commonly used in the ED and are generally safe but may lower the seizure threshold and worsen serotonin toxicity, neuroleptic malignant syndrome (NMS), or alcohol/GABA-A/B withdrawal.

Exposure allows the clinician to fully evaluate the patient's skin which may point to certain etiologies with cutaneous manifestations such as in the case of carbon monoxide, methemoglobin inducers, and certain metals. Investigation of patient belongings may reveal the implicated agent in the patient's clothing or personal effects.

The challenge arises, in rapidly synthesizing information from the patient, or more often, collateral providers of history, prehospital care, vital signs, physical examination, and key clinical data and determining potential toxicologic causes while not overlooking nontoxicological causes. **Fig. 1** summarizes a potential initial approach to the unknown toxicologic patient. The tables below provide common examples of findings but are not exhaustive.

The Toxidrome

The term *toxidrome* is taken from the words *toxic* and *syndrome* and is used to describe the constellation of signs and symptoms that typically result from exposure to a particular class of toxic agents. Toxidromes are best described by a combination of vital signs and appreciable effects on the body. **Table 2** highlights classic toxidromes along with some of their implicated etiologies. Notably, of the millions of different naturally occurring and man-made agents in existence, the vast majority do not have a specific toxidrome. In fact, many present with a combination of these signs and symptoms or have nonspecific findings common to many illnesses. However, when present, certain expanded toxidromes or organ system-based patterns of illness can suggest certain etiologies or at least help to exclude others (**Table 3**). This is further complicated by drugs that may mimic certain classes of drugs, multi-drug/chemical exposures, and the plethora of emerging synthetic illicit drugs acting on multiple receptors and clinically manifesting nonspecifically (see **Tables 2** and **3**).[7]

History

The patient who presents with a possible toxicologic emergency may not be able to participate in the history taking process. It is important to obtain collateral information from as many sources as possible in these circumstances. This starts with obtaining on-scene information:

- Substances present and any material information that may have been collected (eg, pill bottles, paraphernalia, and chemical bottles)
- Potential route of exposure
- Number of victims
- Scene situation (eg, indoor/outdoor space, correctional facility, residential vs nonresidential site)

Emergency Medical Services may also have information about any on-site environmental testing conducted, such as ambient carbon monoxide or hydrogen sulfide levels. If an occupational exposure occurred, contacting the facility for all potential chemical exposures is paramount. Contacting family and friends, when possible, can elucidate relevant past medical, medication, and social history. When medication history is unreliable, contacting the patient's pharmacy or reviewing the state Prescription Drug Monitoring Program may reveal the most recent prescriptions a patient filled. Using electronic medical records and more global systems that allow multi-institution integration may also prove useful in these scenarios. Furthermore, some

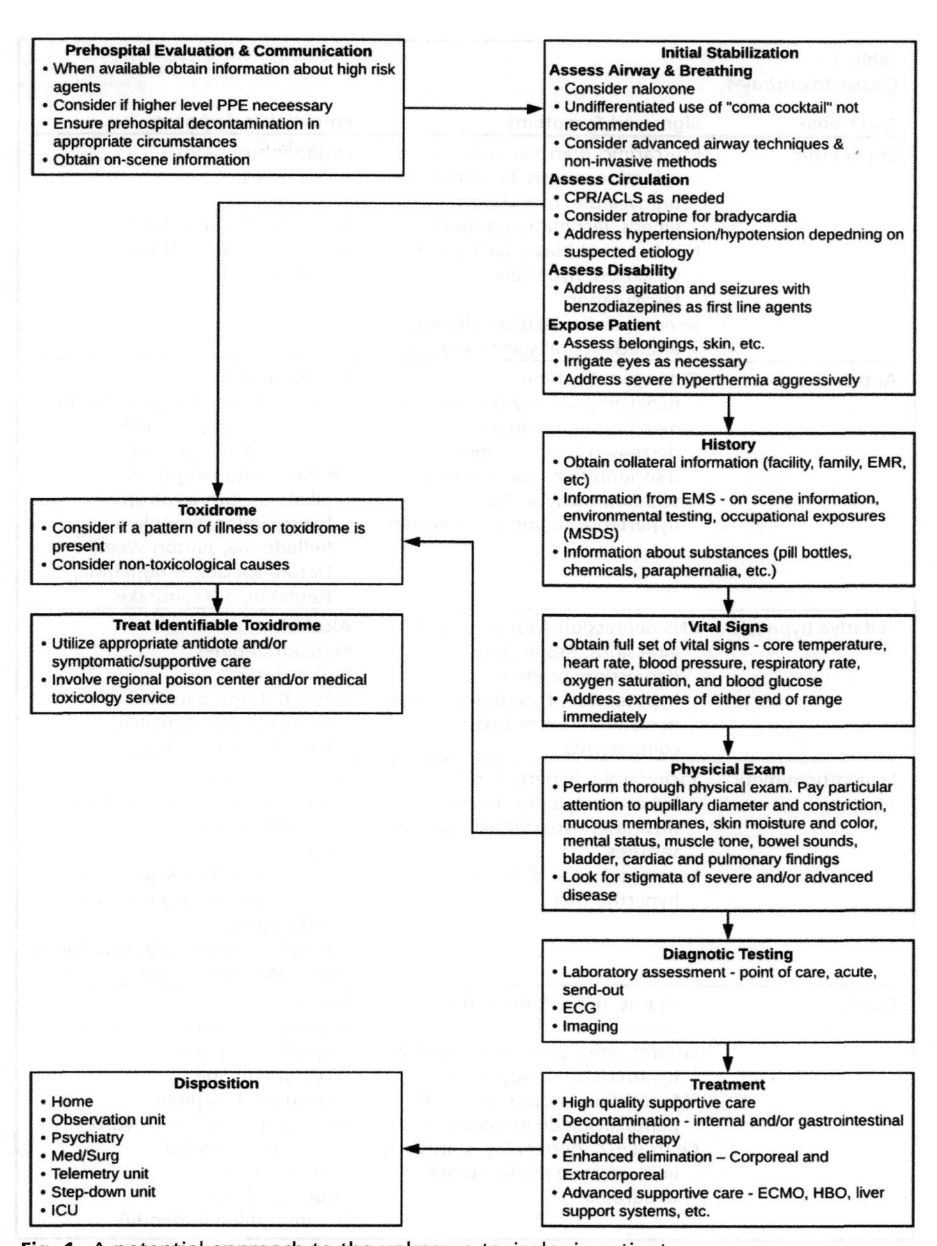

Fig. 1. A potential approach to the unknown toxicologic patient.

regional poison centers may have previous poisoning encounters documented for the same patient which may contribute to the overall current picture of the patient.

Vitals Signs

Vitals sign assessment is naturally entrenched into the initial evaluation and stabilization of a patient in the ED, as it is into the initial formulation of differential diagnosis and

Table 2
Classic toxidromes

Toxidrome	Signs and Symptoms	Potential Toxic Agent
Cholinergic	Muscarinic: diarrhea, diaphoresis, urination, miosis, bronchorrhea, bradycardia, bronchospasm, emesis, lacrimation, salivation Nicotinic: mydriasis, tachycardia, weakness, hypertension, fasciculation Severe: cardiovascular collapse, altered mental status, seizures	Organophosphates Carbamates Nicotine Neonicotinoid insecticides Medicinal carbamates (eg, physostigmine)
Anticholinergic	Cutaneous flushing, hyperthermia, dry skin/mucous membranes, mydriasis, decreased bowel sounds, disorientation, hallucination, seizures, tachycardia, hypertension, urinary retention	Antihistamines (diphenhydramine, cimetidine, meclizine, and so forth) Tricyclic antidepressants Herbals containing tropane alkaloids such as atropine, hyoscyamine, scopolamine: Belladonna, Jimson Weed/ Datura species, Brugmansia, Henbane, or Mandrake
Sedative hypnotic	CNS depression with preserved vital signs. Respiratory depression, bradycardia, hypotension, hypothermia may occur with severe toxicity or coingestants	Alcohols Benzodiazepines Barbiturates GABA B drugs: gamma-hydroxybutyrate (GBH), baclofen, and so forth
Sympathomimetic	Tachycardia, hypertension, hyperthermia, diaphoresis, mydriasis, hyperreflexia, anxiety, seizures Severe: agitated delirium, hyperthermia	Amphetamines (methamphetamine, ecstasy, MDMA, Molly) Cocaine Cathinones (Khat) & synthetic cathinones (bupropion, bath salts, flakka) Synthetic cannabinoids (K2, Spice) Ma Huang (ephedrine)
Opioid	Lethargy, miosis[a], respiratory depression. Severe: coma, pulmonary edema, hypotension, bradycardia [a]Meperidine, propoxyphene & pentazocine do not cause miosis Central α-2 agonists (eg, clonidine, imidazolines) mimic opioid toxidrome	Heroin Fentanyl, methadone & other synthetic opioids OTC: loperamide, dextromethorphan Prescription: codeine, hydro/ oxycodone, hydro/ oxymorphone Buprenorphine Desomorphine (krokodil)

evaluation for possible toxidromes. It is, therefore, extremely important to have a full set of initial vital signs which include core temperature, heart rate, blood pressure, respiratory rate, oxygen saturation, and blood glucose. **Table 3** highlights some considerations that can be made based on abnormal vital signs.[8] It should be noted that a high temperature (greater than 106°C) is more consistent with a toxic or environmental etiology than an infectious cause. The management of severe hyperthermia should be a priority in the management of the poisoned patient. Ice water immersion has been

Table 3
Table 2. Patterns of illness and potential toxic etiologies

Other Toxic Patterns of Illness	Signs and Symptoms	Potential Toxic Agent
Hallucinogen	Disorientation, hallucination, panic, altered mental status. Vital signs are usually normal.	Lysergic acid diethylamide (LSD) Phencyclidine (PCP) Peyote Psilocybin mushrooms Lysergic acid-containing plants: Morning Glory, Hawaiian Woodrose
Withdrawal/ Discontinuation Syndromes	Specific to the mechanism of action of the withdrawn agent	GABA-A agents (benzodiazepines, ethanol) GABA-B agents (barbiturates, baclofen, GBH, and so forth) Neuroleptics [a]Opioids [a]Cocaine/amphetamines (washout) [a]Cannabinoid [a]SSRI/SNRI
Hyperthermia	Elevated core temperature, altered mental status, multi-organ injury (acute liver injury, acute kidney injury, rhabdomyolysis, coagulopathy, myocardial injury, and so forth)	Serotonin toxicity Neuroleptic malignant syndrome Malignant hyperthermia Stimulant toxidrome Anticholinergic toxidrome GABA-A/B withdrawal Oxidative phosphorylation uncouplers (salicylates, dinitrophenol)
Cardiovascular	Hypotension ± Bradycardia, ECG changes, +/– CNS depression, glucose derangements	Central α agonists β antagonists Calcium channel blockers Cardiac glycosides Sodium channel modulators (veratrum alkaloids, grayanotoxin, aconite, and so forth) Antidysrhythmics

(continued on next page)

Table 3
(*continued*)

Other Toxic Patterns of Illness	Signs and Symptoms	Potential Toxic Agent
Cellular hypoxia	Airway toxicity: Cough, hoarseness, dyspnea, chest tightness, hemoptysis, dizziness, wheezing or rales, cyanosis, hypoxemia, pulmonary edema	Phosgene Ricin Ammonia Chlorine Phosphine gas Nitrogen oxides Organofluorine (Teflon) pyrolysis
	Dyshemoglobinemia: Nausea, headache, dizziness, dyspnea, confusion, coma, convulsions	Methemoglobinemia-inducing agents (nitrates, dapsone, aniline dyes, and so forth) Carbon monoxide
	Mitochondrial toxicity: Mild - nausea, vomiting, headache, dizziness, weakness Severe - altered mental status, dyspnea, hypotension, seizures, metabolic acidosis, cardiovascular collapse	Cyanide Sodium monofluoroacetate Carbon monoxide Hydrogen sulfide Sodium azide Phosphine, phosphides
Gastrointestinal illness	Abdominal pain, vomiting, profuse diarrhea (possibly bloody), dehydration, hypotension, possibly followed by multisystem organ failure	Arsenic Phosphine Dinitrophenol Colchicine Ricin Metal salts (barium, iron, copper) Cyclopeptide poisoning (eg, Amanita and Galerina mushrooms) GI Irritant mushrooms (eg, Chlorophyllum spp) Monomethylhydrazine poisoning (eg, Gyromitra mushrooms) Shigatoxin (eg, ground beef, raw vegetables) Ciguatoxin poisoning (tropical reef fish) Shellfish poisonings (mussels, clams, and so forth) Scombrotoxic fish poisoning (tuna, mackerel, bonito, and so forth)

(*continued on next page*)

Table 3
(*continued*)

Other Toxic Patterns of Illness	Signs and Symptoms	Potential Toxic Agent
Peripheral neuropathy and/or neurocognitive effects	Muscle weakness and atrophy, "glove and stocking" sensory loss, depressed or absent deep tendon reflexes, neurocognitive effects (memory loss, delirium, ataxia, and encephalopathy)	Methyl bromide (fumigant, toxic gas) Mercury (organic) Arsenic (inorganic) Thallium Lead Hexane Acrylamide Nitrous oxide Organophosphate-induced delayed polyneuropathy
	Paresthesias of face or mouth/arms/legs, headache, dizziness, nausea, and muscle incoordination	Saxitoxin - Paralytic shellfish poisoning (eg, "red tide" associated mussels, and so forth) Tetrodotoxin (eg, pufferfish) Neurotoxic shellfish poisoning (eg, oysters, clams, mussels) Ciguatoxin
	Diffuse weakness; proximal > distal dysphagia, dysarthria, ptosis, extra-ocular muscle weakness	Botulinum toxin (eg, home-canned foods, honey, and so forth) Elapid envenomation Tick paralysis
	Inebriation, hallucinations, manic behavior, delirium, deep sleep	Ibotenic acid- muscimol poisoning (eg, Amanita and Tricholoma mushrooms) Psilocybin poisoning (eg, Psilocybe and other mushrooms)
Seizures	Predominant or primary feature of poisoning: Seizures (due to direct CNS effect and not as a secondary effect such as cellular hypoxia)	Bupropion and other cathinones Sympathomimetics (cocaine, MDMA, amphetamines, and so forth) Ketamine/Phencyclidine Tetramine (Du-Shu-quiang rodenticide) Hydrazine (INH, gyromitrin) Camphor Organochlorines (Lindane) Picrotoxin Pyrethrins and pyrethroids Plants (eg, water hemlock) Methylxanthines Salicylates TCAs, diphenhydramine Severe lead exposures

(*continued on next page*)

Table 3
(continued)

Other Toxic Patterns of Illness	Signs and Symptoms	Potential Toxic Agent
Oropharyngeal pain and ulcerations	Lip, mouth, and pharyngeal ulcerations and burning pain	Paraquat Diquat Caustics (acids and alkalis) Metal salts Mustards (eg, sulfur)
Nonimmune-mediated hemolysis	Symptoms caused by massive hemolysis: malaise, dyspnea, hemoglobinuria (reddish, heme-positive urine that is often acellular), bronze discoloration of skin	Arsine (toxic industrial gas) Copper sulfate Dinitrophenol Chlorates and bromates Acetic acid Other oxidant stressors (aniline dyes, large quantities of acetaminophen, dapsone)

[a] Non life-threatening.

shown to be the most effective cooling method for environmental and toxicologic etiologies of severe hyperthermia.[9] An apparently normal oxygen saturation may in fact be falsely elevated due to specific toxicologic etiologies (**Table 4**). In general, the hallmark of sedative-hypnotic intoxication is CNS depression with the maintenance of normal vital signs; however, in severe toxicity or with certain coingestants, vital signs may be in the lower range. Furthermore, in mixed intoxications, vital sign abnormalities may change with time reflecting the mechanisms of action and pharmacokinetics of each agent.

Physical Examination

A toxicologic physical examination is also naturally incorporated into the initial stabilization of a patient, but a secondary assessment paying particular attention to certain organ systems may elucidate clues into the possible toxic etiology observed in the patient. These include:

- Pupillary diameter
- Nystagmus
- Mucous membranes
- Skin moisture and color
- Mental status
- Muscle tone
- Reflexes
- Clonus
- Bowel sounds
- Bladder, if distended

Table 5 provides a detailed list of findings in each of these systems.[10] Although odors associated with toxins are oft mentioned, odors tend to be nonspecific in actual practice and not generally useful in ED management. It should be noted that patients presenting in extremis with such findings as CNS depression, stigmata of cardiogenic (CHF) or noncardiogenic pulmonary edema (ARDS), coagulopathy from DIC, and anuria due to acute renal failure may be a manifestation of a severe toxic exposure with poor prognosis.

Table 4
Vital sign patterns and possible toxic etiologies

Vital Sign	Temperature	Heart Rate	Blood Pressure	Respiratory Rate	Oxygen Saturation	Blood Glucose
Elevated	Serotonin toxicity NMS Malignant hyperthermia Stimulants (cocaine, amphetamines, cathinones) Anticholinergic toxidrome GABA A/B withdrawal Oxidative phosphorylation uncouplers (salicylates, DNP)	Stimulants (cocaine, amphetamines, cathinones) Nicotinic agents Methylxanthines (caffeine, theophylline) β agonists Anticholinergics TCAs Bupropion GABA-A/B withdrawal	Stimulants (cocaine, amphetamines, cathinones) Nicotinic agents Methylxanthines (caffeine, theophylline) β agonists Anticholinergics TCAs Bupropion Early α2 agonists (clonidine, imidazolines) GABA-A or GABA-B withdrawal	Oxidative phosphorylation uncouplers (salicylates, DNP) Serotonin toxicity NMS\Stimulants (cocaine, amphetamines, cathinones) Pulmonary toxins (irritants, HCs, paraquat, OPs) GABA A/B withdrawal	[a]Carbon Monoxide [a]Cyanide	CCBs Methylxanthines (caffeine, theophylline) β agonists Glucagon Octreotide Stimulants (cocaine, amphetamines, cathinones)
Decreased	Sedative hypnotics (ethanol, GABA A/B) Opioids Cardiac toxins (α antagonists/ agonists, BB, CCB) Sulfonylureas α2 agonists (clonidine, imidazolines)	α2 agonists (clonidine, imidazolines) β antagonists Nondihydropyridine CCB (diltiazem, verapamil Cardiac glycosides Sodium channel modulators (veratrum alkaloids, grayanotoxin, aconite, and so forth) Antidysrhythmics Organophosphates	α2 agonists (clonidine, imidazolines) β antagonists CCBs Cardiac glycosides Sodium channel modulators (veratrum alkaloids, grayanotoxin, aconite, and so forth) Antidysrhythmics TCAs Sedative hypnotics (severe) Opioids (severe)	Opioids Sedative hypnotics (severe) Sulfonylureas α2 agonists (clonidine, imidazolines) Neurotoxins (elapid envenomation, botulinum toxin, tetrodotoxin)	Methemoglobinemia Opioid Sedative hypnotics (severe) α2 agonists (clonidine, imidazolines) Neurotoxins (elapid envenomation, botulinum toxin, tetrodotoxin)	Insulin Sulfonylureas Ethanol Salicylates (neuroglycopenia in the setting of normal BG)

[a] Falsely elevated or normal.

Table 5
Examination findings by organ systems and possible toxicologic etiologies

Organ System	Examination Finding & Possible Etiology
Ophthalmologic	Mydriasis: Stimulants, Anticholinergics Miosis: Opioids, cholinergics, α2 agonists (clonidine, imidazolines) Nystagmus: Dextromethorphan, PCP, Ketamine, scorpion envenomations, lithium, serotonin toxicity Ophthalmoplegia: Neurotoxins (elapid envenomation, botulinum toxin, tetrodotoxin) Vision loss: Methanol, caustics, quinine
ENT	Anosmia: Intranasal decongestants/zinc, hydrogen sulfide (olfactory fatigue) Dysgeusia: chemotherapeutics, radiation, caustics, radiation Tinnitus: Salicylates, NSAIDs, quinine, platinum chemotherapeutics Hearing loss: Opioids, aminoglycosides, platinum chemotherapeutics
Integumentary	Skin color change: blue (methemoglobin inducers, colloidal silver), red (carbon monoxide, cyanide), yellow (hepatotoxic drugs, carotene containing plants, tanning pills) Blistering: vesicants, chemotherapeutics, caustic burns Chemical dermatitis: caustics, hair dye components (p-Phenylenediamine), urushiol plants (poison ivy/oak/sumac), nickel Photodermatitis: Psoralen plant (lime, celery), amiodarone, 5FU, NSAIDs TEN: NSAIDs, nitrofurantoin, phenytoin, trimethoprim–sulfamethoxazole Vasculitis (purpura, breakdown): levamisole contaminated illicit drugs, NSAIDs, cephalosporins, OCPs, phenytoin Mees lines: lead, other metals, cyclophosphamide
Neurologic	CNS depression: opioid, sedative hypnotic (ethanol, GABA A/B), β antagonists, cocaine washout Generalized excitability: stimulants, anticholinergics, GABA A/B withdrawal Psychosis: glucocorticoids, stimulants Parkinson-like: carbon monoxide, hydrogen sulfide, cyanide, dopamine antagonists, dopamine agonist withdrawal, MPTP, manganese Ascending paralysis: tetrodotoxin, saxitoxin Descending paralysis: botulinum toxin, elapid envenomation Generalized paralysis: curare-like agents, cholinergics Peripheral neuropathy: Solvents (TCE, toluene, methylene chloride), ciguatoxin, vincristine/vinblastine
Cardiovascular	Murmur (valvulopathy): fenfluramine (fen-phen), ergot alkaloids (methysergide, pergolide), MDMA Stigmata of heart failure: cyclophosphamide, taxanes (paclitaxel), anthracyclines (doxorubicin), anabolic steroids, cocaine, ethanol Pericardial effusion: anticoagulants, isoniazid, carbamazepine, immune modulators (methotrexate, TNF-α drugs, sulfasalazine)
Pulmonary	Bronchospasm: cholinergics, pulmonary irritants (ammonia, chlorine), caustics Chest wall rigidity: tetanus, fentanyl, malignant hyperthermia Chest wall weakness: Neurotoxins (elapid envenomation, botulinum toxin, tetrodotoxin), curare-like agents, cholinergics Stigmata of pneumothorax: nitrous oxide, nasal insufflation of illicit drugs

(*continued on next page*)

Table 5
(continued)

Organ System	Examination Finding & Possible Etiology
Gastrointestinal	Epigastric tenderness (gastritis/PUD): caustics, NSAIDs, chemotherapeutics, ethanol, isopropyl alcohol Diarrhea: chemotherapeutics, radiation, mushrooms, many plants (calcium oxalate containing, pokeweed), colchicine, cholinergics Stigmata of liver injury: acetaminophen, many bodybuilding/weight loss supplements, amoxicillin-clavulanate, green tea extract, amatoxin
Genitourinary	Priapism: antidepressants (trazodone, bupropion), prazosin, cocaine, nitric oxide modulators (amyl nitrate "poppers," sildenafil) Enlarged bladder: Anticholinergic, antihistamines, antipsychotics, opioids Urine discoloration: milky (propofol), orange (fluoresceine, pyridium, rifampin), red (hydroxocobalamin), green/blue (propofol, methylene blue)

Additional Sources

In the initial stages of information gathering after an unknown toxicologic patient has been stabilized, there are some additional support and sources of information that are helpful to the clinician in the ED. There are significant data to support the early involvement of a regional poison center. It has been shown not only to reduce overall health care dollars but also hospital-based decrease in cost, length of stay, and patient outcome. The same is true of the involvement of a bedside medical toxicology service when available.[11,12]

If an occupational exposure had occurred, reviewing the available SDS (safety data sheet) information is invaluable. The SDS contain information on specific hazardous chemicals contained along with brief health effects and first aid instructions. These are also available online if a physical copy was not brought with the patient. When household products may be involved, having first responders gather the products from the field is also helpful. When relaying this information to the regional poison center, having the exact brand and/or active ingredients in the chemicals is important. In cases whereby pesticides were potentially involved, the Federal Insecticide,

Table 6
Toxicologic causes of elevated anion gap acidosis, according to serum lactate

Lactate Predominant	Nonlactate Predominant
Isoniazid	Ketoacidosis: alcoholic, starvation, diabetic
Iron	Methanol
Metformin	Ethylene glycol[a]
Seizures, Simple asphyxia	Acetaminophen
Ethylene glycol[a]	Toluene
Cyanide	Salicylate
Carbon Monoxide	
Thiamine deficiency	
Ibuprofen, NSAIDS	
Salicylate	

Salicylate poisoning may cause a modestly elevated lactate, but acidosis is not lactate predominant.
[a] Ethylene glycol toxicity does not cause elevated serum lactate, but glycolic acid metabolite may interfere with some analytical methods of detecting lactate and cause a false elevation.

Fungicide, and Rodenticide Act (FIFRA) mandates strict information keeping of regulated pesticides on any site.

At times, a pill or a botanic sample may be brought in with a patient. There are multiple pill identifiers available freely online and as mobile applications. The basis for identification, however, is the National Drug Code (NDC) which is etched into an untampered pill. There is also a plethora of mobile applications available as well as Facebook groups that can aid in the quick identification of botanic samples; however, regional poison centers work with local botanists and mycologists who can provide the most definitive identification.

DIAGNOSTIC TESTING

Laboratory Assessment

Following the initial assessment and stabilization, focused laboratory evaluation may yield important clues as to the etiology of illness. Although blood glucose should be measured immediately, the next phase of laboratory evaluation should include electrolytes, blood gas, and co-oximetry, and should also incorporate the calculation of the anion gap. The presence of an anion gap metabolic acidosis is a common toxicologic entity with a discrete list of potential diagnoses, which can be further narrowed to states with elevated or normal blood lactate (**Table 6**). These highlighted distinctions are not always exact, but help to frame diagnostic decision making.

A common pitfall in the initial evaluation of unknown poisoning is overreliance on the urine drug screen. Sometimes termed the "drugs of abuse" screen, this method uses immunoassay techniques to detect prototypes in several drug classes: opioids, benzodiazepines, barbiturates, phencyclidine, amphetamines, cocaine, and cannabis. However, there are frequent false positives and false negatives, and few answers which cannot be otherwise obtained through careful history and physical examination. **Table 7** highlights errors in urine drug screening.[13]

In the patient for whom either carbon monoxide poisoning is suspected, or who appears on clinical examination to be cyanotic and therefore may have methemoglobinemia, blood co-oximetry should be performed. Co-oximeters detect wavelengths reflected from hemoglobin, and in contrast to transcutaneous pulse oximetry which measures only the absorption spectra of oxy- and deoxyhemoglobin, can also

Table 7
Pitfalls in urine drug immunoassay screening

Analyte	Potential Errors
Tetrahydrocannabinol (THC, cannabis)	May be detected many days to weeks after use. Some false positives due to interference.
Benzodiazepines	Detects oxazepam, diazepam. Does not detect newer agents lorazepam, alprazolam, clonazepam
Barbiturates	Few false positives including NSAIDs and phenytoin
Cocaine	Few false positives. Detects benzoylecgonine, the presence of which may be fleeting
Phencyclidine	Many false positives due to dextromethorphan, others
Opiates	Detects morphine and natural alkaloids only (codeine, heroin). Does not detect synthetic opioids (oxycodone, fentanyl, buprenorphine) and exhibits poor reactivity with semisynthetic opioids (hydrocodone, hydromorphone)
Amphetamine	Many false positives. Detects prescription and illicit amphetamines. Does not detect some recreational amphetamines such as MDMA.

Table 8
Quantitative drug levels which may assist in the unknown poisoning patient

Drug	Reference Range (therapeutic or nonaction)
Acetaminophen	10–30 mcg/mL
Carbamazepine	4–12 mg/L
Digoxin	0.8–2 ng/mL
Ethanol	No therapeutic level
Ethylene glycol	No therapeutic level; action level >25 mg/dL
International normalized ratio (Warfarin)	1.0
Lithium	0.6–1.2 mEq/L
Methanol	No therapeutic level: action level >25 mg/dL
Phenobarbital	15–40 mg/L
Salicylates	15–30 mg/dL
Valproic acid	50–120 mg/L

measure that of carboxyhemoglobin and methemoglobin. More advanced machines may detect other rarer hemoglobin abnormalities. Of note, point-of-care transcutaneous measurement of carboxyhemoglobin is not as reliable as blood co-oximetry and should not be used as a substitute.[14]

Quantitative measurement of specific substances is indicated if the clinical picture suggests exposure. While it is common practice to empirically obtain a blood acetaminophen and salicylate concentration in the patient presenting with an intentional overdose, other quantitative levels should only be obtained if there is a suspicion of a given exposure. **Table 8** highlights commonly obtained quantitative drug concentrations.

Heavy metal testing may be considered in the patient with unexplained new-onset organ failure or clinical findings characteristic of a specific metal. For example, the patient with lead poisoning may exhibit abdominal pain and peripheral motor neuropathy with hypochromic microcytic anemia. Arsenic poisoning may cause electrocardiographic abnormalities, marked gastrointestinal distress, and later cause peripheral neuropathy, hair loss, and pancytopenia. Patients exposed to a variety of metals exhibit skin, hair, and nail abnormalities along with organ injury and neuropathy. In these cases, 24-hour urine collection for metals as well as a blood lead level may be obtained depending on the specific metal suspected.

Advanced testing may be obtained in cases of unknown exposure in which there is a concern for a novel agent or public health concern. This includes specialty laboratory analysis of unusual drugs of abuse such as fentanyl analogs, synthetic cannabinoid receptor agonists, novel psychoactives, and suspected adulterants of recreational drugs including clenbuterol, xylazine, levamisole, quinine, and others. However, these results are not obtained in clinically meaningful time frames, and generally take days to weeks. More comprehensive open-ended toxicology testing using advanced methods such as mass spectrometry may also be performed in cases of severe unexplained illness or death investigation.

The Electrocardiogram

After initial stabilization, the ECG is a key piece of clinical data in the early diagnosis and management of unknown toxicologic patient. Therefore, obtaining an ECG should be prioritized immediately after patient stabilization, and if possible, concurrently. **Table 9** summarizes important ECG findings that may point toward a possible toxicologic etiology.

Table 9
ECG effects and potential toxic causes. ECGs courtesy of Dr. De Voogt and ECGpedia.org

ECG Effect	Pathophysiology & Manifestation	Potential Toxic Agent	Examples
QRS	Sodium channel blockade manifesting as prolonged QRS interval, RBBB pattern, terminal R wave in AvR. QRS prolongation will also prolong QT interval.	Class Ia & Ic antidysrrythmics Tricyclic antidepressants Diphenhydramine Cyclobenzaprine Bupropion	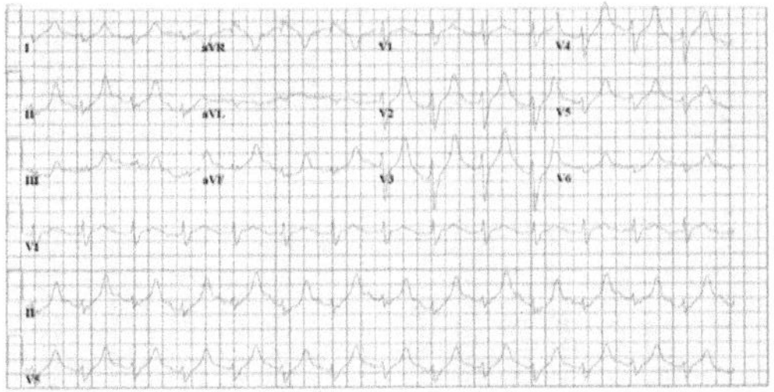
QT	QT prolongation as a result of QRS prolongation, Potassium channel blockade, hypocalcemia. Can progress to Torsades de Pointes	Class III antidysrrhythmics Antipsychotics Loperamide Antiemetics (ondanstron) Many antibiotics (azithromycin) Agents causing K+, Ca2+, or Mg2+ abnormalities (diuretics, insulin, ethylene glycol, barium salts)	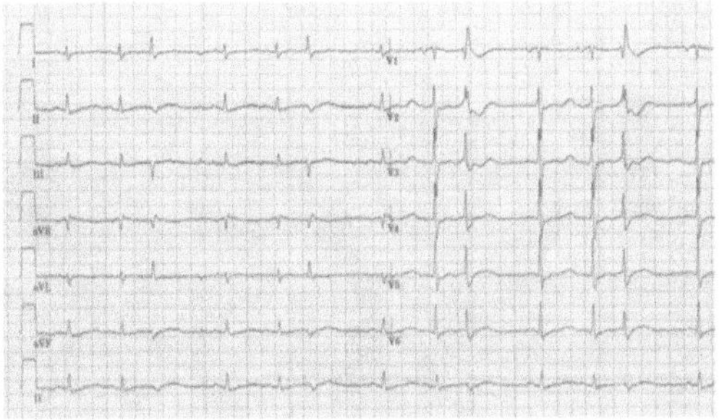

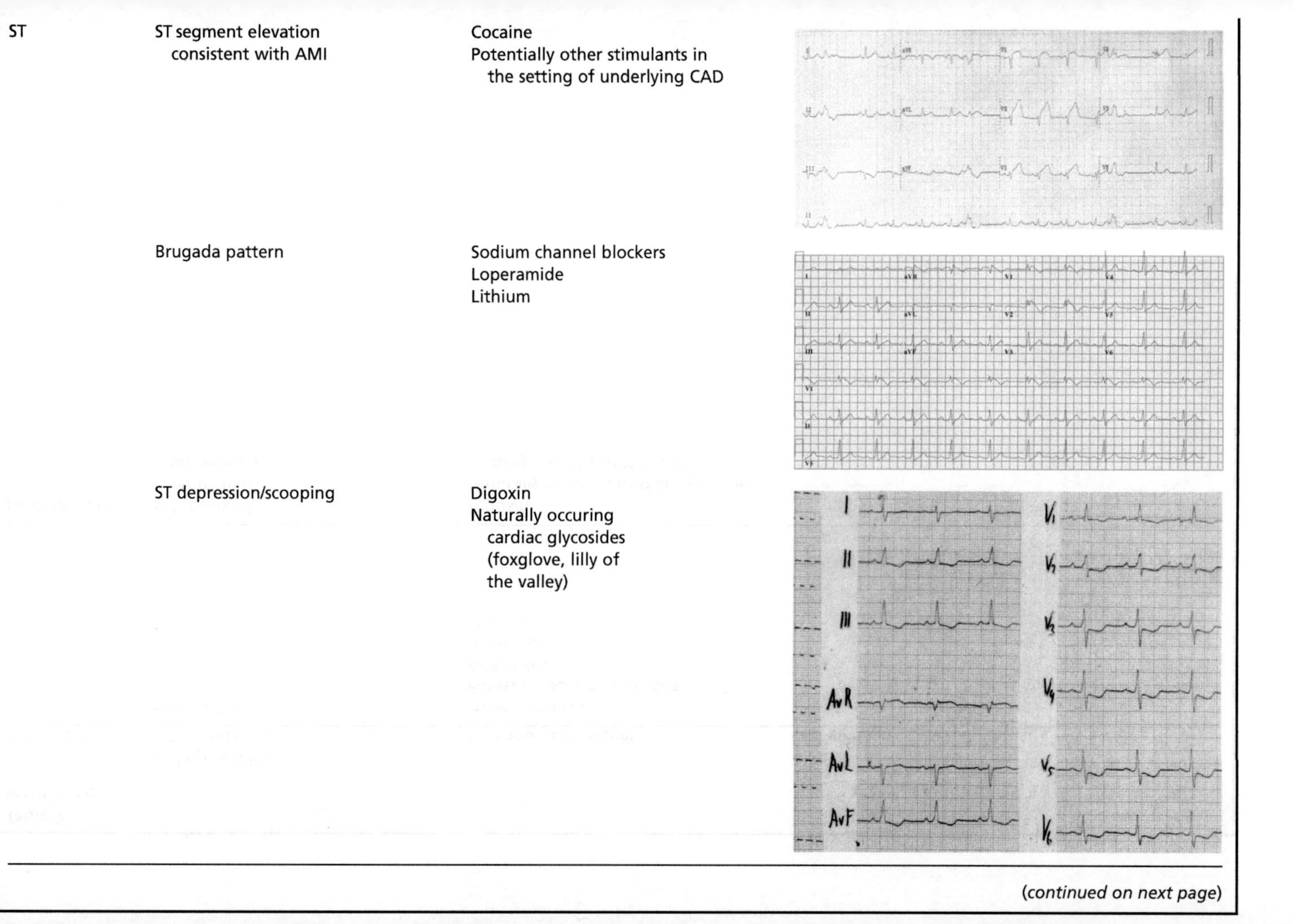

ST	ST segment elevation consistent with AMI	Cocaine Potentially other stimulants in the setting of underlying CAD	
	Brugada pattern	Sodium channel blockers Loperamide Lithium	
	ST depression/scooping	Digoxin Naturally occuring cardiac glycosides (foxglove, lilly of the valley)	

(continued on next page)

Table 9
(continued)

ECG Effect	Pathophysiology & Manifestation	Potential Toxic Agent	Examples
T wave	Peaked T waves	Hyperkalemia due to: Potassium sparing diuretics ACEI/ARBs Arsine gas Fluoride	
Dysrrhythmias	Bidirectional ventricular tachycardia	Digoxin Naturally occuring cardiac glycosides (foxglove, lilly of the valley)	

Torsades de Pointes	QT prolonging drugs	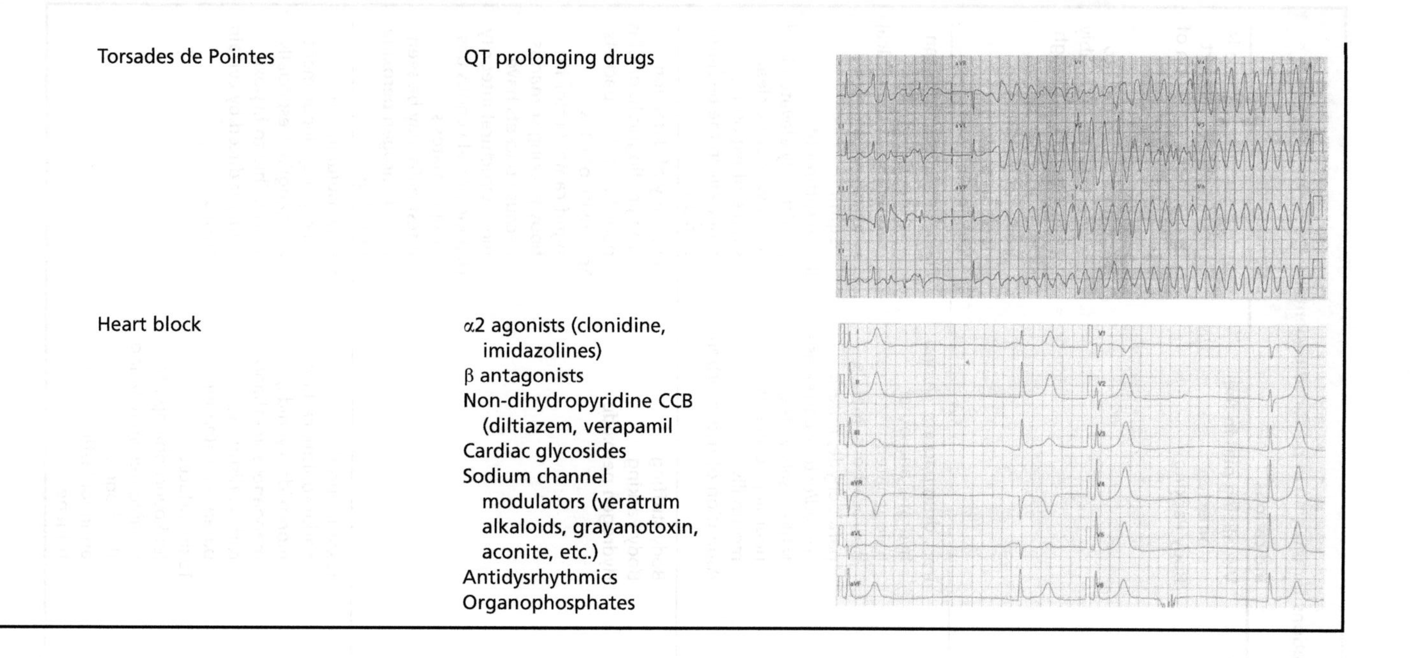
Heart block	α2 agonists (clonidine, imidazolines) β antagonists Non-dihydropyridine CCB (diltiazem, verapamil Cardiac glycosides Sodium channel modulators (veratrum alkaloids, grayanotoxin, aconite, etc.) Antidysrhythmics Organophosphates	

Table 10
Indications and considerations for imaging in poisoned patients

Modality	Indications	Consideration
Point of Care Ultrasound (POCUS)	Visualizing pills in the stomach Body Packing	unclear sensitivity. There is no evidence to support its use in the detection of pill ingestion or pharmacobezoar. There are limited data to support its use in reliably detecting pills, although there are reports of utility in guiding the decision to do gastric lavage and WBI
Plain radiographs	Iron, drug packets, chloral hydrate, and other halogenated hydrocarbons, metals, paraldehyde, enteric coated/extended-release tablets, salicylates, neuroleptic agents, mothballs Aspiration of hydrocarbons	Plain film radiographs can be obtained for the completion of the clinical workup but are rarely helpful In the setting of persistently elevated lead levels without a clear source of exposure, especially in the pediatric patient
Computed Tomography (CT) (Abdominal)	Body stuffing Body Packing Hydrogen peroxide	Sensitivity of detection using radiographs or CT is poor for stuffed packets Sensitivity of CT is significantly better in body packing scenarios because packets have more structural integrity Hepatic portal venous gas or pneumatosis intestinalis may be seen after hydrogen peroxide ingestion
Magnetic Resonance Imaging (MRI)	Toxin-induced parkinsonism: carbon monoxide, cyanide, manganese, methanol, carbon disulfide, paraquat, rotenone Toxin induced leukoencephalopathy: inhaled heroin (chasing the dragon), antineoplastic agents, toluene	Rarely useful in the emergency department Basal ganglia is especially susceptible to hypoxic injury induced by certain toxins

Imaging

Current imaging modalities may be useful in the right clinical context with the unknown toxicologic patient in the ED. **Table 10** lists imaging modalities, potential utility, and considerations/limitations of their use.[15–21]

TREATMENT

As evaluation unfolds, the emergency medicine clinician must also consider simultaneous therapies which may prevent or reverse toxicity. Attention to the basics of airway, breathing, and circulation is paramount at the outset, after which consideration can be given to treatment of the specific poisoning.

Supportive Care

Supportive care is the cornerstone of all management options in the poisoned patient. This includes addressing and correcting any clinical abnormalities when possible, and may consist of oxygen administration for hypoxia, intravenous fluids for hypovolemia, vasopressors for hypotension, intravenous dextrose for hypoglycemia, and other therapies. It is essential to abide by the practice of consistently providing supportive care while elucidating the diagnosis and considering other targeted therapies.

Supportive care may also involve providing care for sedation or agitation. Several sedation/agitation scales may be useful to quickly evaluate this for both documentation and communication purposes. These scales include but are not limited to the Richmond Agitation-Sedation Scale (RASS), Delirium Detection Scale (DDS), and Ramsay Sedation Scale (RSS).[22]

Decontamination

Decontamination—either external (for dermal or ocular exposures) or internal (for ingestions)—can prevent absorption and resultant injury if performed in a timely fashion. Patients who have been exposed to a toxin and/or hazardous material to the skin should undergo decontamination using the following methods:[23]

- Removal of contaminated clothing and irrigation. Copious irrigation can remove and dilute toxins before dermal absorption.
- Water-based solutions are generally suitable
- Certain rare exposures may require specialized irrigation solutions and are beyond the scope of this discussion.
- Ocular exposures must be immediately irrigated to avoid delicate tissue penetration by concentrated xenobiotics. Contact lenses must be removed beforehand.

Gastrointestinal decontamination is performed selectively and often in consultation with the regional poison center and/or medical toxicologist with the aim of limiting the absorption of an ingested toxin. The use of these techniques has declined significantly over the past 20 years. Gastrointestinal decontamination can be accomplished by attempting to empty the gastric contents via orogastric lavage, by the administration of activated charcoal to adsorb toxin, or by whole bowel irrigation with polyethylene glycol solution to hasten gastrointestinal transit. **Table 11** provides a summary of gastrointestinal decontamination methods.[24]

Antidotes

Although many poisonings will require supportive care only, specific antidotes can be useful or essential in certain exposures. Antidotes may work via several mechanisms:

1. Competitive inhibition at the target receptor, such as the use of atropine for acetylcholinesterase inhibitors
2. Binding of the toxin so it is not able to reach target tissues, such as antivenom, digoxin-specific antibody fragments, and chelators
3. Cellular repair and detoxification of metabolites, such as n-acetylcysteine for acetaminophen
4. Displacing the toxin from its intended target via higher receptor or enzyme affinity, such as buprenorphine or naloxone, and
5. Blockade of metabolism to more toxic compounds, such as fomepizole for toxic alcohols

Table 12 describes the indications, mechanisms of action, and dosing of some commonly used antidotes. In years past, patients with an altered sensorium presenting to the ED may have been reflexively given a "coma cocktail" consisting usually of naloxone, thiamine, and dextrose. However, such a a shotgun approach was seen to be counterproductive, wasteful, and cause significant adverse effects as point of care assessments and techniques in acute resuscitation advanced. As with any antidote, a thorough risk-benefit analysis should be made before use. Inappropriate use may distract clinicians away from other indicated therapies and adverse effects can occur.[25]

Enhanced Elimination – Corporeal and Extracorporeal

Once a toxin is absorbed, hastening removal from the body can improve outcomes. This includes methods that take place inside (*corporeal* removal) the body or outside (*extracorporeal* removal). **Table 13** provides examples of substances in which enhanced elimination may be used.[26–29]

Corporeal

removal takes place from within the body. These techniques include:

- Multiple-dose activated charcoal (MDAC) begins with the same aim as single-dose charcoal, but with multiple doses alsodraws toxin from enterohepatic circulation back into the intestine, and as such is described as "intestinal dialysis." It is ideal for drugs in which there is erratic absorption or significant enterohepatic circulation.
- Urinary alkalinization can be used to increase the elimination of certain weakly acidic toxins by trapping them in the urine in the ionized state.

Extracorporeal

removal includes:

- Hemodialysis is the most effective for rapid clearance of many toxins, provided the substance is dialyzable.
- Charcoal hemoperfusion allows for removal of larger molecules and substances avidly bound to charcoal (such as amatoxin) but is logistically difficult due to poor cartridge availability.
- Exchange transfusion may be used in the young infant in whom hemodialysis may be difficult
- Plasmapheresis removes large molecules and proteins a standard hemodialysis circuit cannot.

Table 11
Indications and contraindications for gastrointestinal decontamination methods

Method	Dose	Indications	Contraindications	Other Considerations
Orogastric lavage	250 mL aliquots of saline through large-bore tube (36–40Fr)	Recent ingestion (within 1–2 h) high-lethality ingestions which may be refractory to other treatments	Ingestion of corrosive substances Risk of hemorrhage or GI perforation due to pathology or recent surgery	Difficult to perform - difficulty finding equipment, lack of experience with procedure If performed inappropriately after caustic ingestion, risk of esophageal or pharyngeal perforation Scant studies have failed to show benefit, although the methodology in existing studies is lacking due to the difficulty in studying poisoned patients
Activated charcoal (single dose)	1g/kg PO or NG (PO preferred), with or without cathartic	Substance binds to AC Ideal time is within 1–2 h, delayed gastric emptying in some exposures may extend the window for administration	Caustic or hydrocarbon ingestion Metals, salts, and alcohols do not bind effectively	Caution for aspiration in patients with current or impending altered mental status and/or seizure
Whole bowel irrigation	1–2 L/h of polyethylene glycol, NG	Ingestion of sustained-release tablets or patches of a consequential substance Removal of drug packets Large ingestion of metals	Ileus, patients who cannot tolerate NGT placement Compromise of GI tract Intractable vomiting	Large amount of PEG ingestion may not be well tolerated, NGT may be necessary. Conflicting studies on efficacy in nonpoisoned subjects May be combined with AC

Table 12
Antidotes: Indications, Mechanism of action, and Dosing

Antidote	Indication	Mechanism of Action	Dosing and Administration (Adult)[b]
Antivenom	Various snakes, scorpions, spiders	Forms venom-antibody complexes, inactivating venom at target tissue	Product-dependent
Atropine	Cholinergic crisis	Competitive inhibition at acetylcholine receptor	1–2 mg IV, doubled every 3–5 min until "atropinization" (improvement of bronchorrhea)
Botulinum antitoxin	Botulism	Forms toxin-antibody complexes, inactivating toxin at the target tissue	According to the package insert for Botulism Antitoxin Heptavalent or Baby-BIG product
Bromocriptine	Neuroleptic malignant syndrome	Dopamine D2 receptor agonist	2.5 mg (through nasogastric tube) every 6–8 h, titrated up to a maximum dose of 45 mg/d
Chelating Agents	Metal poisoning	Forms complex around metal species, creating an excretable compound	Examples: succimer (given PO), $CaNa_2EDTA$ (IV), British Antilewisite (BAL), Penicillamine
Cyproheptadine	Serotonin toxicity	Competitive antagonist at $5HT_{1A/2A}$ receptors	12 mg orally initially, then 2 mg given every 2 h if patient remains symptomatic. Maximum dose 32 mg in 24 h
Dantrolene	Malignant Hyperthermia	Inhibits ryanodine receptor-dependent muscle contractility	2.5 mg/kg IV bolus; may repeat until full resolution up to 10 mg/kg
Deferoxamine	Iron poisoning	Binds iron moiety, creating excretable compound	5 mg/kg/h continuous IV infusion, titrate up as tolerated to 15 mg/kg/h
Digoxin-Specific Antibody Fragments	Digoxin toxicity	Forms digoxin-antibody complexes, inactivating drug at target tissue	Digoxin concentration x weight (Kg)/100 = number of 40 mg vials; Empiric dosing up to 10 vials
Flumazenil	Benzodiazepine overdose	Competitive antagonist at GABA-A receptor	Initial dose is 0.2 mg IV over 30 s. Can give additional 0.3 mg IV over 30 s if the desired response does not occur within 30 s.

(*continued on next page*)

Table 12
(continued)

Antidote	Indication	Mechanism of Action	Dosing and Administration (Adult)[b]
			Repeat doses of 0.5 mg IV may be given at 1-min intervals as needed up to 3 mg total dose
Fomepizole[c]	Ethylene glycol, methanol[a]	Competitive inhibitor of alcohol dehydrogenase reducing the formation of toxic metabolites	15 mg/kg over 30 min, followed by 10 mg/kg IV every 12 h for 4 doses, increase to 15 mg/kg every 12 h for subsequent doses.
Glucagon	Beta blocker-induced hypotension	Bypasses beta-receptor blockade through glucagon receptor on cardiac myocyte	2–5 mg IV over 5–10 min; repeat as needed for hypotension. Emesis is a common adverse effect.
High-Dose Insulin	Circulatory collapse from calcium channel antagonists, beta-blockers	Enhances metabolism of cardiac myocyte for increased inotropy	1 unit/kg IV bolus followed by 1 u/kg/h, titrate upwards to effect. Concomitant dextrose infusion and frequent blood sugar/K+ monitoring essential
Hydroxocobalamin	Cyanide poisoning	Binds cyanide to create nontoxic cyanocobalamin	5 g IV over 15 min[d]
Hyperbaric Oxygen	Carbon monoxide poisoning	Enhances elimination of CO from blood, may prevent lipid peroxidation in brain	100% oxygen at pressures >1 atm; multiple sessions may be performed
L-carnitine	Valproic acid-induced hyperammonemia	Replenishes deficient substrate for fatty acid metabolism	100 mg/kg IV over 30 min, followed by 15 mg/kg every 6 h
Lipid Emulsion	Refractory circulatory collapse Local anesthetics	Unclear: may form "lipid sink" phase of drug, rendering it inactive to target tissues	1–2 mL/kg IV infusion over 30 min, followed by 0.25 mL/kg/min over 60 min for 1–2 h
Methylene Blue	Methemoglobinemia, shock	Generates reduction of MetHb species, inhibits nitric oxide synthase	1 mg/kg of 1% solution IV over 5 min

(continued on next page)

Table 12 (*continued*)

Antidote	Indication	Mechanism of Action	Dosing and Administration (Adult)[b]
N-acetylcysteine[c]	Prevention of acetaminophen hepatotoxicity	Detoxification of NAPQI metabolite	150 mg/kg over 1 h IV, followed by 50 mg/kg over 4 h, followed by 100 mg/kg over 16 h; package insert for solution preparation and pediatric dosing[d]
Naloxone	Opioid overdose	Displacement of opioids from mu receptor	0.04 mg IV, repeat or increase as needed
Physostigmine	Anticholinergic delirium	Acetylcholinesterase inhibition	1–2 mg IV over 5 min
Pralidoxime	Acetylcholinesterase inhibition (nerve agents, organophosphorus pesticides)	Pulls organophosphate compound off acetylcholinesterase enzyme, preventing aging	30 mg/kg over 15–30 min followed by 8–10 mg/kg/h
Pyridoxine	Isoniazid, *Gyromitra* mushroom	Increased glutamate conversion into GABA	1 g per g of isoniazid up to maximum 5 g IV infusion at 0.5 g/min until seizures stop, remainder infused over 4–6 h
Sodium Bicarbonate	Salicylism, tricyclic antidepressant poisoning, phenobarbital	Salicylism: enhances ionized state to limit CNS distribution and promote excretion TCAs: alters sodium channel conformation to limit binding of drug	Salicylates: administration until target serum pH 7.45–7.55 and urine pH > 7.5 reached TCAs: 1–2 mEq/kg IV push, repeat as needed for QRS widening Frequent K+ monitoring is essential
Sodium nitrite and sodium thiosulfate	Cyanide poisoning	Induces methemoglobinemia reducing cyanide's binding capability and conversion to nontoxic metabolite thiocyanate	Sodium Nitrite: 300 mg (10 mL) intravenously (IV) at a rate of 2.5–5 mL/min Sodium Thiosulfate: 12.5 g (50 mL), slow IV, immediately following sodium nitrite administration

[a] Emerging evidence for use in acetaminophen poisoning, not yet established.
[b] Pediatric dosing may vary, consultation advised.
[c] Dose adjustment needed during hemodialysis.
[d] IV solution, dilution, and reconstitution instructions per package insert.

Table 13
Substances amenable to enhanced elimination by modality

Hemodialysis[a]	Multiple Dose Activated Charcoal	Urinary Alkalinization
Salicylates	Carbamazepine	Salicylates
Lithium	Theophylline	Methotrexate
Theophylline, caffeine	Amatoxin (cyclopeptide mushroom)	Phenobarbital
Valproic acid	Colchicine	
Ethylene glycol, methanol, diethylene glycol	Phenobarbital	**Plasmapheresis**
Acetaminophen (massive overdose)	Dapsone	Digoxin-antibody complexes (anuric patient)
Phenobarbital	Quinine	
Baclofen[b]	Salicylates	
Thallium	Other concretion-forming drugs	
Electrolyte salts (Na, K, Ca, and so forth)		

[a] For specific recommendations, see https://www.extrip-workgroup.org/recommendations.
[b] In the presence of kidney impairment.

- Continuous renal replacement therapy has little benefit in rapid toxin removal but may be used in between dialysis sessions or if the patient is too unstable to perfuse a hemodialysis circuit.

ADVANCED SUPPORTIVE CARE

In the critically ill patient with suspected poisoning, advanced measures may be of additional benefit along with the care described above. Venoarterial extracorporeal membrane oxygenation (ECMO) and ventricular assist devices can provide circulatory support in a patient with refractory cardiogenic shock while the toxic syndrome resolves. Venovenous ECMO can support a patient with severe respiratory failure. Targeted temperature management (therapeutic hypothermia) in the postcardiac arrest patient is used in an attempt to reduce the risk of secondary tissue injury. In hepatic failure, artificial liver support such as albumin dialysis (eg, the Molecular Adsorbent Recirculating System) may be used as a potential bridge to transplant.[30,31]

DISPOSITION

While the acutely unstable patient with unknown poisoning clearly needs an intensive care unit setting, some patients who are awake, protecting the airway, and do not have impending cardiovascular collapse may be watched on an inpatient unit. If there is potential for worsening ECG abnormalities, telemetry is advised. If the patient is stable but being watched for the development of more concerning findings, an observation unit may be suitable. Discharge should be considered only when clinical and laboratory abnormalities are resolved and there is no concern for further harm.

SPECIAL CONSIDERATIONS

Certain groups of patients have unique physiology warranting a tailored approach.

- Pediatrics: the young child may be more susceptible to inhaled or dermal exposures, due to increased minute ventilation and surface area:weight ratio. In addition, a small dose ingested may be a high mg/kg amount. Children develop drug-metabolizing enzyme activity throughout childhood, which can alter pharmacokinetics and influence the length of observation recommended. Generally, the child with exploratory poison exposure will have a good outcome but vigilance is essential.
- Pregnancy: many substances pass from the mother to the fetus via placental circulation with untoward effects. These can be chronic (in the case of teratogens) or pose an acute fetal risk, particularly if the mother is critically ill. The first line of therapy is to treat maternal poisoning to ensure the best fetal outcome, but specialty consultation is advised.
- Geriatrics: the metabolism and elimination of drugs and toxins may be affected in older patients, and the high incidence of polypharmacy in this population can complicate assessment and care. A detailed medication list and medical history is vital.
- Brain death: Rarely a patient may present to the ED with indications of brain death but in the poisoned patient this may be confounded by the presence of xenobiotics which may mimic brain death. These include baclofen, barbiturates, neurotoxic snake venom (in endemic areas), antidepressants, and other agents. Medical toxicology consultation is strongly encouraged to ensure accurate assessment of these patients.[32,33]

SUMMARY

There is a seemingly endless array of considerations in the patient with unknown poisonings. Careful attention to history, physical examination, and evolving clues will reveal the next steps in the astute clinician. Approaching the diagnosis and management in a strategic yet simultaneous fashion will maximize the likelihood of the best clinical outcome.

CLINICS CARE POINTS

- The management of severe hyperthermia should be a priority in the management of the toxicological patient. Ice water immersion has been shown to be the most effective cooling method for environmental and toxicological etiologies of severe hyperthermia.
- For any patient with hypertension due to poisoning, benzodiazepines are a reasonable first line agent to improve hemodynamic status.
- Norepinephrine is generally a good first line agent for the undifferentiated toxicological patient in shock.
- Urine drug screens are immunoassays with frequent false positives and false negatives with may be misleading in the clinical care of a patient.
- Scant studies regarding orogastric lavage have failed to show benefit, although the methodology in existing studies is lacking due to the difficulty in studying poisoned patients.

DISCLOSURE

The authors have nothing to disclose.

REFERENCES

1. Gummin DD, Mowry JB, Beuhler MC, et al. 2019 Annual Report of the American Association of Poison Control Centers' National Poison Data System (NPDS): 37th Annual Report. Clin Toxicol 2020;58:1360–541.
2. Brent, J. & Burkhart, Keith & Dargan, Paul & Hatten, B. & Megarbane, Bruno & Palmer, R. & White, J. (2017). The critically poisoned patient. In: Critical Care Toxicology: Diagnosis and Management of the Critically Poisoned Patient.
3. Turgut K, Yavuz E. Comparison of non-invasive CPAP with mask use in carbon monoxide poisoning. Am J Emerg Med 2020;38(7):1454–7.
4. Lange RA, Cigarroa RG, Flores ED, et al. Potentiation of cocaine-induced coronary vasoconstriction by beta-adrenergic blockade. Ann Intern Med 1990; 112(12):897–903.
5. McCord J, Jneid H, Hollander JE, et al. American Heart Association Acute Cardiac Care Committee of the Council on Clinical Cardiology. Management of cocaine-associated chest pain and myocardial infarction: a scientific statement from the American Heart Association Acute Cardiac Care Committee of the Council on Clinical Cardiology. Circulation 2008;117(14):1897–907.
6. Clifford C, Sethi M, Cox D, et al. First-Line Vasopressor and Mortality Rates in ED Patients with Acute Drug Overdose. J Med Toxicol 2021;17(1):1–9.
7. Holstege CP, Borek HA. Toxidromes. Crit Care Clin 2012;28(4):479–98.
8. Nelson LS, Howland M, Lewin NA, , et al. Initial evaluation of the patient: vital signs and toxic syndromes. In: Nelson LS, Howland M, Lewin NA, Smith SW, Goldfrank LR, Hoffman RS. eds. Goldfrank's toxicologic Emergencies, 11th edition. McGraw-Hill; Accessed June 2, 2021.
9. Laskowski LK, Landry A, Vassallo SU, et al. Ice water submersion for rapid cooling in severe drug-induced hyperthermia. Clin Toxicol (Phila) 2015;53:181–4.
10. Nelson LS, Howland M, Lewin NA, et al. Principles of Managing the Acutely Poisoned or Overdosed Patient. In: Nelson LS, Howland M, Lewin NA, Smith SW, Goldfrank LR, Hoffman RS, editors. Goldfrank's toxicologic Emergencies. 11th edition. McGraw Hill; 2019. Accessed October 14, 2021.
11. Friedman LS, Krajewski A, Vannoy E, et al. The association between U.S. Poison Center assistance and length of stay and hospital charges. Clin Toxicol (Phila) 2014;52(3):198–206.
12. Legg RG, Little M. Inpatient toxicology services improve resource utilization for intoxicated patients: a systematic review. Br J Clin Pharmacol 2019;85(1):11–9.
13. Moeller KE, Lee KC, Kissack JC. Urine drug screening: practical guide for clinicians. Mayo Clin Proc 2008;83(1):66–76.
14. Wolf SJ, Byyny R, Carpenter CR, et al. ACEP Clinical Policy: critical issues in the evaluation and management of adult patients presenting to the emergency department with acute carbon monoxide poisoning. Ann Emerg Med 2017; 74(4):e41–74.
15. Bajaj T, Nelson M, Lehman V. Initiation of gastric lavage in a patient with acute overdose after visualization of pills in stomach using bedside ultrasound. J Clin Toxicol 2016;6:331.
16. Schwartz DT. Principles of diagnostic imaging. In: Nelson LS, Howland M, Lewin NA, Smith SW, Goldfrank LR, Hoffman RS. eds. Goldfrank's Toxicologic Emergencies, 11th edition New York: McGraw-Hill; Accessed July 11, 2021.
17. Savitt DL, Hawkins HH, Roberts JR. The radiopacity of ingested medications. Ann Emerg Med 1987;16(3):331–9.

18. Flach PM. “Drug mules” as a radiological challenge: sensitivity and specificity in identifying internal cocaine in body packers, body pushers and body stuffers by computed tomography, plain radiography and Lodox. Eur J Radiol 2012;81: 2518–26.
19. Woolf AD, Goldman R, Bellinger DC. Update on the clinical management of childhood lead poisoning. Pediatr Clin North Am 2007;54(2):271–94, viii.
20. Kim Y, Kim JW. Toxic encephalopathy. Saf Health Work 2012;3(4):243–56.
21. Filley CM, Kleinschmidt-DeMasters BK. Toxic leukoencephalopathy. N Engl J Med 2001;345(6):425–32.
22. Sessler CN. Sedation scales in the ICU. Chest 2004;126(6):1727–30.
23. Lucyk S. Decontamination principles: prevention of dermal, ophthalmic, and inhalational absorption. In: Nelson LS, Howland M, Lewin NA, et al. eds. Goldfrank's toxicologic Emergencies, 11th edition. McGraw-Hill; Accessed June 2, 2021.
24. Position statement: gastric lavage. J Toxicol Clin Toxicol 1997;35:711–9.
25. Sivilotti ML. Flumazenil, naloxone and the ‘coma cocktail’. Br J Clin Pharmacol 2016;81(3):428–36.
26. Position statement and practice guidelines on the use of multi-dose activated charcoal in the treatment of acute poisoning. American Academy of Clinical Toxicology; European Association of Poisons Centres and Clinical Toxicologists. J Toxicol Clin Toxicol 1999;37(6):731–51.
27. Proudfoot AT, Krenzelok EP, Vale JA. Position Paper on urine alkalinization. J Toxicol Clin Toxicol 2004;42(1):1–26.
28. Ghannoum M, Hoffman RS, Gosselin S, et al. Use of extracorporeal treatments in the management of poisonings. Kidney Int 2018 Oct;94(4):682–8.
29. Executive Summar of Recommendations. EXTRIP: The extracorporeal treatments in poisoning workgroup. Available at. https://www.extrip-workgroup.org/recommendations. Accessed September 4, 2021.
30. Eyer F. The Assessment and Management of Hypotension and Shock in the Poisoned Patient. In: Brent J, Burkhart K, Dargan P, et al, editors. Critical care toxicology. Cham (Switzerland): Springer; 2017. https://doi-org.proxy.libraries.rutgers.edu/10.1007/978-3-319-17900-1_55.
31. Upchurch C, Blumenberg A, Brodie D, et al. Extracorporeal membrane oxygenation use in poisoning: a narrative review with clinical recommendations. Clin Toxicol (Phila) 2021 Oct;59(10):877–87.
32. Murphy L, Wolfer H, Hendrickson RG. Toxicologic Confounders of Brain Death Determination: A Narrative Review. Neurocrit Care 2021;34(3):1072–89.
33. Neavyn MJ, Stolbach A, Greer DM, et al. ACMT position statement: determining brain death in adults after drug overdose. J Med Toxicol 2017;13(3):271–3.

The Management of Agitated Toxidromes

Sophie Gosselin, MD, FRCPC, CSPQ[a,b,c,*], Robert S. Hoffman, MD, FRCP Edin, FEAPCCT[d]

KEYWORDS

- Agitation • Sedation • Hyperthermia • Cooling • Intoxication

KEY POINTS

- Agitated patients are medical emergencies with potential life-threatening conditions and must be evaluated in a critical care area to rapidly control their behavior.
- Physical restraints are temporizing measures to provide patient and staff safety while pharmacologic sedation is achieved to promptly allow a thorough physical examination.
- Complete vital signs including capillary glucose and core temperature are needed within minutes of arrival to detect and treat hyperthermia or hypoglycemia and other life-threatening conditions.
- Fast-acting benzodiazepines are preferred for unknown agitated patients while parenteral droperidol is a safe and effective option whereby available.
- Specific antidotal therapy is rarely indicated in the initial management of agitated patients.

INTRODUCTION

The assessment and treatment of patients with psychomotor agitation is a common clinical situation in emergency medicine. These patients are often challenging in that some are gravely ill, and many pose a significant threat not only to their own safety but also to the safety of other patients in the emergency department as well as the hospital staff. Health care teams need to develop a rapid, organized, and safe approach to the behavioral control, diagnosis, and management of agitated patients.

Historically, the care of agitated patients was relegated to psychiatry services and included practices such as seclusion, prolonged use of full-body restraints with strait-jackets or other devices, and in the 1970s large doses of potent and long-acting antipsychotics.[1] These practices often neglected underlying medical conditions or

[a] Centre Intégré de Santé et de Services Sociaux (CISSS), Montérégie-Centre Emergency Department, Hôpital Charles-Lemoyne, 3120 Boulevard Taschereau, Greenfield Park, Québec J4V 2H1, Canada; [b] Centre Antipoison du Québec, Québec, Canada; [c] Department of Emergency Medicine, McGill University, Montreal, Québec, Canada; [d] Division of Medical Toxicology, Ronald O. Perelman Department of Emergency Medicine, NYU Grossman School of Medicine, 455 First Avenue Room 123, New York, NY 10016, USA
* Corresponding author. 3120 Boulevard Taschereau, Greenfield Park, Québec, Canada.
E-mail address: sgosselinmd@gmail.com

Emerg Med Clin N Am 40 (2022) 223–235
https://doi.org/10.1016/j.emc.2022.01.009

allowed patients to suffer complications and even death from hyperthermia, fluid and electrolyte abnormalities, and oversedation with subsequent aspiration pneumonitis. Even in the modern era, inappropriate pharmacotherapy for agitation that produced lethal serotonin toxicity reshaped graduate medical education in the United States[2,3] and shifted the focus of care of agitated patients to emergency physicians.

It is noteworthy that in many of the foundational studies that address the appropriate pharmacologic options for agitated patients, a large percentage are ultimately diagnosed with toxicologic conditions, most commonly alcohol intoxication or sympathomimetic toxicity.[4–11] However, because the initial diagnosis of many patients is unclear or completely unknown, their abnormal behavior should be approached as an emergency and dealt with in an appropriate acute care area such as the resuscitation bay. In this way life-threatening conditions such as hypoglycemia, hyperthermia, or epidural hematoma can be rapidly identified and treated. While this article focuses on the diagnosis and treatment of agitated toxicology patients, it also discusses safe and effective strategies for patients with undifferentiated agitation. For the purposes of this article, we use the following definitions:

- Agitation: A psychomotor abnormality that results in physical behavior that is either harmful to the patient or staff or prevents a rapid thorough medical assessment.
- Undifferentiated agitation: Patients for whom the etiology of their agitation is not conclusive based on history and a rapid physical assessment and for whom laboratory investigations and other tests are usually warranted.

The differential diagnosis for agitation is extensive and includes infectious, metabolic, toxicologic, psychiatric, traumatic, electrolyte, and endocrine abnormalities among others. An extensive discussion of the mechanisms for each of these possibilities is beyond the scope of this article. Rather we will focus on the common toxicologic causes (**Table 1**).

ASSESSMENT

Traditionally, the medical evaluation begins with obtaining a complete history followed by physical examination. However, agitated patients are often unable to provide much (if any) history, and behavioral control followed by a rapid physical assessment must take precedence for the safety of both the patient and hospital personnel. When multiple members of the health care team are available, one member should be assigned to obtain any possible collateral information about the patient from family, friends, emergency services personnel, or police, who accompany the patient to the hospital. Additional sources such as the electronic medical record should be queried for evidence of substance use disorders, psychiatric illness, pharmacotherapy, or medical comorbidities.

Patients should be brought immediately to a critical care area, such as a resuscitation bay. Doing so offers many advantages:

Table 1
Common toxicologic causes of agitation

Amphetamines	Ethanol intoxication
Anticholinergics	Ethanol and sedative hypnotic withdrawal
Cocaine	Ketamine and phencyclidine
Dissociative (ketamine and phencyclidine)	Serotonin toxicity

- It heightens the team's awareness that a life-threatening emergency may be occurring
- It provides access to monitoring and resuscitation equipment and in certain settings, imaging studies.
- It facilitates the rapid initial use and prompt the titration of intravenous sedation medications to achieve the desired behavioral effect.
- It allows sufficient space for multiple members to care for the patient in a safe environment.
- It removes the patient from the main emergency department to limit stress on other patients, family members, and providers.

The assessment of all patients begins with a full set of vital signs that includes blood pressure, heart rate, respiratory rate, core temperature, oxygen saturation, and a bedside determination of the blood glucose concentration. Agitated toxicology patients are most commonly hypertensive, tachycardic, tachypneic, and hyperthermic. The extent of these vital sign abnormalities is multifactorial and relate to the toxin, the individual and their preexisting conditions, the duration of the event, and ambient environmental conditions. Although no patient should ever be considered too agitated to obtain all vital signs, pharmacologic intervention is often required to measure a core temperature. Also, while abnormalities of blood pressure and heart rate can be dramatic, clinicians should be aware that unrecognized and or untreated hyperthermia likely poses the most immediate life threat. Although data are not available for all etiologies in the differential diagnosis noted above, the most illustrative data address the cause of lethality in cocaine toxicity. In a conscious animal model, rapid control of temperature was the single most important factor contributing to survival.[12] Additional support comes from epidemiologic evidence that demonstrates an increase in the fatality rate from cocaine as ambient temperatures climb.[13,14] Presumably this represents an inability to dissipate the heat generated during agitation as ambient temperature (and likely humidity) increase. As such, rather than defining behavioral control as the main outcome, we set the goals for a successful initial assessment as follows and divide our standard into 2 time frames:

- The first 10 minutes from presentation
  - o Achieve physical control
  - o Determine of vital signs including a bedside glucose measurement
  - o Assure the adequacy of the airway, breathing, and circulation
  - o Exclude trauma
  - o Insert an intravenous catheter and if the IV is not successful after 1 to 2 attempts, expose an area for intramuscular administration
  - o Begin pharmacologic sedation to achieve behavioral control
  - o Treat hypoglycemia if present
  - o Attach the patient to a cardiac monitor and continuous pulse oximetry and observe the rhythm strip
- The first 20 minutes
  - o Obtain necessary blood specimens; electrolytes can be requested on a blood gas analyzer to rapidly exclude MDMA induced hyponatremia *before* fluid boluses
  - o Begin treatment of hyperthermia if present
  - o Obtain a 12-lead electrocardiogram if indicated
  - o Begin volume resuscitation if indicated
  - o Restore the patient to a clinical state in which physical restraint is no longer needed

It is essential to recognize that physical restraints are only indicated as a temporizing measure until behavioral control can be achieved by pharmacologic intervention. Prolonged physical restraint without adequate chemical sedation is inhumane and can lead to mechanical complications as well as severe psychological distress.

A complete physical assessment is necessary to help identify clues to traumatic injuries and medical disorders. The toxicologic physical examination focuses on skin, eyes, bowel, bladder, and muscle tone. **Table 2** highlights how an assessment of these organ systems can help differentiate among patients who, on initial evaluation may seem similar.

Individualized laboratory testing is recommended and often includes a complete blood count, electrolytes, hepatic and kidney function testing, creatine phosphokinase, and troponin. Targeted toxicology testing of co-ingestants (such as acetaminophen, ethanol, and known psychoactive medications) is also recommended in cases of suspected self-harm. In contrast, however, we discourage the routine use of urine testing for common drugs of abuse because turn-around times for testing are, in some settings, too long to influence acute management,[15] there are significant false positive and false negative results[16] that are too often misinterpreted by clinicians, and when studied these tests rarely if ever impact on acute patient care.[17–20] Many of our psychiatric colleagues use the results of urine drug testing to engage a conversation with patients with the dual diagnoses of substance use disorders and psychiatric illness. Because the results of urine drug testing rarely change over a short period of time, urine testing can be deferred until a time that the psychiatric team can evaluate its benefit in their intervention and recommend a more precise assay if available.

Similarly, the indications for neuroimaging should be individualized rather than included as part of the mandatory initial assessment. Sending patients prematurely for neuroimaging despite the lack of focal findings or signs of significant trauma while life-threatening hyperthermia, hypoglycemia, or hyponatremia are left untreated is dangerous. Neuroimaging should be deferred until the patient's ABCs are stabilized, and other immediately life-threatening abnormalities are addressed. When infectious central nervous system processes are highly suspected, administration of empirical antimicrobials is indicated, and lumbar puncture should only be performed when the patient can be positioned safely considering that modern PCR techniques improve the accuracy of delayed diagnosis.

Table 2
Common differentiating findings on physical examination

Organ System	Characteristic Findings
Skin	*Diaphoretic* with sympathomimetics, serotonin toxicity and ethanol and sedative hypnotic withdrawal *Dry* with anticholinergic toxicity
Eyes	*Mydriatic and briskly responsive to light* with sympathomimetics *Mydriatic and poorly responsive to light* with anticholinergics *Vertical and rotatory nystagmus* with phencyclidine and ketamine
Bowel sounds	*Active* with sympathomimetics, serotonin toxicity, and ethanol and sedative hypnotic withdrawal *Quiet or absent* with anticholinergic toxicity
Bladder	*Urinary retention* with anticholinergics, ketamine and phencyclidine
Muscle tone	*Spontaneous and inducible clonus* that is more pronounced in the legs than in the arms with serotonin toxicity

THERAPEUTIC INTERVENTIONS

Sedation

Perhaps there is no greater controversial topic in the treatment of the agitated patient than the choice of pharmacologic agents for behavioral control. Therapeutic options generally fall into one of the 3 categories: benzodiazepines (diazepam, lorazepam, midazolam), antipsychotics (haloperidol, droperidol, olanzapine) and dissociatives (ketamine). When the nature of the agitation is reasonably clear the literature supports optimal pairing of intervention with the disorder (**Table 3**).

However, when patients truly have undifferentiated agitation or possibly multiple concomitant causes of agitation the therapeutic option should be selected based on the preferred route of administration, the onset and duration of the effect, and the risk of adverse reactions. The following statements present evidence-based corrections to common misstatements conveyed in multiple scientific discussions:

- *Droperidol and risk of QT prolongation. Evidence: The use of droperidol in acutely agitated patients is not commonly associated with clinically significant QT interval prolongation.*[11]
- *Antipsychotic drugs lower seizure threshold. Evidence: Antipsychotics do not appear to lower seizure threshold or impair heat dissipation to a clinically degree in patients with sympathomimetic toxicity.*[21]
- *Olanzapine increases the risk of benzodiazepine-induced respiratory depression. Evidence:* Although the US FDA recently changed the labeling of olanzapine because of adverse drug events reported during postmarketing surveillance,[22] this is not supported by systematic review or prospective evaluations.[23–26]

Whenever possible, the use of intravenous administration is preferred over intramuscular administration. The faster onset of action and guaranteed systemic absorption allow more precise titration compared with the longer and erratic intramuscular absorption. The additional benefits of secured intravenous access allow for prompt laboratory testing and glucose or fluid administration. Knowledge of the pharmacokinetics and pharmacodynamic properties of each medication will guide the appropriate dose and interval of administration. Some general guidelines are provided in the following discussion.

Benzodiazepines

Three parenteral benzodiazepines are generally used; diazepam, lorazepam, and midazolam. For all indications, diazepam should never be used intramuscularly as the absorption is incomplete and unpredictable.[27–29] The pharmacodynamics of these drugs differ by indication in terms of relative times to peak and durations of effect. When used parenterally as an anticonvulsant all 3 drugs have a fairly rapid onset of action with midazolam showing some clinical superiority with regard to terminating seizures

Table 3
Potential Initial intervention for patients with known toxicologic diagnoses[a]

Diagnosis	Initial Intervention
Alcohol withdrawal	Benzodiazepine
Alcohol intoxication	Antipsychotic
Anticholinergic	Physostigmine
Cocaine	Benzodiazepine

[a] For diagnoses not listed in this table, data are insufficient to recommend one specific pharmacologic intervention over the others.

in adults,[30] whereas in children both lorazepam and midazolam have similar efficacy.[31] For seizure control, lorazepam also has the longest duration of action. However, with regard to sedation, these drugs behave quite differently. Midazolam and lorazepam are both predictably absorbed by the intramuscular route. The onset and peak effect of midazolam is fast, whereas the onset of action of lorazepam is slower, and the peak effect of lorazepam is delayed up to about 20 minutes regardless of the route of administration.[32–35] The sedation from lorazepam lasts longer than midazolam. Following a single dose, sedation from lorazepam may last for as long as 4 hours[36] compared with 1 hour for midazolam.[37] Repeated dosing or continuous infusion delays the time to the restoration of consciousness. Following the termination of a 1 to 2-day continuous infusion, sedation lasted 8.7 hours from lorazepam versus 3.0 hours from midazolam.[38] Because of the delayed to peak effect of lorazepam there is a tendency to over-sedate patients when repeated dosing is necessary. This occurs because the peak effect has not occurred from the first dose at a time when subsequent doses are being given. Midazolam is preferable when rapid behavioral control or possible titration is necessary. Although the short duration of effect requires frequent repeat administration, this also allows clinical reevaluation and helps prevent oversedation. As the cause of agitation is properly diagnosed over time, other medications can be administered with longer duration of effects.

Antipsychotics

In multiple controlled trials parenteral olanzapine, haloperidol, droperidol, and ziprasidone safely and effectively produce rapid control of agitated patients in an emergency department setting.[4,9–11] While the differences among these medications often reach statistical significance the clinical relevance of these differences are uncertain. Some distinctions are worth mentioning. The effects of midazolam are generally appreciated sooner than antipsychotics but are shorter in duration. As single therapies, droperidol and olanzapine have pharmacodynamic profiles that are more desirable than haloperidol or ziprasidone.

Controlled data do not support the preferential use of haloperidol at the typical doses studied. Most initial studies were performed in psychiatric patients in an era when adverse effects of oversedation were overlooked. Many clinicians still use relatively large doses of haloperidol. It should be noted, however, that based on studies that analyze dopamine receptor occupancy, parenteral doses of haloperidol of 5 mg are generally sufficient to maximize sedation in the average adult,[39] with greater doses only increasing the likelihood of extrapyramidal symptoms. Smaller adults likely warrant lower doses.

Ketamine

Success with the prehospital use of ketamine for trauma patients stimulated interest in ketamine use for agitation. While it is clear that ketamine produces rapid behavioral control, patients treated with ketamine are more likely to be admitted to the hospital and more likely to require endotracheal intubation than patients treated with other medications when a fixed standard dose of ketamine is administered irrespective of weight.[7,8,40] Because admission to an intensive care unit is a precious resource, the use of intramuscular ketamine as initial therapy should be reserved for situations in which insufficient personnel exist to safely physically restrain patients for intravenous access and/or situations for which the use of other medications are undesirable (eg, end-stage COPD or high BMI for benzodiazepines, hyperthermic patients and antipsychotic or borderline hypotension for both drug classes). When other medications have failed, there is sufficient literature support for the use of ketamine as a second-line or “rescue” medication.[41]

Combination Therapies

The choice to begin with combination therapies (usually an antipsychotic plus a benzodiazepine) is again rooted in the treatment of patients on psychiatric wards making a distinction between rapid tranquilization (ie, behavioral control) and rapid neuroleptization (ie, psychiatric control).[42] This practice is based on a theory of a broad spectrum pharmacologic approach that limits the doses of each medication to maximize individual adverse-effect profiles and gave rise to the common practice of "5 and 2" (5 mg of haloperidol combined with 2 mg of lorazepam). It does, however, increase the risks of an adverse interaction between the 2 therapies. We want to reiterate that the use of midazolam is superior to lorazepam in patients who require rapid behavioral control and that the practice of combined lorazepam and antipsychotic therapy predates the wider availability of midazolam. One study comparing the intramuscular use of 10 mg of midazolam to either 10 mg of droperidol intramuscularly or the combined use of 5 mg of each drug supported this practice noting a similar time to achieve behavioral control in all groups and more adverse airway effects (desaturation or airway obstruction) in the midazolam only group.[11] Additionally, the routine use of diphenhydramine or another anticholinergic is discouraged because of concerns of QRS and QT interval prolongation and the false pharmacologic claim that it prevents dystonic reactions (which are usually delayed by at least 24 hours) when coadministered with antipsychotics.

Existing Guidelines

Guidance exists from white papers,[43] best practice statements in emergency medicine,[44] and consensus statements from psychiatry,[45] and psychopharmacology.[46] These statements do not provide convincing evidence to support any particular pharmacologic approach in patients with undifferentiated agitation and are therefore only included for completeness.

Cooling

Untreated hyperthermia can lead to cerebral edema, myocardial dysfunction, and disseminated intravascular coagulopathy (DIC). It is common for patients who are insufficiently cooled to survive the acute event only to develop these complications 12 to 48 hours after presentation.[47] As the core temperature increases a cascade of events leads to increased intestinal permeability to endotoxin[48] resulting in a clinical syndrome that resembles gram-negative sepsis.

There is a critical time and temperature beyond which irreversible damage is likely to occur. In animal models of heatstroke this varies by species studied and ranges from 12 minutes at 43.5 °C in rabbits[49] to 23 minutes at 42 °C in rats[50] and 68 minutes at 44 °C in dogs.[51] For obvious reasons, data on human toxicology patients are lacking, but heatstroke references often use critical core temperatures of 40 °C[52] to 40.5 °C[52,53] When considering the animal data and recognizing that patients usually become hyperthermic in the prehospital setting; activation of emergency services and transport to the hospital take some time; and that patients must then be assessed before hyperthermia is confirmed, cooling must begin rapidly and proceed as efficiently as possible. Thus from the time of recognition, the goal should be to cool the patient to a near-normal core temperature in 20 minutes or less. This requires an organized and practiced approach to cooling.

Debate continues over optimal cooling methods, with physicists supporting evaporative cooling and others championing immersion in cold water. In a human volunteer model of exertional heatstroke a specialized evaporative cooling device produced cooling rates as rapid as 0.30 °C/min which was better than the 0.19 °C/min rate in a tepid water bath.[54] However, when used in real-world conditions, many of the sickest patients required more than 1 hour to cool to a normal temperature.[55] In contrast, immersion of hyperthermic volunteers in water at 2 °C produced a mean cooling rate of 0.35 °C/min) and was not associated with shivering.[56] By comparison, cooling rates in 2 agitated hyperthermic toxicology patients who were placed in ice baths were 0.18 °C/min and 0.28 °C/min[57] These rates are not achievable with ice blankets, customized external cooling devices, or endovascular devices designed for postresuscitation care. In fact, one recent systematic review of the treatment of exertional heatstroke concluded that cooling rates faster than 0.15 °C/min were positively associated with increased survival and that cold water immersion was essential to reduce complications and maximize survival.[53] Another systematic review of both exertional and nonexertional heatstroke concluded that ice water immersion was the most efficient cooling technique.[52]

In practice, agitated patients with core temperatures in excess of 40.5 °C require sedation (see section above on the choice of sedatives) and occasionally paralysis postintubation based on their clinical condition and immersion in an ice and water bath as previously described.[57] Continuous monitoring of vital signs are maintained and core temperature is measured via a flexible rectal probe or one included as part of a urinary catheter. Patients are maintained in the bath until their core temperature approaches 38 °C at which point they are removed, dried, and placed on a stretcher. This generally prevents hypothermia as patients continue to cool during the moving and drying process. Recurrent hyperthermia is uncommon as long as sedation is maintained until the physiologic effects of the toxin resolve.

For settings in which ice and water bath immersion or cooling devices are not available, another option is to cover both the back, thorax, abdomen, and limbs of the patient in towels submerged in ice water and change the towels frequently. The addition of a fan is desirable.

Antidotes for Toxin-Specific Receptor Antagonism

Physostigmine

Although the cholinesterase inhibitor physostigmine was once used reflexively in the empiric treatment of poisoned patients with altered mental status,[58] this practice fell out of favor when several authors reported serious and sometimes lethal adverse effects when physostigmine was given to patients with tricyclic antidepressant poisoning.[59–61] Subsequent confusion over the risks, benefits, indications, and contraindications resulted in a near abandonment of physostigmine use. Fortunately, several retrospective studies suggested that the judicious use of physostigmine in patients with suspected anticholinergic poisoning could safely reverse agitation, delirium and reduce unnecessary testing.[62–65] Recently, a small randomized controlled trial demonstrated that when compared with lorazepam, patients given physostigmine had better control of their agitation and anticholinergic delirium.[66]

The life-threatening manifestations of isolated antimuscarinic toxicity (ie, anticholinergic toxicity in the absence of cardiovascular complications from anticholinergic drugs such as tricyclic antidepressants) generally relate to psychomotor agitation and its complications namely hyperthermia and rhabdomyolysis. As such, the generic approach to sedation and proactive care of agitated toxicology patients discussed above is more than sufficient to protect patients from the complications of antimuscarinic toxicity. However, when that approach is selected many of these patients will become deeply sedated, require critical care admissions, and be subjected to unnecessary testing such as CT scans and lumbar punctures as they will often be hyperthermic and altered. Physostigmine should be used in selected patients who are clinically antimuscarinic, have a normal QRS duration on their ECG, and would otherwise need physical restraint followed by chemical sedation. For these patients, physostigmine will not only confirm the diagnosis but also awaken the patient to allow thorough history taking, a psychiatric interview if necessary, and reduce unnecessary testing. Consultation with a regional poison center or a local medical toxicologist can help with this assessment.

Cyproheptadine

Serotonin toxicity results from single or combined use of drugs that stimulate mostly the 5-HT_{2A} and also possibly the 5-HT_{1A} receptors. Drugs that increase presynaptic stores (MAO inhibitors), promote release (amphetamines) or block reuptake (SSRIs, cocaine, meperidine) of serotonin are commonly implicated. Experimental animal models[67] and human case reports[68,69] suggest a potential role for cyproheptadine as an adjunct in the care of these patients. However, given that the major life threats are agitation and hyperthermia, that cyproheptadine is not available in a parenteral formulation, and that in select acute overdoses gastrointestinal decontamination with activated charcoal might be warranted, cyproheptadine's role is limited but is reasonable for mild cases of serotonin toxicity.

Dantrolene

Dantrolene is the drug of choice for malignant hyperthermia, a rare genetic disorder of the ryanodine receptor that leads to hyperthermia after exposure to inhalation anesthetics, succinylcholine, and other even less common drugs and conditions. Simply because a condition results in temperature elevation and adverse outcomes it is not always "malignant hyperthermia" and treatment with dantrolene is not indicated by analogy.[70,71] Attempts to find and administer dantrolene to patients who do not have malignant hyperthermia can lead to delays in life-saving interventions, specifically sedation and cooling. Dantrolene is, therefore, not indicated as a first-line therapy in patients with a low likelihood of malignant hyperthermia based on historical considerations. It can, however, be administered after sedation and cooling are started if malignant hyperthermia is suspected and muscle relaxation is refractory to neuromuscular blockade.

SUMMARY

Patients with agitated toxidromes span severities of illness from conditions as benign as alcohol intoxication to sympathomimetic toxicity with life-threatening hyperthermia. Even when the etiology seems toxicologic in nature these patients not only have the ability to sustain trauma but also by their behavior injure health care providers, other patients, and their families, and disrupt an entire emergency department. Emergency departments need to develop organized protocols for the assessment and treatment of these patients that recognize the potential for a high-acuity condition, provide a safe environment for all involved, minimize the use and duration of physical restraints, and immediately identify and treat life-threatening conditions. When the etiology is clearly known, specific interventions can be directed at the underlying pathology such as the preferred use of benzodiazepines in patients with alcohol withdrawal. When the etiology is undifferentiated the choice of pharmacotherapy is largely driven by provider experience and institutional protocols. The available data suggest that the differences in the onset and duration of behavioral control could be tailored to the individual needs of the patient. Understanding the pharmacokinetics and pharmacodynamics of these drugs is essential to such an approach. The goal of behavioral control should not be limited to the restoration of a calm state, but rather to the time to attain a full set of vital signs including a core temperature and a rapid glucose concentration, establish intravenous access and send desired laboratory investigations, perform a focused physical examination, and begin resuscitation and cooling if needed.

CLINICS CARE POINTS

- Hyperthermia from sympathomimetics is most quickly treated with immersion in bath water.
- Physostigmine is safe to use in a pure anticholinergic toxidrome.
- Intravenous use of sedatives achieves behavioral control faster than intramuscular administration and should be preferred in severely agitated patients.

DISCLOSURE

The authors have nothing to disclose.

REFERENCES

1. Donlon PT, Hopkin J, Tupin JP. Overview: efficacy and safety of the rapid neuroleptization method with injectable haloperidol. Am J Psychiatry 1979;136(3):273–8.
2. Asch DA, Parker RM. The Libby Zion case. One step forward or two steps backward? N Engl J Med 1988;318(12):771–5.
3. Patel N. Learning lessons: the Libby Zion case revisited. J Am Coll Cardiol 2014;64(25):2802–4.
4. Klein LR, Driver BE, Miner JR, et al. Intramuscular midazolam, olanzapine, ziprasidone, or haloperidol for treating acute agitation in the emergency department. Ann Emerg Med 2018;72(4):374–85.
5. Martel ML, Driver BE, Miner JR, et al. Randomized double-blind trial of intramuscular droperidol, ziprasidone, and lorazepam for acute undifferentiated agitation in the emergency department. Acad Emerg Med 2021;28(4):421–34.
6. Cole JB, Stang JL, DeVries PA, et al. A prospective study of intramuscular droperidol or olanzapine for acute agitation in the emergency department: a natural experiment owing to drug shortages. Ann Emerg Med 2021;78(2):274–86.
7. Cole JB, Moore JC, Nystrom PC, et al. A prospective study of ketamine versus haloperidol for severe prehospital agitation. Clin Toxicol (Phila) 2016;54(7):556–62.
8. Cole JB, Klein LR, Nystrom PC, et al. A prospective study of ketamine as primary therapy for prehospital profound agitation. Am J Emerg Med 2018;36(5):789–96.
9. Martel M, Sterzinger A, Miner J, et al. Management of acute undifferentiated agitation in the emergency department: a randomized double-blind trial of droperidol, ziprasidone, and midazolam. Acad Emerg Med 2005;12(12):1167–72.
10. Calver L, Drinkwater V, Gupta R, et al. Droperidol v. haloperidol for sedation of aggressive behaviour in acute mental health: randomised controlled trial. Br J Psychiatry 2015;206(3):223–8.
11. Isbister GK, Calver LA, Page CB, et al. Randomized controlled trial of intramuscular droperidol versus midazolam for violence and acute behavioral disturbance: the DORM study. Ann Emerg Med 2010;56(4):392–401 e1.
12. Catravas JD, Waters IW. Acute cocaine intoxication in the conscious dog: studies on the mechanism of lethality. J Pharmacol Exp Ther 1981;217(2):350–6.

13. Bohnert AS, Prescott MR, Vlahov D, et al. Ambient temperature and risk of death from accidental drug overdose in New York City, 1990-2006. Addiction 2010; 105(6):1049–54.
14. Marzuk PM, Tardiff K, Leon AC, et al. Ambient temperature and mortality from unintentional cocaine overdose. JAMA 1998;279(22):1795–800.
15. Wu AH, McKay C, Broussard LA, et al. National academy of clinical biochemistry laboratory medicine practice guidelines: recommendations for the use of laboratory tests to support poisoned patients who present to the emergency department. Clin Chem 2003;49(3):357–79.
16. Moeller KE, Kissack JC, Atayee RS, et al. Clinical interpretation of urine drug tests: what clinicians need to know about urine drug screens. Mayo Clin Proc 2017;92(5):774–96.
17. Kellermann AL, Fihn SD, LoGerfo JP, et al. Impact of drug screening in suspected overdose. Ann Emerg Med 1987;16(11):1206–16.
18. Eisen JS, Sivilotti ML, Boyd KU, et al. Screening urine for drugs of abuse in the emergency department: do test results affect physicians' patient care decisions? CJEM 2004;6(2):104–11.
19. Tenenbein M. Do you really need that emergency drug screen? Clin Toxicol (Phila) 2009;47(4):286–91.
20. Lager PS, Attema-de Jonge ME, Gorzeman MP, et al. Clinical value of drugs of abuse point of care testing in an emergency department setting. Toxicol Rep 2018;5:12–7.
21. Connors NJ, Alsakha A, Larocque A, et al. Antipsychotics for the treatment of sympathomimetic toxicity: A systematic review. Am J Emerg Med 2019;37(10): 1880–90.
22. Marder SR, Sorsaburu S, Dunayevich E, et al. Case reports of postmarketing adverse event experiences with olanzapine intramuscular treatment in patients with agitation. J Clin Psychiatry 2010;71(4):433–41.
23. Chan EW, Taylor DM, Knott JC, et al. Intravenous droperidol or olanzapine as an adjunct to midazolam for the acutely agitated patient: a multicenter, randomized, double-blind, placebo-controlled clinical trial. Ann Emerg Med 2013;61(1):72–81.
24. Cole JB, Moore JC, Dolan BJ, et al. A prospective observational study of patients receiving intravenous and intramuscular olanzapine in the emergency department. Ann Emerg Med 2017;69(3):327–336 e2.
25. Martel ML, Klein LR, Rivard RL, et al. A large retrospective cohort of patients receiving intravenous olanzapine in the emergency department. Acad Emerg Med 2016;23(1):29–35.
26. Williams AM. Coadministration of intramuscular olanzapine and benzodiazepines in agitated patients with mental illness. Ment Health Clin 2018;8(5):208–13.
27. Dundee JW, Gamble JA, Assaf RA. Letter: Plasma-diazepam levels following intramuscular injection by nurses and doctors. Lancet 1974;2(7894):1461.
28. Hung OR, Dyck JB, Varvel J, et al. Comparative absorption kinetics of intramuscular midazolam and diazepam. Can J Anaesth 1996;43(5 Pt 1):450–5.
29. Korttila K, Linnoila M. Absorption and sedative effects of diazepam after oral administration and intramuscular administration into the vastus lateralis muscle and the deltoid muscle. Br J Anaesth 1975;47(8):857–62.
30. Silbergleit R, Durkalski V, Lowenstein D, et al. Intramuscular versus intravenous therapy for prehospital status epilepticus. N Engl J Med 2012;366(7):591–600.
31. Welch RD, Nicholas K, Durkalski-Mauldin VL, et al. Intramuscular midazolam versus intravenous lorazepam for the prehospital treatment of status epilepticus in the pediatric population. Epilepsia 2015;56(2):254–62.

32. Greenblatt DJ, Comer WH, Elliott HW, et al. Clinical pharmacokinetics of lorazepam. III. Intravenous injection. Preliminary results. Research Support, U.S. Gov't, Non-P.H.S. J Clin Pharmacol 1977;17(8–9):490–4.
33. Greenblatt DJ, Ehrenberg BL, Gunderman J, et al. Pharmacokinetic and electroencephalographic study of intravenous diazepam, midazolam, and placebo. Clin Pharmacol Ther 1989;45(4):356–65.
34. Greenblatt DJ, Ehrenberg BL, Gunderman J, et al. Kinetic and dynamic study of intravenous lorazepam: comparison with intravenous diazepam 1989;250(1): 134–40.
35. Greenblatt DJ, Joyce TH, Comer WH, et al. Clinical pharmacokinetics of lorazepam. II. Intramuscular injection. Research Support, U.S. Gov't, Non-P.H.S. Clin Pharmacol Ther 1977;21(2):222–30.
36. File SE, Bond AJ. Impaired performance and sedation after a single dose of lorazepam. Psychopharmacology (Berl) 1979;66(3):309–13.
37. Reves JG, Fragen RJ, Vinik HR, et al. Midazolam: pharmacology and uses. Anesthesiology 1985;62(3):310–24.
38. Barr J, Zomorodi K, Bertaccini EJ, et al. A double-blind, randomized comparison of i.v. lorazepam versus midazolam for sedation of ICU patients via a pharmacologic model. Anesthesiology 2001;95(2):286–98.
39. Lim HS, Kim SJ, Noh YH, et al. Exploration of optimal dosing regimens of haloperidol, a D2 Antagonist, via modeling and simulation analysis in a D2 receptor occupancy study. Pharm Res 2013;30(3):683–93.
40. Riddell J, Tran A, Bengiamin R, et al. Ketamine as a first-line treatment for severely agitated emergency department patients. Am J Emerg Med 2017; 35(7):1000–4.
41. Isbister GK, Calver LA, Downes MA, et al. Ketamine as rescue treatment for difficult-to-sedate severe acute behavioral disturbance in the emergency department. Ann Emerg Med 2016;67(5):581–7.e1.
42. Battaglia J, Moss S, Rush J, et al. Haloperidol, lorazepam, or both for psychotic agitation? A multicenter, prospective, double-blind, emergency department study. Am J Emerg Med 1997;15(4):335–40.
43. ACEP Excited Delirium Task Force. White paper report on excited delirium syndrome. 2009;
44. Roppolo LP, Morris DW, Khan F, et al. Improving the management of acutely agitated patients in the emergency department through implementation of Project BETA (Best Practices in the Evaluation and Treatment of Agitation). J Am Coll Emerg Physicians Open 2020;1(5):898–907.
45. Garriga M, Pacchiarotti I, Kasper S, et al. Assessment and management of agitation in psychiatry: expert consensus. World J Biol Psychiatry 2016;17(2):86–128.
46. Wilson MP, Pepper D, Currier GW, et al. The psychopharmacology of agit ation: consensus statement of the american association for emergency psychiatry project Beta psychopharmacology workgroup. West J Emerg Med 2012;13(1):26–34.
47. Bouchama A, Knochel JP. Heat stroke. N Engl J Med 2002;346(25):1978–88.
48. Shapiro Y, Alkan M, Epstein Y, et al. Increase in rat intestinal permeability to endotoxin during hyperthermia. Eur J Appl Physiol Occup Physiol 1986;55(4):410–2.
49. Shih CJ, Lin MT, Tsai SH. Experimental study on the pathogenesis of heat stroke. J Neurosurg 1984;60(6):1246–52.
50. Yang TH, Shih MF, Wen YS, et al. Attenuation of circulatory shock and cerebral ischemia injury in heat stroke by combination treatment with dexamethasone and hydroxyethyl starch. Exp Transl Stroke Med 2010;2(1):19.

51. Shapiro Y, Rosenthal T, Sohar E. Experimental heatstroke. A model in dogs. Arch Intern Med 1973;131(5):688–92.
52. Douma MJ, Aves T, Allan KS, et al. First aid cooling techniques for heat stroke and exertional hyperthermia: a systematic review and meta-analysis. Resuscitation 2020;148:173–90.
53. Filep EM, Murata Y, Endres BD, et al. Exertional heat stroke, modality cooling rate, and survival outcomes: a systematic review. Medicina (Kaunas) 2020;56(11):589.
54. Weiner JS, Khogali M. A physiological body-cooling unit for treatment of heat stroke. Lancet 1980;315(8167):507–9.
55. Khogali M, Weiner JS. Heat stroke: report on 18 cases. Lancet 1980;316(8189): 276–8.
56. Proulx CI, Ducharme MB, Kenny GP. Effect of water temperature on cooling efficiency during hyperthermia in humans. J Appl Physiol 1985;94(4):1317–23.
57. Laskowski LK, Landry A, Vassallo SU, et al. Ice water submersion for rapid cooling in severe drug-induced hyperthermia. Clin Toxicol (Phila) 2015;53(3):181–4.
58. Hoffman RS, Goldfrank LR. The poisoned patient with altered consciousness. Controversies in the use of a 'coma cocktail. JAMA 1995;274(7):562–9.
59. Shannon M. Toxicology reviews: physostigmine. Pediatr Emerg Care 1998;14(3): 224–6.
60. Pentel P, Peterson CD. Asystole complicating physostigmine treatment of tricyclic antidepressant overdose. Ann Emerg Med 1980;9(11):588–90.
61. Tong TG, Benowitz NL, Becker CE. Tricyclic antidepressant overdose. Drug Intell Clin Pharm 1976;10:711–2.
62. Burns MJ, Linden CH, Graudins A, et al. A comparison of physostigmine and benzodiazepines for the treatment of anticholinergic poisoning. Ann Emerg Med 2000;35(4):374–81.
63. Watkins JW, Schwarz ES, Arroyo-Plasencia AM, et al. The use of physostigmine by toxicologists in anticholinergic toxicity. J Med Toxicol 2015;11(2):179–84.
64. Arens AM, Shah K, Al-Abri S, et al. Safety and effectiveness of physostigmine: a 10-year retrospective review. Clin Toxicol (Phila) 2017;13:1–7.
65. Boley SP, Olives TD, Bangh SA, et al. Physostigmine is superior to non-antidote therapy in the management of antimuscarinic delirium: a prospective study from a regional poison center. Clin Toxicol (Phila) 2019;57(1):50–5.
66. Wang GS, Baker K, Ng P, et al. A randomized trial comparing physostigmine vs lorazepam for treatment of antimuscarinic (anticholinergic) toxidrome. Clin Toxicol (Phila) 2020;1–13. https://doi.org/10.1080/15563650.2020.1854281.
67. Nisijima K, Yoshino T, Yui K, et al. Potent serotonin (5-HT)(2A) receptor antagonists completely prevent the development of hyperthermia in an animal model of the 5-HT syndrome. Brain Res 2001;890(1):23–31.
68. Graudins A, Stearman A, Chan B. Treatment of the serotonin syndrome with cyproheptadine. J Emerg Med 1998;16(4):615–9.
69. Lappin RI, Auchincloss EL. Treatment of the serotonin syndrome with cyproheptadine. N Engl J Med 1994;331(15):1021–2.
70. Fox AW. More on rhabdomyolysis associated with cocaine intoxication. N Engl J Med 1989;321(18):1271.
71. Hadad E, Cohen-Sivan Y, Heled Y, et al. Clinical review: treatment of heat stroke: should dantrolene be considered? Crit Care 2005;9(1):86–91.

Pediatric Toxicology

Jennifer A. Ross, MD, MPH[a,*], David L. Eldridge, MD[b]

KEYWORDS

- Pediatric toxicology • Toxic single pills and swallows • Essential oils
- Gastrointestinal decontamination • Evaluation of the poisoned patient

KEY POINTS

- All health care practitioners who work with children in any capacity, especially emergency medicine physicians, should be familiar with the general management of the poisoned pediatric patient.
- There is limited evidence of clinical benefit with early gastrointestinal decontamination in the poisoned pediatric patient.
- Small children can be uniquely and severely affected by very small exposures to toxic substances.
- Certain medications have proven fatal to children in ingestions of single tablets or swallows, and health care providers should be cautious when managing children with exposures to these agents.

INTRODUCTION

Pediatrics plays an important role in the field of medical toxicology. According to the most recent annual report from the American Association of Poison Control Centers (AAPCC), pediatric exposures accounted for 58% of all U.S. poison center calls involving human exposures.[1] Poisoned pediatric patients can present unique and complex issues when compared with their adult counterparts. Small children are innately curious, leading to frequent inadvertent exposures to medications and substances. Providers must be aware of substances that have been found to be extremely toxic to children even when only small, accidental ingestions occur.[2–5] The majority of exposures in younger children are unintentional (99% of exposures in children <6 years old), compared with exposures in teenagers that are more commonly intentional (62% of exposures in children 13–19 years old).[1] There also continue to be increased pediatric exposures to essential oils, which remain unregulated by the U.S. Food and Drug Administration (FDA) and can have potentially severe adverse effects in children.[1,6,7] With such a vast array of potential toxic exposures affecting children of all ages, it

[a] Boston Children's Hospital, 300 Longwood Avenue, Boston, MA 02115, USA; [b] Department of Pediatrics, Brody School of Medicine at East Carolina University, 600 Moye Blvd, Greenville, NC 27834, USA

* Corresponding author.

E-mail address: Jennifer.Ross@childrens.harvard.edu

Emerg Med Clin N Am 40 (2022) 237–250
https://doi.org/10.1016/j.emc.2022.01.004 emed.theclinics.com
0733-8627/22/

is important for all health care practitioners who work with children to understand the general management approach to the poisoned pediatric patient.

DISCUSSION

Children comprise the majority of toxic exposures, with 1,236,227 exposures reported in children less than 20 years old in 2019, including 917,512 exposures reported in children 5 years of age and younger.[1] The overwhelming majority of these exposures are not fatal. Based on the National Poison Data System, 100 pediatric fatalities were reported in 2019 to the U.S. poison centers (less than 20 years old).[1] However, pediatric fatalities from toxic exposures in 2019 increased 16.3% when compared with 2018.[1] Even though pediatric poisoning fatalities are rare, certain substances have high potential to cause pediatric morbidity and mortality and warrant special attention and educational efforts.[5]

Approach to Pediatric Poisonings

Poisoned patients should be medically stabilized first, followed by seeking out further information, performing a complete physical examination, and obtaining ancillary testing.[8] While the physical examination and laboratory testing process will be similar in both poisoned children and adults, there are special considerations to be taken in the evaluation and management of the poisoned pediatric patient.[9]

History

Obtaining a history in the setting of potential poisoning can present many difficulties. In the case of an inadvertent exposure in a toddler, the potential exposure may have been unwitnessed and it is often unclear how much of the substance was ingested. On the other hand, adolescents and young adults may choose to withhold information about exposure from health care providers. Additionally, many pediatric patients present to a health care setting already symptomatic and may be too altered or too sedated to answer questions appropriately. It is important that physicians consider poisoning as a potential diagnosis in children who present with symptoms of unclear etiology.[2]

A thorough history should be attempted from the patient, witnesses to the exposure, or household members/social contacts. Specific questions pertinent to toxicologic history should focus on the timing of the exposure, the substance(s) involved, the method of exposure (ingestion, inhalation, injection, dermal absorption, and so forth), and any medications in the household (eg, the patient's prescriptions, household members' prescriptions, over-the-counter medications, and vitamins/supplements).[8] Household members should be asked about whereby such medications are stored, as medications that have been removed from their original containers and transferred into secondary containers (ie, pill organizers) can be a risk factor for unintentional pediatric exposures.[10] Toddlers are more often poisoned by a single agent, as opposed to the multiple agents seen more commonly in intentional ingestions.[5] It is important to separate adolescents and young adults from their caregivers, as they may be more forthcoming about substance use or medication misuse when alone.

Gastrointestinal decontamination

In the majority of pediatric poisonings, supportive care is warranted more than any other specific treatments. There are methods of gastrointestinal decontamination that warrant further discussion, including the administration of activated charcoal, whole bowel irrigation, and gastric lavage. It is important that children with toxic exposures who need further evaluation present to the emergency department (ED) immediately and that prehospital transport is not delayed for gastrointestinal decontamination.[2] These techniques have limited indication, carry risk, and should never be routine. We also recommend that these gastrointestinal decontamination techniques be conducted through consultation with a medical toxicologist or local poison control center.[11–13]

Activated charcoal. Activated charcoal therapy involves the oral or nasogastric administration of activated charcoal to adsorb toxin and prevent systemic absorption.[11] Activated charcoal was administered in only 0.5% of exposures in children less than 6 years old in 2019 according to the data associated with U.S. poison centers.[1] As there is no definitive evidence that activated charcoal administration improves clinical outcomes, it should not be administered routinely in poisoned pediatric patients.[11] We recommend that health care providers call the poison center immediately on the recognition of potential pediatric poisoning and discuss the utility of activated charcoal administration on a case-by-case basis.

Whole bowel irrigation. Whole bowel irrigation involves the administration of large amounts of polyethylene glycol electrolyte solution to cleanse the bowel and reduce systemic absorption of toxins.[12] While there is no conclusive evidence that it leads to improved clinical outcomes in poisoned patients, it has the potential to be beneficial in specific situations.[14] In 2019, whole bowel irrigation was performed in 85 cases of pediatric exposures in children less than 6 years old according to data associated with U.S. poison centers.[1] We recommend that whole bowel irrigation not be performed routinely in poisoned pediatric patients and not without guidance from a poison center or a medical toxicologist.

Lavage. Fifty years ago, gastric lavage was used routinely for patients with oral overdoses.[15] However, since that time there have been numerous reports documenting the risks and complications associated with its administration.[13,15] In 2019, gastric lavage was rarely used in the pediatric population according to the data associated with U.S. poison centers (eg, used in only 14 cases of pediatric exposures in children <6 years old).[1] Administration of gastric lavage likely has no clinical benefit in most cases of pediatric poisoning.

Urine drug screen

The history and physical examination is often sufficient to dictate management in the poisoned pediatric patient, but in certain cases, ancillary work-up can provide further clues.[5] Urine drug screens, while commonly obtained in cases of suspected toxicologic exposures, have numerous limitations.[16,17] False-positive results occur due to cross-reactivity with drugs having similar structures, while false negatives occur due to cut-off levels whereby the drug is present but in too low of an amount to be detected, or due to contaminants interfering with the test.[18] It is impossible for any screening test to evaluate for all possible toxicologic exposures, especially with the plethora of substances entering into society via the Internet.[5,18] Urine drug screens must be interpreted with caution and, if questions arise, the provider should request the assistance of your health systems' laboratory clinical chemist and/or a medical toxicologist. The management of symptomatic patients should be determined by clinical presentation regardless of urine drug screen results.

Medications and Substances that Are Toxic to Small Children in Small Amounts

Young children, especially those less than 6 years of age, are susceptible to toxic effects from small exposures due to their low body mass and less developed metabolic pathways.[19] In addition, their developmental age may increase their likelihood of exploratory consumption.[5,19] Certain medications are dangerous in ingestions as small as a single pill or swallow.[2–5] As new drugs are manufactured, especially those in higher doses and extended-release formulations, the list of substances that are toxic to children in small amounts continues to expand.[20] **Box 1** lists some of the drugs and substances that are particularly dangerous to small children. Much of the concern with the agents listed in **Box 1** is based largely on case reports or case series whereby small amounts were reportedly ingested and severe effects occurred. The strength of this evidence is often not rigorous. However, these reports recur consistently enough that the treating physician should be particularly cautious when managing pediatric exposures to these agents in small children. Instilling this caution is the core objective of this section. We will briefly discuss some of these medications and the available evidence of significant toxicity in children exposed to small amounts (usually only 1 or 2 doses). Recognition of this potential danger, and not the management, is the focus of this discussion.[21]

Antimalarials

Chloroquine and hydroxychloroquine are classically recognized as antimalarial, but also have FDA indications for lupus erythematosus and rheumatoid arthritis.[20,22] In 2020, due to reports of their potential benefit in the prevention and treatment of COVID-19 as well as a temporary emergency use authorization by the FDA, chloroquine and hydroxychloroquine received increased media attention.[23,24] This led to increased exposures in the general population and reiterated the need for physicians to be familiar with the toxicity associated with chloroquine and hydroxychloroquine.[25] In 2019, there were 187 antimalarial exposures in children less than 20 years old, with 114 of those exposures in children less than 6 years old.[1]

Chloroquine and hydroxychloroquine have a narrow therapeutic index and can lead to significant multi-system organ toxicity in overdose, including ventricular arrhythmias, conduction blockade, cardiovascular collapse, seizures, and hypokalemia.[20,22–24] The minimum potential fatal dose per body weight is 20 mg/kg for both chloroquine and hydroxychloroquine.[3] Hydroxychloroquine is available in 200 mg tablets, and chloroquine is available in 500 mg tablets; ingestion of 1 tablet of either hydroxychloroquine or chloroquine could be potentially fatal in a toddler.[3] There are

Box 1
Drugs that are potentially highly toxic to small children in small amounts

Antiarrhythmics

Antimalarials

Antipsychotics

Benzocaine

Beta-blockers

Calcium channel blockers

Opioids

Sulfonylureas

Tricyclic antidepressants

Data from the following references.[2–5,8]

numerous pediatric case reports of fatalities associated with ingestions of 1 or 2 tablets of chloroquine in children less than 6 years of age, with reports of fatalities after ingestions as small as 300 mg.[19,22,26] There are fewer case reports of pediatric exposures to hydroxychloroquine in the literature; however, ingestions should be considered similar to chloroquine and regarded with extreme caution.[22]

Calcium channel blockers

Calcium channel blockers (CCBs) are used for a variety of indications including hypertension, angina pectoris, coronary artery disease, atrial fibrillation, and migraine headaches.[27–29] CCBs work by inhibiting the flow of calcium through voltage-dependent L-type calcium channels located in smooth muscle, myocardium, and the pancreas.[27–30] This blockade leads to decreased intracellular calcium, causing peripheral vasodilation, decreased cardiac conduction and contractility, as well as a hypoinsulinemic state leading to hyperglycemia.[27–31]

There are multiple CCBs available in the US, including dihydropyridines such as amlodipine and nifedipine, and non-dihydropyridines such as verapamil and diltiazem.[4,27–29,31] It is believed that in CCB overdose the drug's pharmacologic selectivity is lost and thus all classes of CCBs can lead to significant toxicity, including profound bradycardia, hypotension, dysrhythmias, conduction disturbances, and cardiovascular collapse.[28,31] CCBs are manufactured in both immediate-release and modified-release preparations, with ingestions of the latter requiring an extended observation period due to the potential for delayed adverse effects.[4,27]

In 2019, CCBs were associated with the sixth largest number of exposure-related fatalities according to U.S. poison center data, with CCBs alone responsible for 1198 exposures in children less than 6 years old.[1] Nifedipine and verapamil are most often associated with symptomatic ingestions.[31,32] The minimal potential fatal dose per body weight is 15 mg/kg for nifedipine, verapamil, and diltiazem.[3] Diltiazem is available in tablets as large as 420 mg, verapamil is available in tablets as large as 360 mg, and nifedipine is available in tablets as large as 90 mg.[3,33] There are numerous reports of pediatric fatalities associated with verapamil and nifedipine, in some cases after the ingestion of only 1 or 2 pills.[4,19,27,31,34] There is at least one case report of a pediatric fatality after the ingestion of an unknown amount of diltiazem.[31] In a review of pediatric amlodipine ingestions using the U.S. National Poison Data System, there were no fatalities, but there were noted clinical effects with ingestions as small as 2.5 mg.[35] Consultation with a poison control center is strongly recommended for any ingestions involving CCBs. Unless there is a clear asymptomatic presentation and dosing can be confirmed at subtherapeutic amounts, immediate referral to the ED is recommended.[27]

Essential oils

There are numerous essential oils that can cause toxicity in pediatric patients, often due to inadvertent ingestions. Unfortunately, consumers frequently use these oils unaware of their potential toxicities.[6,36] In the 2019 annual U.S. poison center report, essential oils were responsible for the sixteenth most common exposures in pediatric patients less than 6 years of age, contributing to 17,394 exposures (~2% of exposures in this age range).[1] **Box 2** lists examples of essential oils that have been associated with pediatric toxicity. Some of the most toxic essential oils are discussed in further detail .

Camphor. Camphor was initially derived from *Cinnamonum camphora*, the camphor tree, but today is synthetically produced.[20,37–39] In the past it has been used as a contraceptive, abortifacient, analeptic, aphrodisiac, antiseptic, lactation suppressant, and

Box 2
Essential oils with reports of significant pediatric toxicity

Camphor

Cinnamon oil

Clove oil

Comfrey

Eucalyptus

Lavender oil

Nutmeg

Oil of wintergreen

Pennyroyal

Peppermint oil

Pine oil

Tea tree oil

Data from the following references.[2,4,5,9,20]

cold remedy.[2,40,41] Currently, there are numerous nonprescription products containing camphor such as essential oils and topical medications, including rubs, balms, gels, ointments, creams, sprays, patches, and chapsticks.[37,41,42] Reports of camphor toxicity have appeared in the literature for over 100 years.[38] Toxicity generally occurs due to the oral ingestion of topical products, likely due to toddlers' exploratory natures, and can lead to rapid onset of effects within 5 to 15 minutes.[2,37,38,40–42] There are also case reports of toxicity due to camphor inhalation or dermal exposure.[41] In 2019, camphor alone was responsible for 7321 exposures in children less than 6 years old.[1] It is important that health care providers be aware of camphor toxicity due to its continued availability in over-the-counter and unregulated products, many of which lack child-resistant packaging.[20,40]

Mild camphor toxicity may present with gastrointestinal symptoms such as nausea and vomiting in addition to a feeling of warmth, while severe toxicity produces neurologic effects such as confusion, myoclonus, seizures, or coma.[20,37–40,42,43] Neurologic symptoms generally appear within 4 hours of ingestion.[2] There is a case report of delayed onset seizure 9 hours postingestion of Vicks VapoRub (4.8% camphor).[44] The minimal potential fatal dose per body weight is reported as 100 mg/kg.[3] Ingestions of amounts of camphor as small as 500 mg have resulted in pediatric fatalities due to respiratory failure or status epilepticus.[2,37,38,45] The FDA has regulated that products cannot contain more than 11% camphor.[37,41] However, with products such as Tiger Balm containing 11% camphor and Campho-Phenique containing 10.8% camphor, ingestions of less than 5 mL can still reach the potentially fatal amount of 500 mg.[2,5,37,39] Per a 2008 practice guideline from the AAPCC, patients who have ingested more than 30 mg/kg of a camphor-containing product should be referred to an ED.[41]

Oil of wintergreen. Oil of wintergreen is a concentrated essential oil that often contains nearly 100% methyl salicylate.[2,4,46] Methyl salicylate is found in many household products including creams, oils, lotions, liniments, ointments, and analgesic balms.[29,46] If inadvertently ingested, methyl salicylate is metabolized to salicylic acid.[46] Oil of wintergreen is high risk to young children who might inadvertently drink this pleasant-smelling and palatable essential oil.[2,4,36,40] Toxicity occurs quickly after ingestion and is identical to poisoning from other forms of salicylates.[2,40] In 2019, methyl salicylate alone was responsible for 2965 exposures in children less than 6 years old.[1] The FDA has regulated that all products containing more than 5% methyl salicylate must contain a warning about potential toxicity.[36]

Symptoms of methyl salicylate toxicity may include such findings as respiratory alkalosis, metabolic acidosis, nausea, vomiting, tachypnea, tinnitus, dehydration, diaphoresis, fever, lethargy, seizures, coma, and cardiovascular collapse.[2,4,29,40,46] Methyl salicylate has a minimal potential fatal dose per body weight of 200 mg/kg.[3] As 1 mL of 98% oil of wintergreen contains 1400 mg of salicylate, exposure to less than a teaspoon (7000 mg of salicylate) can be a potentially fatal ingestion.[4,5,29,46] Case reports endorse that small ingestions (4–15 mL) of oil of wintergreen can be fatal in children less than 6 years of age.[46–48] Fatalities are often secondary to pulmonary or cerebral edema.[2] All children suspected to have ingested oil of wintergreen should be immediately referred to the ED due to their acute risk of decompensation.[2,40,46]

Lindane

Lindane, or gamma-hexachlorocyclohexane, is an organochlorine used for the treatment of lice and scabies.[49,50] Organochlorines are highly toxic, with many products banned throughout the United States.[51] Commercial lindane pesticide products were banned by the FDA in 2007.[52] Pharmaceutical use of lindane was banned in the state of California in 2002 due to concerns over lindane's effects on water quality.[49,50] In other states, lindane continues to be used in lotions and shampoos, and in 2003 the FDA mandated that these products have a black box warning label on their potential neurotoxic effects.[53] In 2007, the FDA sent a letter to Morton Grove pharmaceuticals (the U.S. manufacturer of lindane products), citing them for false safety claims, and in 2009 the lindane warning label was changed to note that seizures and deaths had been reported with its use.[54,55]

Lindane is absorbed across both intact and abraded skin, and younger children with more skin surface area per weight may absorb more lindane systemically.[49,53] Lindane toxicity can manifest as nausea, vomiting, abdominal pain, oral irritation, cough, dyspnea, headache, confusion, central nervous system (CNS) depression, and seizures.[5,56,57] Of these symptoms, neurotoxicity is the most frequently reported and is often described in infants and young children.[57,58] Toxicity has occurred after both excessive dermal exposures and inadvertent ingestions of topical agents.[58–60] After lindane product use, an infant fatality was found attributable to lindane toxicity, and other reported deaths have been associated with lindane use.[54,57,61]

Opioids

As the opioid epidemic worsens and expands, deaths due to opioid exposures continue to increase.[62] The Centers for Disease Control and Prevention (CDC) reported that opioids were involved in 28.7% of suspected overdoses treated in EDs among persons aged 15 to 24 years in 2019.[63] Pharmaceutical and illegal opioid preparations were responsible for the second most fatalities reported to poison centers in 2019, contributing to 9.2% of all deaths.[1] There were 2913 exposures attributed to pharmaceutical and illegal opioids in children less than 6 years old.[1] Opioid exposures present a high risk of toxicity in the pediatric population, with certain opioids causing fatalities in ingestions of single pills or swallows.[2–4,8,64] Exposures to these drugs can lead to the opioid toxidrome of miosis, CNS depression, and respiratory depression, in addition to dizziness, hypotension, hypothermia, and ileus.[2,4,8,29] Opioids are high risk to children in small doses and include such agents as buprenorphine, codeine, diphenoxylate, fentanyl, hydrocodone, methadone, morphine, oxycodone, propoxyphene, and tramadol.[2,3] Highlighting the danger, there is a published case report example of a pediatric fatality in a 3 year old after the ingestion of two 2 mg hydromorphone tablets.[65]

In 2019, methadone was responsible for 123 single agent and combination exposures in children less than 6 years old.[1] Significant pediatric toxicity has been reported after ingestions as small as 5 mg.[66] The minimal potential fatal dose per body weight is 1 mg/kg, with methadone tablets available in doses up to 40 mg.[3] There have been numerous cases of methadone ingestions that have led to fatalities, some after ingestions of a single methadone tablet or single teaspoon of methadone suspension.[66,67] All children ingesting any amount of methadone should be referred to an ED.[66]

Lomotil (diphenoxylate-atropine)

Lomotil is an antidiarrheal medication consisting of diphenoxylate and atropine.[2,4,5,40,64,68] Diphenoxylate is used to decrease gastrointestinal motility, with atropine added to deter potential diphenoxylate misuse.[20,68,69] The presence of atropine may lead to gut slowing due to anticholinergic effects, and thus there is potential for delayed diphenoxylate absorption and prolonged opioid effects.[2,4,5,40] Severe toxicity has occurred in children after ingestions as small as half a tablet of Lomotil, and there are numerous case reports of Lomotil exposures resulting in fatalities.[64,68–72] It should be noted that some health care providers believe that children ingesting 1 tablet or less can remain at home, while others argue that there is not enough data to reach this conclusion.[64,73] Due to often unclear histories of exposures and unclear correlations between amount ingested and toxicity, we recommend referring all diphenoxylate-atropine exposures in children less than 6 years of age to an ED.[69–71]

Sulfonylureas

Sulfonylureas are hypoglycemic agents commonly used in the treatment of diabetes mellitus.[2,4,29] Agents in this class include such drugs as acetohexamide, chlorpropamide, glimepiride, glipizide, glyburide, tolazamide, and tolbutamide.[2,29,74] These medications work on the pancreatic beta cells to release insulin independent of the systemic glucose concentration and induce hypoglycemia.[2,4,74] As sulfonylureas are commonly prescribed and present in numerous households, there is large potential for inadvertent exposures in young children.[29,74]

In 2019, sulfonylureas were responsible for 595 single agent and combination exposures in children less than 6 years old.[1] Ingestions of sulfonylureas in children can lead to delayed and profound hypoglycemia in part due to children's small size, limited synthesis of glucose, and increased glucose utilization.[2,8,75,76] Hypoglycemia can present with a variety of symptoms including diaphoresis, tachycardia, headache, confusion, sedation, weakness, irritability, seizures, and coma.[4,8,74] It is widely reported that pediatric ingestions of 1 or 2 sulfonylurea tablets can cause severe toxicity including delayed life-threatening hypoglycemia.[2,4,5,74–76] The minimal potential fatal dose per body weight is 0.1 mg/kg for glyburide, glipizide, and glimepiride, and 27 mg/kg for chlorpropamide; ingestions of 1 or 2 tablets of these medications could reach a potentially fatal dose in toddlers.[3] There is a reported pediatric fatality of a 2 year old who was found playing with an extended-release glipizide and benazepril, developed seizures, and died secondary to cerebral edema.[74,77] Due to the potential risk for severe toxicity after ingestions of even a single pill, all exposures to sulfonylureas in pediatric patients should be referred to the ED for admission and observation.

Topical anesthetics

Topical anesthetics, such as lidocaine, dibucaine, and benzocaine, can be found in a variety of products.[78] These products can be both prescription and over-the-counter, and are used for multiple indications such as teething gels, thrush, otitis externa, vaginitis, diaper rash, and hemorrhoid creams.[78] In 2019, anesthetics were the fifth most involved substance category contributing to pediatric fatalities in children less than 6 years of age (5.13% of fatalities in this age range).[1] Between 1983 and 2003, there were 7 deaths reported from topical anesthetics in children less than 6 years old.[78] Topical anesthetics can be divided into 2 classes: the amides and the esters. Each class has different potential toxic effects.

Amide anesthetics. Amide anesthetics include lidocaine, EMLA (lidocaine and prilocaine), dibucaine, and bupivacaine.[78] The amide anesthetics block voltage-gated sodium channels and can cause significant toxicity including CNS depression, seizures, and dysrhythmias.[78,79] These effects, specifically seizures, can occur after small ingestions in pediatric patients.[78,80] In 2019, lidocaine was responsible for 621 exposures and dibucaine was responsible for 11 exposures reported to U.S. poison centers in children less than 6 years old.[1] Dibucaine, while prescribed less often, is reported to be 10 times more potent than lidocaine.[78] Oral ingestions of lidocaine and dibucaine have led to death in pediatric patients.[19,78,81]

Ester anesthetics. Ester anesthetics include benzocaine, tetracaine, and procaine.[78] Benzocaine is frequently found in over-the-counter teething gels, mouth rinses and throat lozenges, first aid ointments for burns and dermatitis, hemorrhoid creams, and vaginal creams.[2,40,78] Exposures are often secondary to unintentional ingestions due to exploratory behavior by toddlers or mucosal absorption after topical application.[5,40,82] Benzocaine is known to cause methemoglobinemia, occurring in pediatric patients after topical, oral, and rectal administration.[5,40,78,83] Children with benzocaine toxicity and resulting methemoglobinemia may have a variety of symptoms including emesis, headache, dyspnea, central cyanosis, hypoxia, tachycardia, metabolic acidosis, and somnolence.[2,20,40] Benzocaine can be toxic in small exposures especially in young children, with potential life-threatening consequences.[2,5,40,78,84] Products containing benzocaine are often not found in child-resistant containers.[84] In 2011 and 2018, the FDA released drug safety communications on the toxic effects of benzocaine products and warned consumers not to use these products in children less than 2 years old, but exposures continue to occur.[82,85,86]

Tricyclic antidepressants

Tricyclic antidepressants (TCAs) have numerous mechanisms of action, including sodium channel blockade, potassium channel blockade, alpha-adrenergic blockade, biogenic amine reuptake inhibition, antihistamine properties, and anticholinergic properties.[4,87–89] These mechanisms lead to a complex picture of toxicity, which can include anticholinergic symptoms, QRS prolongation, QTc prolongation, dysrhythmias, hypotension, delirium, coma, and seizures, among other symptoms.[4,5,19,87,89]

The first reported TCA overdoses occurred in 1959.[89,90] In 2019, TCAs were responsible for the twentieth largest number of exposure-related fatalities.[1] The minimum potential fatal dose is reported as 15 mg/kg for amitriptyline, imipramine, and desipramine.[3,88] As all 3 of these medications are supplied in a 150 mg tablet, a 10 kg toddler could ingest the potentially fatal amount with just 1 pill.[5] Death is generally due to cardiotoxicity and CNS toxicity.[4] There are several case reports in the literature of fatalities associated with ingestions of 1 or 2 tablets of a TCA.[19,88] However, it should be noted that some toxicologists argue that single pill ingestions of TCAs are unlikely to cause child fatalities, with the majority of such exposures resulting in benign outcomes.[91] Per an evidence-based consensus published in 2007, ingestions of TCAs (apart from desipramine, nortriptyline, trimipramine, and protriptyline, which have their own guidelines) less than or equal to 5 mg/kg can be monitored at home.[92] In general, TCA exposures should be regarded with extreme caution, and pediatric exposures that are unwitnessed or of unclear amounts will likely need to be referred to a health care facility for evaluation, with guidance from the local poison center. If a child remains asymptomatic 6 hours postingestion, they are unlikely to develop signs of TCA toxicity after this time.[4,29,89,92]

SUMMARY

Pediatric poisonings comprise most of the toxic exposures reported to poison control centers. Exposures to certain substances have high potential to cause pediatric morbidity and mortality in extremely small amounts. These toxins include certain prescription medications, over-the-counter medications, and essential oils. With such a vast array of potential toxic exposures affecting children of all ages, it is important for health care practitioners who work with children to understand the general management approach to the poisoned pediatric patient.

CLINICS CARE POINTS

- All health care practitioners who work with children in any capacity, especially emergency medicine physicians, should be familiar with the general management of the poisoned pediatric patient.
- There is limited evidence of clinical benefit with early gastrointestinal decontamination in the poisoned pediatric patient.
- Small children can be uniquely and severely affected by very small exposures to toxic substances.
- Certain medications have proven fatal to children in ingestions of single tablets or swallows, and health care providers should be cautious when managing children with exposures to these agents.

DISCLOSURE

The authors have nothing to disclose.

REFERENCES

1. Gummin D, Mowry J, Beuhler M, et al. Annual report of the American Association of Poison Control Centers' National Poison Data System (NPDS): 37th annual report. Clin Toxicol 2020;58(12):1360–541. https://doi.org/10.1080/15563650.2020.1834219.
2. Eldridge D, Mutter K, Holstege C, et al. An evidence-based review of single pills and swallows that can kill a child. Pediatr Emerg Med Pract 2010;7(3):1–14.
3. Koren G, Nachmani A. Drugs that can kill a toddler with one tablet or teaspoonful: A 2018 updated list. Clin Drug Investig 2019;39:217–22.
4. Michael J, Sztajnkrycer M. Deadly pediatric poisons: nine common agents that kill at low doses. Emerg Med Clin North Am 2004;22.
5. Osterhoudt K. The toxic toddler: drugs that can kill in small doses. Contemp Pediatr 2000;3(73).

6. Woolf A. Essential oil poisoning. J Toxicol Clin Toxicol 1999;37(6):721–7.
7. Crumley N. Essential oils, hand sanitizers, OTC drugs, and more. AAP News. 2020. https://www.aappublications.org/news/2020/11/01/healthalerts110120. Accessed May 22, 2021.
8. McGregor T, Parkar M, Rao S. Evaluation and management of common childhood poisonings. Am Fam Physician 2009;79(5):397–403.
9. Olson KR, Anderson IB, Benowitz NL, et al. Poisoning & drug overdose. 7th edition. McGraw-Hill Education; 2018.
10. Wang G, Hoppe J, Brou L, et al. Medication organizers (pill minders) increase the risk for unintentional pediatric ingestions. J Emerg Med 2017;55:897–901.
11. American Academy of Clinical Toxicology and European Association of Poisons Centres and Clinical Toxicologists. Position paper: single-dose activated charcaol. Clin Toxicol 2005;43(2):61–87.
12. American Academy of Clinical Toxicology and European Association of Poisons Centres and Clinical Toxicologists. Position paper: whole bowel irrigation. Clin Toxicol 2004;42(6):843–54.
13. Benson B, Hoppu K, Troutman W, et al. Position paper update: gastric lavage for gastrointestinal decontamination. Clin Toxicol 2013;51(3):140–6.
14. Tenebein M. Whole bowel irrigation for toxic ingestions. J Toxicol Clin Toxicol 1985;23(2–3):177–84.
15. Kulig K, Rosen P. Lavage redux. J Emerg Med 2017;52(5):758–9.
16. Belson MG, Simon HK. Utility of comprehensive toxicologic screens in children. Am J Emerg Med 1999;17(3):221–4.
17. Eldridge DL, Dobson T, Brady W, et al. Utilizing Diagnostic Investigations in the Poisoned Patient. Med Clin North Am 2005;89(6):1079–105.
18. Kale N. Urine drug tests: ordering and interpretation. Am Fam Physician 2019; 99(1):33–9.
19. Gresham C, Buller SJ. Pediatric single-dose fatal ingestions. Medscape 2020;. https://emedicine.medscape.com/article/1011108.
20. Emery D, Singer JI. Highly toxic ingestions for toddlers: when a pill can kill. Pediatr Emerg Med Rep 1998;3(12):111.
21. Eldridge DL, Van Eyk J, Kornegay C. Pediatric Toxicology. Emerg Med Clin North Am 2007;25(2):283–308.
22. Smith ER, Klein-Schwartz W. Are 1-2 dangerous? chloroquine and hydroxychloroquine exposure in toddlers. J Emerg Med 2005;28(4):437–43.
23. Doyno C, Sobieraj DM, Baker WL. Toxicity of chloroquine and hydroxychloroquine following therapeutic use or overdose. Clin Toxicol 2021;59(1):12–23.
24. Megarbane B. Chloroquine and hydroxychloroquine to treat COVID-19: between hope and caution. Clin Toxicol 2021;59(1):70–1.
25. Erickson T, Chai P, Boyer E. Chloroquine, hydroxychloroquine and COVID-19. Toxicol Commun. 2020;4(1):40–2. https://doi.org/10.1080/24734306.2020.1757967.
26. Kelly J, Wasserman G, Bernard W, et al. Chloroquine poisoning in a child. Ann Emerg Med 1990;19(1):47–50.
27. Olson KR, Erdman AR, Woolf AD, et al. Calcium Channel Blocker Ingestion: An Evidence-Based Consensus Guideline for Out-of-Hospital Management. Clin Toxicol 2005;43(7):797–822.
28. Bartlett JW, Walker PL. Management of Calcium Channel Blocker Toxicity in the Pediatric Patient. J Pediatr Pharmacol Ther 2019;24(5):378–89.
29. Henry K, Harris CR. Deadly Ingestions. Pediatr Clin North Am 2006;53(2): 293–315.

30. Vaghy PL, Williams JS, Schwartz A. Receptor pharmacology of calcium entry blocking agents. Am J Cardiol 1987;59(2):A9–17.
31. Ranniger C, Roche C. Are One or Two Dangerous? Calcium Channel Blocker Exposure in Toddlers. J Emerg Med 2007;33(2):145–54.
32. Passal DB, Crespin FH. Verapamil poisoning in an infant. Pediatrics 1984;73(4): 543–5.
33. Diltiazem Hydrochloride. In: IBM Micromedex drug Ref. 2021. Available at: www.micromedexsolutions.com. Accessed June 21, 2021.
34. Lee DC, Greene T, Dougherty T, et al. Fatal nifedipine ingestions in children. J Emerg Med 2000;19(4):359–61.
35. Benson BE, Spyker DA, Troutman WG, et al. Amlodipine Toxicity in Children Less Than 6 Years of Age: A Dose-Response Analysis Using National Poison Data System Data. J Emerg Med 2010;39(2):186–93.
36. U.S. Food and Drug Administration. Code of Federal Regulations, 21CFR201.303, revised April 1, 2020. 2020. Available at: https://www.accessdata.fda.gov/scripts/cdrh/cfdocs/cfcfr/CFRSearch.cfm?fr=201.303. Accessed June 4, 2021.
37. Love JN, Sammon M, Smereck J. Are one or two dangerous? camphor exposure in toddlers. J Emerg Med 2004;27(1):49–54.
38. Commitee on Drugs. Camphor: who needs it? Pediatrics 1978;62(3):404–6.
39. Phelan WJ. Campor poisoning: over-the-counter dangers. Pediatrics 1976;57(3): 428–31.
40. Liebelt EL, Shannon MW. Small doses, big problems: a selected review of highly toxic common medications. Pediatr Emerg Care 1993;9(5):292–7.
41. Manoguerra AS, Erdman AR, Wax PM, et al. Camphor Poisoning: an Evidence-Based Practice Guideline for Out-of-Hospital Management. Clin Toxicol 2006; 44(4):357–70.
42. Committee on Drugs. Camphor revisited: focus on toxicity. Pediatrics 1994;94(1): 127–8.
43. Khine H, Weiss D, Graber N, et al. A Cluster of Children With Seizures Caused by Camphor Poisoning. Pediatrics 2009;123(5):1269–72.
44. Ruha A, Graeme K, Field A. Late seizure following ingestion of Vicks VapoRub. Acad Emerg Med 2003;10(6):691.
45. Smith A, Margolis G. Camphor poisoning. Am J Pathol 1954;30(5):857–68.
46. Davis JE. Are one or two dangerous? Methyl salicylate exposure in toddlers. J Emerg Med 2007;32(1):63–9.
47. Stevenson C. Oil of wintergreen (methyl salicylate) poisoning: report of three cases, one with autopsy, and a review of the literature. Am J Med Sci 1937; 193:772–88.
48. Litovitz TL, Bailey K, Schmitz B, et al. 1990 annual report of the American Association of Poison Control Centers National Data Collection System. Am J Emerg Med 1991;9(5):461–509.
49. Roberts JR, Karr CJ, Council on Environmental Health. Pesticide Exposure in Children. Pediatrics 2012;130(6):e1765–88.
50. Humphreys EH, Janssen S, Heil A, et al. Outcomes of the California Ban on Pharmaceutical Lindane: Clinical and Ecologic Impacts. Environ Health Perspect 2008;116(3):297–302.
51. Jayaraj R, Megha P, Sreedev P. Review Article. Organochlorine pesticides, their toxic effects on living organisms and their fate in the environment. Interdiscip Toxicol 2016;9(3–4):90–100.

52. U.S. Environmental Protection Agency. Lindane; cancellation order. Fed Regist 2006;71(239):74905–7.
53. FDA issues advisory regarding labeling changes for Lindane products. AAP News 2003;22(3):209.
54. Abrams TW. Warning letter. In: U.S. Food and Drug Administration. 2007. Available at: https://web.archive.org/web/20080104154942/https://www.fda.gov/foi/warning_letters/s6604c.htm. Accessed June 1, 2021.
55. Tucker ME. In: Medscape, editor. FDA rejects NRDC petition to ban lindane. 2012. Available at: https://www.medscape.com/viewarticle/7756900. Accessed June 25, 2021.
56. Unintentional topical lindane ingestions - United States, 1998-2003. Morb Mortal Wkly Rep 2005;54(21):533–5.
57. Nolan K, Kamrath J, Levitt J. Lindane Toxicity: A Comprehensive Review of the Medical Literature: Lindane Toxicity. Pediatr Dermatol 2012;29(2):141–6.
58. Singal A, Thami G. Lindane neurotoxicity in childhood. Am J Ther 2006;13(3):277–80.
59. Ramabhatta S, Sunilkumar G, Somashekhar C. Lindane toxicity following accidental oral ingestion. Indian J Dermatol Venereol Leprol 2014;80(2):181.
60. Lifshitz M, Gavrilov V. Acute lindane poisoning in a child. Isr Med Assoc J 2002;4:731–2.
61. Sudakin DL. Fatality after a single dermal application of lindane lotion. Arch Environ Occup Health 2007;62(4):201–3.
62. Mattson C, Tanz L, Quinn K, et al. Trends and geographic patterns in drug and synthetic opioid overdose deaths - United States, 2013-2019. Morb Mortal Wkly Rep 2021;70(6):202–7. https://doi.org/10.15585/mmwr.mm7006a4.
63. Liu S, Scholl L, Hoots B, et al. Nonfatal drug and polydrug overdoses treated in emergency departments - 29 states, 2018-2019. Morb Mortal Wkly Rep. 2020;69(34):1149–55. https://doi.org/10.15585/mmwr.mm6934a1.
64. Thomas TJ, Pauze D, Love JN. Are One or Two Dangerous? Diphenoxylate-Atropine Exposure in Toddlers. J Emerg Med 2008;34(1):71–5.
65. Cantrell FL, Sherrard J, Andrade M, et al. A pediatric fatality due to accidental hydromorphone ingestion. Clin Toxicol 2017;55(1):60–2.
66. Sachdeva DK, Stadnyk JM. Are one or two dangerous? Opioid exposure in toddlers. J Emerg Med 2005;29(1):77–84.
67. Smialek JE, Monforte JR, Aronow R, et al. Methadone deaths in children: a continuing problem. J Am Med Assoc 1977;238(23):2516–7.
68. Ginsburg CM, Angle CR. Diphenoxylate-Atropine (Lomotil) Poisoning. Clin Toxicol 1969;2(4):377–82.
69. Curtis J, Goel K. Lomotil poisoning in children. Arch Dis Child 1979;54:222–5.
70. Rumack BH, Temple AR. Lomotil poisoning. Pediatrics 1974;53(4):495–500.
71. McCarron MM, Challoner KR, Thompson GA. Diphenoxylate-atropine (Lomotil) overdose in children: an update (report of eight cases and review of the literature). Pediatrics 1991;87(5):694–700.
72. Penfold D, Volans G. Overdose from lomotil. Br Med J 1977;2(6099):1401–2.
73. Farmer BM, Prosser JM, Hoffman RS. Re: "Are One or Two Dangerous? Diphenoxylate-Atropine Exposure in Toddlers. J Emerg Med 2010;38(3):384.
74. Little GL, Boniface KS. Are one or two dangerous? Sulfonylurea exposure in toddlers. J Emerg Med 2005;28(3):305–10.
75. Quadrani DA, Spiller HA, Widder P. Five Year Retrospective Evaluation of Sulfonylurea Ingestion in Children. J Toxicol Clin Toxicol 1996;34(3):267–70.

76. Szlatenyi C, Capes K, Wang R. Delayed hypoglycemia in a child after ingestion of a single glipizide tablet. Ann Emerg Med 1998;31(6):773–6.
77. Litovitz TL, Klein-Schwartz W, Dyer KS, et al. 1997 annual report of the American Association of Poison Control Centers Toxic Exposure Surveillance System. Am J Emerg Med 1998;16:443–97.
78. Curtis LA, Dolan TS, Seibert HE. Are One or Two Dangerous? Lidocaine and Topical Anesthetic Exposures in Children. J Emerg Med 2009;37(1):32–9.
79. Jonville AP, Barbier P, Blond MH, et al. Accidental lidocaine overdosage in an infant. J Toxicol Clin Toxicol 1990;28(1):101–6.
80. Garrettson LK, McGee EB. Rapid Onset of Seizures Following Aspiration of Viscous Lidocaine. J Toxicol Clin Toxicol 1992;30(3):413–22.
81. Amitai Y, Whitesell L, Lovejoy FH. Death Following Accidental Lidocaine Overdose in a Child. N Engl J Med 1986;314(3):182–3.
82. Vohra R, Huntington S, Koike J, et al. Pediatric Exposures to Topical Benzocaine Preparations Reported to a Statewide Poison Control System. West J Emerg Med 2017;18(5):923–7.
83. Goluboff N. Methemoglobinemia due to benzocaine. Pediatrics 1958;21(2): 340–1.
84. Calello DP. Benzocaine: Not Dangerous Enough? Pediatrics 2005;115(5):1452.
85. U.S. Food and Drug Administration. FDA drug safety communication: reports of a rare, but serious and potentially fatal adverse effect with the use of over-the-counter (OTC) benzocaine gels and liquids applied to the gums or mouth. Available at: https://www.fda.gov/drugs/drug-safety-and-availability/fda-drug-safety-communication-reports-rare-serious-and-potentially-fatal-adverse-effect-use-over. Accessed June 1, 2021.
86. U.S. Food and Drug Administration. Risk of serious and potentially fatal blood disorder prompts FDA action on oral over-the-counter benzocaine products used for teething and mouth pain and prescription local anesthetics. 2018. Available at: https://www.fda.gov/drugs/drug-safety-and-availability/risk-serious-and-potentially-fatal-blood-disorder-prompts-fda-action-oral-over-counter-benzocaine. Accessed June 1, 2021.
87. Kerr G, McGuffie A, Wilkie S. Tricyclic antidepressant overdose: a review. Emerg Med J 2001;18(4):236–41.
88. Rosenbaum TG, Kou M. Are one or two dangerous? tricyclic antidepressant exposure in toddlers. J Emerg Med 2005;28(2):169–74.
89. Frommer D, Kulig K, Marx J, et al. Tricyclic antidepressant overdose. J Am Med Assoc 1987;257(4):521–6.
90. Lancaster N, Foster A. Suicide attempt by imipramine overdose. BMJ 1959;1: 338–9.
91. Mullins M, Fishburn S. Comment on: "drugs that can kill a toddler with one tablet or teaspoonful: a 2018 updated list. Clin Drug Investig 2019;39:821–2.
92. Woolf A, Erdman A, Nelson L, et al. Tricyclic antidepressant poisoning: an evidence-based consensus guideline for out-of-hospital management. Clin Toxicol 2007;45(3):203–33.

Metabolic Acidosis

Differentiating the Causes in the Poisoned Patient

Bryan S. Judge, MD[a,b,*]

KEYWORDS

• Metabolic acidosis • Poisoned patients • Toxins • Drugs • Overdose

KEY POINTS

- Metabolic acidosis can arise from a multitude of drugs and toxins through a variety of mechanisms.
- Differentiating the causes of metabolic acidosis in the poisoned patient is an indispensable skill in clinical emergency medicine practice.
- Comprehension of toxin-induced metabolic acidosis, combined with a thorough history, physical examination, appropriate use of laboratory tests, and a stepwise approach should aid the clinician in determining the cause of metabolic acidosis in the poisoned patient.

INTRODUCTION

Metabolic acidosis can be an important consequence of several toxins. Determining which drugs or toxins might be responsible for metabolic acidosis in a patient with an accidental exposure, unknown ingestion, or from therapeutic drug use can present daunting diagnostic and therapeutic challenges. More importantly, vital cellular functions and metabolic processes become impaired with increasing acidosis.[1] Therefore, it is paramount that a clinician recognize those substances that can result in metabolic acidosis so that timely and appropriate therapy can be instituted.

Metabolic acidosis is defined as a process that lowers serum bicarbonate (HCO_3^-) levels less than 24 mEq/L and occurs when H^+ ion production exceeds the body's ability to adequately compensate through buffering or increased minute ventilation. Acidemia should not be confused with acidosis. Acidemia refers to a blood pH less than 7.40 and does not depict the processes that resulted in the derangement in

[a] Department of Emergency Medicine, Division of Medical Toxicology, Michigan State University College of Human Medicine, 15 Michigan Ave NE, Grand Rapids, MI 49503, USA; [b] Spectrum Health Butterworth Emergency Department MC 49, 100 Michigan NE, Grand Rapids, MI 49503, USA

* Corresponding author. Spectrum Health Butterworth Emergency Department MC 49, 100 Michigan NE, Grand Rapids, MI 49503, USA
E-mail address: bryan.judge@spectrumhealth.org

Emerg Med Clin N Am 40 (2022) 251–264
https://doi.org/10.1016/j.emc.2022.01.002
emed.theclinics.com

pH. Comprehensive discussion of acid-base disturbances is beyond the scope of this article and the reader is referred elsewhere for further information.[1,2]

APPROACH TO THE POISONED PATIENT WITH METABOLIC ACIDOSIS

Evaluating a poisoned patient can present myriad challenges to the treating clinician. Poisoned patients often present with altered mental status, substantially limiting the ability to take an adequate history. Significant clues at the scene suggestive of the nature of the overdose may be absent, may be overlooked by medical first responders and family members, and/or may be inadequately conveyed to health care providers. Family members and/or friends who are often able to provide critical information may not immediately accompany the patient to the hospital or be able to be present in the emergency department due to pandemic-related visitor restrictions. However, the exposure history can be enhanced by specific findings on the physical examination. The patient may have a characteristic toxidrome (eg, anticholinergic, cholinergic, opioid, serotonergic, or sympathomimetic), odor, track marks, or other physical examination clues suggesting a poisoning as the cause for the clinical presentation.

Because many poisoned patients are unable or unwilling to provide an accurate history, laboratory evaluation is essential. Diagnostic tests such as a comprehensive metabolic panel and 12-lead electrocardiography should be obtained because they provide invaluable information regarding end-organ toxicity and may assist with diagnosis and treatment, gauge the gravity of the toxicologic process, as well as provide insight into potential deterioration in a patient's medical condition.[3] A quantitative test, if available, for such drugs and toxins as acetaminophen, carboxyhemoglobin, ethylene glycol, iron, methanol, salicylate, or valproate may delineate the cause of an elevated anion gap (AG) metabolic acidosis. An arterial blood gas serves as a useful adjunct in differentiating acid-base disturbances; however, serum HCO_3^- level remains an important initial diagnostic test because a depressed level is an early indicator of many metabolic toxins.

The routine use of available urine drugs screens in the acutely poisoned patient is rarely beneficial in determining the true cause of a poisoning. Urine drug screens only test for a few common drugs; a negative screen does not exclude drugs or other substances as the illness cause. A positive result on the urine drug screen may confirm exposure to a particular substance, but that substance may not be the cause of the patient's clinical condition. Few institutions have readily available comprehensive toxicology laboratory services, which delays turnaround time for comprehensive drug testing.[4] Furthermore, the results of comprehensive drug screens rarely impact either treatment or outcomes while in the emergency department, and often medical decision making is best accomplished through routine diagnostic tests and thoroughly assessing and reassessing the patient's clinical condition.[5,6] Once the comprehensive metabolic panel has been obtained, an AG should be determined using the following equation: $AG = [Na^+] - ([Cl^-] + [HCO_3^-])$. Historically, a normal AG has been 12 ± 4 mEq/L; however, a study by Winter and colleagues[7] suggests that the normal AG should be 7 ± 4 mEq/L, due to an increase in measured chloride from improved instrumentation. Therefore it is important to recognize that the previously accepted range for the AG may not be suitable with newer laboratory technology. If the ingestion of a toxic alcohol (ie, ethylene glycol, isopropanol, methanol) is suspected, osmolarity should be estimated by $osmolarity = 2 \times [Na^+] + [glucose]/18 + [BUN]/2.8$.[8] An osmol gap (OG) can then be determined by subtracting calculated osmolarity from the measured osmolality (OG = measured osmolality – calculated osmolarity). Note that osmolarity refers to the number of particles in 1 L of solution (osmoles/L of solution) and osmolality refers to the number of particles per kilograms of solution (osmoles/kg of solution), but often are used interchangeably because they are nearly equivalent for body fluids.[9]

CLASSIFICATION OF TOXICANTS ASSOCIATED WITH METABOLIC ACIDOSIS

Although there is no ideal way to classify poisons that cause metabolic acidosis, a clinically useful and systematic approach is to differentiate toxins based on whether they are associated with an elevated AG (**Boxes 1** and **2**) or normal AG (**Box 3**). Many medical conditions also are associated with an increased or normal AG metabolic acidosis and should be included in the differential diagnosis. An elevated AG metabolic acidosis occurs when an acid is paired with an unmeasured anion (ie, lactate), whereas a normal AG metabolic acidosis results from a gain of both H^+ and Cl^- ions or loss of HCO_3^- and retention of Cl^-, thus preserving electroneutrality. However, this classification method has several limitations because the AG can be affected by inherent errors in calculation, laboratory anomalies, and numerous non-acid-base disorders and disease states that may disguise an elevated AG or augment a normal AG (**Box 4**).[10] Also, a normal AG acidosis can occur with several of the toxins that produce an AG, therefore a normal AG should not be used to exclude a possible cause of metabolic acidosis.[11]

Many common toxicologic and illness-related causes of an increased AG metabolic acidosis can be remembered with the mnemonic *MUDPILES* (see **Box 1**). There are, however, several other causes (see **Box 2**) for an elevated AG metabolic acidosis that should not be overlooked. In the author's experience substances such as acetaminophen, amphetamines, carbon monoxide, cocaine, toluene, and valproic acid are toxins commonly encountered in the clinical setting that might be contributing to an increased AG metabolic acidosis, but are not listed in the *MUDPILES* mnemonic. Recognizing the many toxins associated with an increased AG metabolic acidosis is vital because the presence of a profoundly elevated AG may help identify specific causes of the acidosis and have prognostic value.[12]

The osmol gap may provide additional information in a patient with an elevated AG acidosis who has ingested a toxic alcohol. Although the OG can be increased in the presence of toxic alcohols, several other medical conditions such as ketoacidosis, renal failure, and shock states can also increase the measured serum osmolality.[13–15] Toxins that elevate the OG can be found in **Box 5**.[9] For simplicity, a "normal" OG is considered to be less than 10 $\pm$ 6 mOsm/L; however, the use of the "normal" range

Box 1
Toxins and disease states associated with an elevated anion gap metabolic acidosis

Methanol, metformin

Uremia

Diabetic ketoacidosis, alcoholic ketoacidosis, starvation ketoacidosis

Propylene glycol

Iron, isoniazid

Lactic acidosis

Ethylene glycol

Salicylates, sympathomimetics

Box 2
Examples of other drugs and medical conditions not listed in MUDPILES mnemonic associated with an elevated anion gap metabolic acidosis

- Acetaminophen
- Aminocaproic acid
- Amphetamines
- Arsenic
- Benzene
- Caffeine
- Carbon monoxide
- Catecholamines
- Citric acid
- Clenbuterol
- Cocaine
- Cyanide
- Didanosine
- Diethylene glycol
- Ephedrine
- Fluoride
- Formaldehyde
- Hydrogen sulfide
- Inborn errors of metabolism
- Nalidixic acid
- Niacin
- Nitroprusside
- Nonsteroidal anti-inflammatory drugs
- Polyethylene glycol
- Propofol
- Pseudoephedrine
- Sodium glucose cotransporter 2 (SGLT2) inhibitors
- Streptozotocin
- Sulfur
- Theophylline
- Thiamine deficiency
- Toluene
- Triethylene glycol
- Valproate
- Zidovudine

for the OG is limited due to wide variability of the OG among the population[16] and errors in calculation and laboratory methodology (ie, freezing point depression should be used to measure serum osmolality and not vapor pressure).[17] Furthermore, the absence of an OG cannot be used to rule out the presence of a toxic alcohol, because patients with a "normal" OG can have toxic and potentially lethal levels of a toxic alcohol.[18] Conversely, a significantly elevated OG (>25 mOsm/L) is a potential indicator of a toxic alcohol ingestion.

MECHANISMS OF TOXIN-INDUCED METABOLIC ACIDOSIS

Toxin-induced metabolic acidosis arises from increased acid production or impaired acid elimination. There are several important and distinct mechanisms by which toxins accomplish either. Increased acid production can occur with toxins that (1) are acidic or have acidic metabolites, (2) produce an imbalance between adenosine triphosphate (ATP) consumption and production, or (3) cause metabolic derangements resulting in the generation of ketone bodies, whereas underlying impairment of renal function or nephrotoxic compounds can lead to diminished acid elimination and the development

Box 3
Drugs and medical conditions associated with a normal anion gap metabolic acidosis

- Acetazolamide
- Acids (ammonium chloride, calcium chloride, hydrochloric acid)
- Cholestyramine
- Diarrhea
- Hyperalimentation
- Magnesium chloride
- Pancreatic fistula
- Posthypocapnia
- Rapid intravenous fluid administration
- Renal tubular acidosis
- Sulfamylon
- Topiramate
- Ureteroenterostomy

Box 4
Conditions affecting the anion gap

Increased anion gap	Decreased anion gap
Carbenicillin	Halides (bromine, iodine)
Dehydration/diarrhea	Hypercalcemia
Hypocalcemia	Hyperkalemia
Hypokalemia	Hyperlipidemia
Hypomagnesemia	Hypermagnesemia
Metabolic acidosis	Hyperparathyroidism
Metabolic alkalosis	Hypoalbuminemia
Nonketotic hyperosmolar coma	Hyponatremia
Respiratory alkalosis	Lithium intoxication
Sodium penicillin	Multiple myeloma
Uremia	Polymyxin

of a metabolic acidosis. Some toxins, such as salicylates, may produce metabolic acidosis through a combination of the aforementioned mechanisms.

TOXINS RESULTING IN INCREASED ACID PRODUCTION

Toxins that Are Acids or that Have Acid Metabolites

Metabolic acidosis can result from the ingestion of a substance that is either an acid or has an acidifying metabolite. Several alcohols (ie, benzyl alcohol, diethylene glycol, ethanol, ethylene glycol, methanol) are not acidifying until they are metabolized to acidic intermediates.[19] Ethylene glycol has several acidic metabolites (ie, glycolic

Box 5
Toxins associated with an elevated osmol gap

Toxic alcohols
- Ethanol
- Isopropanol
- Methanol
- Ethylene glycol

Drugs and excipients
- Mannitol
- Propylene glycol
- Glycerol
- Osmotic contrast dyes

Other chemicals
- Ethyl ether
- Acetone
- Trichloroethane

Disease or illness
- Chronic renal failure
- Lactic acidosis
- Diabetic ketoacidosis
- Alcoholic ketoacidosis
- Starvation ketoacidosis
- Circulatory shock
- Hyperlipidemia
- Hyperproteinemia

acid, glyoxylic acid, oxalic acid); however, glycolic acid is primarily responsible for the metabolic acidosis with ethylene glycol poisoning and formic acid is the metabolite responsible for metabolic acidosis with methanol poisoning.[20] Large ingestions of ethanol can produce metabolic acidosis due to its metabolism to acetic acid. Benzyl alcohol is commonly used as a preservative in intravenous medications. The use of such preparations in neonates has caused gasping respirations, hypotension, hepatic and renal failure, and fatal metabolic acidosis due to benzoic acid and hippuric acid formation, the products of benzyl alcohol metabolism.[21]

Salicylates are weak acids that can produce metabolic acidosis through numerous mechanisms. In toxic concentrations, salicylates interfere with energy production by uncoupling oxidative phosphorylation[22] and can produce renal insufficiency that causes accumulation of phosphoric and sulfuric acids.[23] The metabolism of fatty acids is increased in patients with salicylate toxicity, which generates ketone body formation. These processes all contribute to the development of an elevated AG metabolic acidosis in patients with salicylate poisoning.

Caustic agents, both acid and alkali, can cause significant tissue damage after ingestion and produce metabolic acidosis. In some instances of acid injury, a metabolic acidosis may occur from the absorption of nonionized acid from the gastric mucosa. The ingestion of hydrochloric acid can initially produce a normal AG metabolic acidosis because both H^+ and Cl^- ions are systemically absorbed and accounted for in the measurement of the AG. Other acids, such as sulfuric acid, may produce an increased AG metabolic acidosis, because the sulfate anion is not accounted for in the measurement of the AG.[24]

Toxins Affecting ATP Consumption and Production

Many poisons can interfere with cellular energy production and consumption resulting in metabolic acidosis. Toxins disrupt mitochondrial function and subsequent energy production either by uncoupling oxidative phosphorylation or inhibiting cytochromes of the electron transport chain. Excessive energy consumption can occur from toxins that produce a hyperadrenergic state.

Acetaminophen is a readily available over-the-counter analgesic that is commonly ingested or coingested during a suicide attempt and can cause an increased AG metabolic acidosis.[25] Both a pH less than 7.30 and lactic acidosis are used as indicators for a poor prognosis in acetaminophen-induced hepatotoxicity.[26,27] Although the exact mechanism of acetaminophen-induced metabolic acidosis remains unknown, animal studies suggest that acetaminophen and its hepatotoxic metabolite *N*-acetyl-*p*-benzoquinone imine inhibit oxidative phosphorylation, which subsequently leads to metabolic acidosis.[28]

Human immunodeficiency virus-positive patients taking antiretroviral therapy are at risk for developing lactic acidosis syndrome. Stavudine, zidovudine, and other nucleoside analogue reverse transcriptase inhibitors impair oxidative phosphorylation by inhibiting mitochondrial DNA polymerase γ that can result in hepatic dysfunction and steatosis, lactic acidosis, and death, with mortality ranging between 25% and 57% in patients who develop this condition.[29,30] Patients on chronic antiretroviral therapy can develop hyperlactatemia without acidosis.[31]

Metabolic acidosis is an important consequence of acute valproic acid toxicity because profound acidosis after massive ingestions is a sign of poor prognosis.[32] Once ingested, valproic acid is extensively metabolized by the liver.[33] The net effect of valproic acid metabolites is depletion of intramitochondrial coenzyme A and carnitine, which inhibits the β-oxidation of fatty acids impairing ATP production.[34] In theory, carnitine supplementation may help restore β-oxidation to mitochondria, and, as early as 1996, the Pediatric Neurology Advisory Committee recommended that carnitine be administered to children with acute ingestions of valproic acid.[35] However, owing to lack of controlled studies further research is required to evaluate the exact role and dose of carnitine in valproic acid overdoses.

Metformin is a biguanide that is commonly used to treat diabetes mellitus and polycystic ovarian disease.[36] A potentially fatal metabolic acidosis with an increased lactate concentration can develop after an acute overdose or with therapeutic use.[37] Most cases of lactic acidosis related to therapeutic metformin use have occurred in the presence of a severe underlying disease state, such as renal failure.[38] Metformin is thought to induce metabolic acidosis with an increased lactate concentration by inhibiting gluconeogenesis and complex I of the electron transport chain.[36,39]

Several mitochondrial poisons are responsible for a profound metabolic acidosis that may require prompt antidotal intervention. Examples of such toxins include carbon monoxide, cyanide, hydrogen sulfide, iron, methanol, and salicylates. Carbon monoxide, cyanide, hydrogen sulfide, and the metabolite of methanol (formic acid) impair oxidative metabolism by inhibiting complex IV of the electron transport chain and decoupling oxidative phosphorylation.[40,41] Iron and salicylates hinder energy production by uncoupling oxidative phosphorylation.[22,42] Following toxicity with these agents, cellular energy stores are quickly diminished resulting in disruption of critical electrolyte gradients, ATP-dependent processes, and the H^+ ion consumption in the aerobic synthesis of ATP.[43] Furthermore, many of these toxins (eg, carbon monoxide, cyanide, iron) impair tissue perfusion that disrupts aerobic cellular energy production and worsens metabolic acidosis.

Excessive adrenergic stimulation from agents such as amphetamines, caffeine, cocaine, β-2 agonists (eg, clenbuterol), ephedrine, phencyclidine, and theophylline can result in hyperglycemia, hypokalemia, leukocytosis, and metabolic acidosis.[44–47] In the presence of catecholamines, β-adrenoreceptor stimulation results in the hydrolysis of ATP and augments cyclic adenosine monophosphate activity within cells, which stimulates Na^+K^+-ATPase and causes K^+ ions to shift intracellular. Excess catecholamines also stimulate glycogenolysis and the breakdown of fatty acids resulting in hyperglycemia and metabolic acidosis, respectively. Poisoning with an agent that causes hyperadrenergic stimulation should be strongly suspected in a patient with the aforementioned laboratory abnormalities and a sympathomimetic toxidrome.

Special mention should be made regarding lactic acidosis, because this terminology is misleading and erroneous. When glucose is converted to lactate during anaerobic metabolism to generate 2 molecules of ATP, net H^+ ions are not produced. The production of net H^+ ions occurs when ATP is used as a cellular energy source.[48] The electron transport chain then uses the H^+ ions that are generated from the hydrolysis of ATP in the aerobic synthesis of ATP, thus maintaining a normal pH during typical physiologic conditions.[49] However, metabolic acidosis can ensue in the presence of a toxin or other physiologic derangement that results in an imbalance of ATP hydrolysis and synthesis. The imbalance of ATP hydrolysis and synthesis is acidifying and not the production of lactate. Lactate should only serve as an indicator of anaerobic metabolism.[48]

Metabolic Derangements Causing Increased Acid Production

Certain toxins can cause metabolic derangements resulting in the increased production of ketone bodies (ie, acetoacetate, acetone, β-hydroxybutyrate). The generation of ketoacids can also occur secondary to uncontrolled diabetes, and is a normal response to fasting and prolonged exercise.[50] Alcoholic ketoacidosis (AKA) is a prime example in which toxin-induced (ie, ethanol) metabolic derangements and an acute starvation state result in the production of ketoacids and an elevated AG metabolic acidosis. Patients who develop AKA are usually chronic ethanol abusers who have been binge drinking and develop a gastrointestinal illness (ie, gastritis, hepatitis, pancreatitis) that limits oral intake.[51] The diagnosis of AKA should be considered in a patient who (1) recently binged on ethanol and has had a decrease in ethanol consumption, (2) has a history of vomiting or decreased oral intake, (3) has a blood glucose level less than 300 mg/dL, and (4) has an elevated AG metabolic acidosis for which other causes have been ruled out.[52]

Isoniazid (INH) poisoning is characterized by refractory seizures, elevated AG metabolic acidosis, and coma. Survival from acute INH toxicity has been reported in a patient with an arterial pH as low as 6.49.[53] The mechanism underlying the development of metabolic acidosis in patients poisoned with INH remains unclear. Plausible explanations include muscular activity from seizures, acidifying INH metabolites, and enhanced fatty acid metabolism that produces ketoacids.[54,55]

The sodium glucose cotransporter 2 (SGLT2) inhibitors (canagliflozin, dapagliflozin, empagliflozin) are a novel class of oral antidiabetic medications that have been associated with ketoacidosis. The therapeutic use of SGLT2 inhibitors can cause a euglycemic ketoacidosis.[56] Because this is one of the newest classes of drugs used for diabetes, overdose data are limited. However, a retrospective review of SGLT2 inhibitor exposures reported to poison centers found that acute ingestions of SGLT2 inhibitors were associated with only minor effects, and no hypoglycemia.[57]

TOXINS IMPAIRING THE RENAL ELIMINATION OF ACIDS

Numerous substances can cause or exacerbate renal insufficiency. Renal dysfunction may lead to the accumulation of parent compounds or toxic intermediates and contribute to or produce a metabolic acidosis. Renal impairment, whether drug-induced or underlying, can result in uremia. Even in the absence of a toxin that produces metabolic acidosis, the buildup of nitrogenous compounds can cause an increased AG metabolic acidosis due to impaired ammonia secretion and retention of unmeasured anions.[12]

Toluene exposure can lead to a metabolic acidosis. This is a result of toluene being metabolized to an acidic metabolite, hippuric acid.[58] The chronic abuse of toluene can result in the development of a clinical picture similar to a distal renal tubular acidosis (RTA) with associated hypokalemia, and metabolic acidosis.[59] The mechanism by which toluene induces this clinical effect has not been fully elucidated. Toluene and hippuric acid are most likely directly toxic to the distal renal tubule[60] and impair H^+ ion secretion. Impaired H^+ ion secretion results in the loss of Na^+ and K^+ ions, inability to acidify the urine, and a normal or increased AG metabolic acidosis.[58,60]

Ethylene glycol is by itself not a nephrotoxin.[61] However, once hepatically metabolized it forms nephrotoxic intermediates. Ethylene glycol-associated renal insufficiency has been attributed to the deposition of calcium oxalate crystals in the renal tubules[62]; however, urinary calcium oxalate crystals are only present in 50% to 65% of patients with ethylene glycol poisoning.[63] Therefore, another mechanism may be responsible or contributing to ethylene glycol-associated renal insufficiency, and the absence of calcium oxalate cyrstalluria cannot be used to rule out ethylene glycol poisoning. Ethylene glycol-associated renal dysfunction can exacerbate the metabolic acidosis produced by the metabolites (glycolic acid, glyoxylic acid, oxalic acid) of this toxic alcohol.

Propylene glycol is commonly used as a diluent and preservative in numerous pharmaceutical preparations including chlordiazepoxide, diazepam, digoxin, esmolol, etomidate, lorazepam, nitroglycerin, phenobarbital, phenytoin, and trimethoprim/sulfamethoxazole. Although considered to be generally safe, problems arise with the prolonged or rapid administration of agents containing propylene glycol, especially in patients with renal insufficiency. Cardiac dysrhythmias, hypotension, conduction abnormalities, and death have occurred with the rapid administration of phenytoin due to the presence of propylene glycol in its intravenous product.[64] Patients receiving continuous infusions of propylene glycol-containing sedatives can develop an elevated AG metabolic acidosis and increased osmolality.[1] These metabolic abnormalities resolve quickly once the offending medication has been discontinued.

TREATMENT CONSIDERATIONS FOR TOXIN-INDUCED METABOLIC ACIDOSIS

The most important measures in treating toxin-induced metabolic acidosis are to recognize and treat the underlying cause, as well as provide excellent supportive care including airway control and fluid resuscitation. Discontinuing the offending agents in a patient who develops metabolic acidosis while taking therapeutic quantities of certain drugs (eg, topiramate, metformin) may be all that is necessary. Many patients who develop a mild metabolic acidosis after an intentional ingestion will experience improvement with close observation and supportive care. However, if poisoned patients have progressive worsening of their metabolic acidosis despite supportive care (ie, fluid resuscitation, oxygen therapy), then more aggressive therapies should be considered or alternative causes of their metabolic acidosis should be sought. Therapy for specific toxin-induced metabolic acidosis is variable with some of the more common management strategies discussed in the following sections.

ROLE OF BUFFER THERAPY

Many clinicians may be inclined to treat toxin-induced metabolic acidosis with a buffer such as sodium bicarbonate to increase serum pH. This practice should be discouraged. The administration of sodium bicarbonate has never been shown to improve outcomes in patients with metabolic acidosis and can be detrimental in some.[65] Paradoxic intracellular acidosis can occur due to increased production of carbon dioxide.[66] Sodium bicarbonate administration may also impair oxygen delivery to tissues by shifting the oxyhemoglobin dissociation curve to the left.[67]

Patients who may benefit from the use of sodium bicarbonate are those poisoned with agents whose elimination may be increased through alkalinization (ie, salicylates) and drugs that cause blockade of cardiac Na^+ channels (ie, cyclic antidepressants). Sodium bicarbonate is useful in decreasing tissue levels of salicylates and in facilitating the elimination of salicylates in the urine.[68] Hemodialysis should be instituted in those salicylate-poisoned patients with altered mental status, pulmonary edema, renal failure, severe electrolyte and metabolic abnormalities, or a salicylate concentration approaching 100 mg/dL after an acute ingestion.[69] Sodium bicarbonate is effective in treating drug-induced cardiac sodium channel blockade.[70] For cyclic antidepressant-induced cardiotoxicity and seizures, for example, 1 to 2 mEq/kg of sodium bicarbonate should be given as an intravenous bolus and repeated as needed until a blood pH of 7.55 is attained.[71]

ANTIDOTAL THERAPY

Ingestion of a toxic alcohol requires antagonism of alcohol dehydrogenase with ethanol or fomepizole and consideration of hemodialysis in patients who are profoundly acidotic or have had a massive ingestion.[69] Neither ethanol nor fomepizole affect the formed toxic metabolites of ethylene glycol or methanol. Complications associated with the administration of ethanol include central nervous system (CNS) depression, hypoglycemia, and fluctuating levels due to patient variability in its metabolism. Advantages of fomepizole are ease of dosing, no monitoring of serum levels, and lack of CNS depressant activity.[63]

Treatment of acute isoniazid toxicity should focus on termination of seizures, reversal of metabolic acidosis, and stabilization of vital signs through supportive measures. Isoniazid causes toxicity by diminishing the synthesis of γ-aminobutyric acid in the CNS through antagonism of the enzyme pyridoxal kinase. The antidote for isoniazid-induced neurotoxicity is pyridoxine in a dose in grams that is equal to the amount of isoniazid that was ingested in grams[72]; however, the pyridoxine dose should not exceed more than 5 g in an adult or 70 mg/kg in a pediatric patient.[73] Pyridoxine rapidly terminates isoniazid-induced seizures, reverses coma, and corrects metabolic acidosis.

Management of patients with cyanide toxicity is complicated by the fact that it is an extremely rapid-acting and potent toxin, thus most victims will succumb to rapid death or are moribund with a severe metabolic acidosis upon presentation. If available, either the cyanide antidote kit containing amyl nitrite, sodium nitrite, and sodium thiosulfate or the antidote hydroxycobalamin should be considered early in the management of toxicity.[74]

SUMMARY

Metabolic acidosis can arise from several drugs and toxins through a variety of mechanisms. Differentiating the causes of metabolic acidosis in the poisoned patient is an indispensable skill in clinical practice. Comprehension of toxin-induced metabolic acidosis, combined with a thorough history, physical examination, appropriate use of laboratory tests, and a stepwise approach should aid the clinician in determining the cause of metabolic acidosis in the poisoned patient. It is imperative when confronted with such a patient that appropriate antidotal therapy is administered when necessary and the patient receives exceptional supportive care.

CLINICS CARE POINTS

- A normal anion gap (AG) acidosis can occur with several of the toxins that produce an AG, therefore a normal AG should not be used to exclude a possible cause of metabolic acidosis.
- The absence of an osmol gap (OG) cannot be used to rule out the presence of a toxic alcohol, whereas a significantly elevated OG (>25 mOsm/L) is a potential indicator of a toxic alcohol ingestion.
- The most important measures in treating toxin-induced metabolic acidosis are to recognize and treat the underlying cause, as well as provide excellent supportive care including airway control and fluid resuscitation.
- Treating a toxin-induced metabolic acidosis with a buffer such as sodium bicarbonate to increase serum pH has never been shown to improve outcomes in patients with metabolic acidosis and can be detrimental in some.

DISCLOSURE

The author has no conflicts of interest, financial or otherwise, to disclose.

REFERENCES

1. Gauthier PM, Szerlip HM. Metabolic acidosis in the intensive care unit. Crit Care Clin 2002;18:289–308.

2. Kraut J, Madias N. Metabolic acidosis: pathophysiology, diagnosis and management. Nat Rev Nephrol 2010;6:274–85.
3. Kirk M, Pace S. Pearls, pitfalls, and updates in toxicology. Emerg Med Clin North Am 1997;15:427–49.
4. College of American pathologists participant summaries: toxicology survey T-B; therapeutic drug monitoring (general) survey set Z-B; urine toxicology survey set UT-B; serum alcohol/volatiles survey set AL2-B; chemistry survey set C4-B. Northfield (IL): College of American Pathologists; 1999.
5. Brett AS. Implications of discordance between clinical impression and toxicology analysis in drug overdose. Arch Intern Med 1988;148:437–41.
6. Sporer KA, Ernst AA. The effect of toxicologic screening on management of minimally symptomatic overdoses. Am J Emerg Med 1992;10:173–5.
7. Winter SD, Pearson JR, Gabow PA, et al. The fall of the serum anion gap. Arch Intern Med 1990;150:311–3.
8. Epstein FB. Osmolality. Emerg Med Clin North Am 1986;4:253–61.
9. Chabali R. Diagnostic use of anion and osmolal gaps in pediatric emergency medicine. Pediatr Emerg Care 1997;13:204–10.
10. Salem MM, Mujais SK. Gaps in the anion gap. Arch Intern Med 1992;152:1625–9.
11. Gabow PA, Anderson RJ, Potts DE, et al. Acid-base disturbances in the salicylate-intoxicated adult. Arch Intern Med 1978;138:1481–4.
12. Ishihara K, Szerlip HM. Anion gap acidosis. Semin Nephrol 1998;18:83–97.
13. Inaba H, Hirasawa H, Mizuguchi T. Serum osmolality gap in postoperative patients in intensive care. Lancet 1987;1:1331–5.
14. Schelling JR, Howard RL, Winter SD, et al. Increased osmolal gap in alcoholic ketoacidosis and lactic acidosis. Ann Intern Med 1990;113:580–2.
15. Sklar AH, Linas SL. The osmolal gap in renal failure. Ann Intern Med 1983;98: 481–2.
16. Hoffman RS, Smilkstein MJ, Howland MA, et al. Osmol gaps revisited: normal values and limitations. J Toxicol Clin Toxicol 1993;31:81–93.
17. Eisen TF, Lacouture PG, Woolf A. Serum osmolality in alcohol ingestions: differences in availability among laboratories of teaching hospital, nonteaching hospital, and commercial facilities. Am J Emerg Med 1989;7:256–9.
18. Glaser DS. Utility of the serum osmol gap in the diagnosis of methanol or ethylene glycol ingestion. Ann Emerg Med 1996;27:343–6.
19. Gabow PA, Clay K, Sullivan JB, et al. Organic acids in ethylene glycol intoxication. Ann Intern Med 1986;105:16–20.
20. Moreau CL, Kerns W 2nd, Tomaszewski CA, et al. Glycolate kinetics and hemodialysis clearance in ethylene glycol poisoning. META Study Group. J Toxicol Clin Toxicol 1998;36:659–66.
21. Gershanik JJ, Boecler G, Ensley H, et al. The gasping syndrome and benzyl alcohol poisoning. N Engl J Med 1982;307:1384–8.
22. Alberti KG, Cohen RD, Woods HF. Lactic acidosis and hyperlactataemia. Lancet 1974;2:1519–60.
23. Insel PA. Analgesic-antipyretic and anti-inflammatory agents and drugs employed in the treatment of gout. In: Harmon JG, Limbird LE, editors. Goodman & Gilman's the pharmacologic basis of therapeutics. 9th edition. New York: McGraw-Hill; 1996. p. 1905.
24. Wightman RS, Fulton JA. Caustics. In: Nelson LS, Howland MA, Lewin NA, et al, editors. Goldfrank's toxicologic emergencies. 11th edition. New York: McGraw-Hill Education; 2019. p. 2070.

25. Flanagan RJ, Mant TG. Coma and metabolic acidosis early in severe acute paracetamol poisoning. Hum Toxicol 1986;5:179–82.
26. O'Grady JG, Alexander GJ, Hayllar KM, et al. Early indicators of prognosis in fulminant hepatic failure. Gastroenterology 1989;97:439–45.
27. Levine M, Stellpflug SJ, Pizon AF, et al. Hypoglycemia and lactic acidosis outperform King's College criteria for predicting death or transplant in acetaminophen toxic patients. Clin Toxicol 2018;56:622–5.
28. Esterline RL, Ray SD, Ji S. Reversible and irreversible inhibition of hepatic mitochondrial respiration by acetaminophen and its toxic metabolite, N-acetyl-p-benzoquinoneimine (NAPQI). Biochem Pharmacol 1989;38:2387–90.
29. Tripuraneni NS, Smith PR, Weedon J, et al. Prognostic factors in lactic acidosis syndrome caused by nucleoside reverse transcriptase inhibitors: report of eight cases and review of the literature. AIDS Patient Care STDS 2004;18:379–84.
30. Mokrzycki MH, Harris C, May H, et al. Lactic acidosis associated with stavudine administration: a report of five cases. Clin Infect Dis 2000;30:198–200.
31. John M, Moore CB, James IR, et al. Chronic hyperlactatemia in HIV-infected patients taking antiretroviral therapy. Aids 2001;15:717–23.
32. Anderson GO, Ritland S. Life-threatening intoxication with sodium valproate. J Toxicol Clin Toxicol 1995;33:279–84.
33. Dupuis RE, Lichtman SN, Pollack GM. Acute valproic acid overdose. Clinical course and pharmacokinetic disposition of valproic acid and metabolites. Drug Saf 1990;5:65–71.
34. Raskind JY, El-Chaar GM. The role of carnitine supplementation during valproic acid therapy. Ann Pharmacother 2000;34:630–8.
35. DeVivo DC, Bohan TP, Coulter DL, et al. e. L-Carnitine supplementation in childhood epilepsy: Current perspectives. Epilepsia 1998;39:1216–25.
36. Bailey CJ, Turner RC. Metformin. N Engl J Med 1996;334:574--9.
37. Dell'Aglio DM, Perino LJ, Kazzi Z, et al. Acute metformin overdose: Examining serum pH, lactate level, and metformin concentrations in survivors versus nonsurvivors: A systematic review of the literature. Ann Emerg Med 2009;54:818–23.
38. Chan NN, Brain HP, Feher MD. Metformin-associated lactic acidosis: a rare or very rare clinical entity? Diabetic Med 1999;16:273–81.
39. Owen MR, Doran E, Halestrap AP. Evidence that metformin exerts its anti-diabetic effects through inhibition of complex 1 of the mitochondrial respiratory chain. Biochem J 2000;3:607–14.
40. Brown SD, Piantadosi CA. In vivo binding of carbon monoxide to cytochrome c oxidase in rat brain. J Appl Physiol 1990;68:604–10.
41. Way JL. Cyanide intoxication and its mechanism of antagonism. Annu Rev Pharmacol Toxicol 1984;24:451–81.
42. Robotham JL, Lietman PS. Acute iron poisoning. A review. Am J Dis Child 1980; 134:875–9.
43. Cao JD, Kleinschmidt KC. Biochemical and metabolic principles. In: Nelson LS, Howland MA, Lewin NA, et al, editors. Goldfrank's toxicologic emergencies. 11th edition. New York: McGraw-Hill Education; 2019. p. 2070.
44. Liem EB, Mnookin SC, Mahla ME. Albuterol-induced lactic acidosis. Anesthesiology 2003;99:505–6.
45. Brown MJ. Hypokalemia from beta 2-receptor stimulation by circulating epinephrine. Am J Cardiol 1985;56:3D–9D.
46. Wong KM, Chak WL, Cheung CY, et al. Hypokalemic metabolic acidosis attributed to cough mixture abuse. Am J Kidney Dis 2001;38:390–4.

47. Bilkoo P, Thomas J, Riddle CD, et al. Clenbuterol toxicity: an emerging epidemic. A case report and review. Conn Med 2007;71:89–91.
48. Mizock BA. Lactic acidosis. DM 1989;35:233–300.
49. Mizock BA. Controversies in lactic acidosis. Implications in critically ill patients. JAMA 1987;258:497–501.
50. Mitchell GA, Kassovska-Bratinova S, Boukaftane Y, et al. Medical aspects of ketone body metabolism. Clin Invest Med Medecine Clinique Experimentale 1995; 18:193–216.
51. Fulop M. Alcoholism, ketoacidosis, and lactic acidosis. Diabetes Metab Rev 1989;5:365–78.
52. Soffer A, Hamburger S. Alcoholic ketoacidosis: a review of 30 cases. J Am Med Womens Assoc 1982;37:106–10.
53. Hankins DG, Saxena K, Faville RJ Jr, et al. Profound acidosis caused by isoniazid ingestion. Am J Emerg Med 1987;5:165–6.
54. Chin L, Sievers ML, Herrier RN, et al. Convulsions as the etiology of lactic acidosis in acute isoniazid toxicity in dogs. Toxicol Appl Pharmacol 1979;49: 377–84.
55. Pahl MV, Vaziri ND, Ness R, et al. Association of beta hydroxybutyric acidosis with isoniazid intoxication. J Toxicol Clin Toxicol 1984;22:167–76.
56. Blau JE, Tella SH, Taylor SI, et al. Ketoacidosis associated with SGLT2 inhibitor treatment: Analysis of FAERS data. Diabetes Metab Res Rev 2017;33:1–14.
57. Schaeffer SE, DesLauriers C, Spiller HA, et al. Retrospective review of SGLT2 inhibitor exposures reported to 13 poison centers. Clin Tox 2018;56:204–8.
58. Carlisle EJ, Donnelly SM, Vasuvattakul S, et al. Glue-sniffing and distal renal tubular acidosis: sticking to the facts. J Am Soc Nephrol 1991;1:1019–27.
59. Kao KC, Tsai YH, Lin MC, et al. Hypokalemic muscular paralysis causing acute respiratory failure due to rhabdomyolysis with renal tubular acidosis in a chronic glue sniffer. J Toxicol Clin Toxicol 2000;38:679–81.
60. Kamijima M, Nakazawa Y, Yamakawa M, et al. Metabolic acidosis and renal tubular injury due to pure toluene inhalation. Arch Environ Health 1994;49:410–3.
61. Cheng JT, Beysolow TD, Kaul B, et al. Clearance of ethylene glycol by kidneys and hemodialysis. J Toxicol Clin Toxicol 1987;25:95–108.
62. Clay KL, Murphy RC. On the metabolic acidosis of ethylene glycol intoxication. Toxicol Appl Pharmacol 1977;39:39–49.
63. Brent J, McMartin K, Phillips S, et al. Fomepizole for the treatment of ethylene glycol poisoning. New Engl J Med 1999;344:424–9.
64. Unger AH, Sklaroff HJ. Fatalities following intravenous use of sodium diphenylhydantoin for cardiac arrhythmias. Report of two cases. JAMA 1967;200:335–6.
65. Stacpoole PW, Wright EC, Baumgartner TG, et al. Natural history and course of acquired lactic acidosis in adults. DCA-Lactic Acidosis Study Group. Am J Med 1994;97:47–54.
66. Nakashima K, Yamashita T, Kashiwagi S, et al. The effect of sodium bicarbonate on CBF and intracellular pH in man: stable Xe-CT and 31P-MRS. Acta Neurol Scand Suppl 1996;166:96–8.
67. Sing RF, Branas CA. Bicarbonate therapy in the treatment of lactic acidosis: medicine or toxin? J Am Osteopath Assoc 1995;95:52–7.
68. Hill JB. Experimental salicylate poisoning: observations on the effects of altering blood pH on tissue and plasma salicylate concentrations. Pediatrics 1971;47: 658–65.
69. King JD, Kern MH, Jaar BG. Extracorporeal removal of poisons and toxins. CJASN 2019;14:1408–15.

70. Hoffman JR, Votey SR, Bayer M, et al. Effect of hypertonic sodium bicarbonate in the treatment of moderate-to-severe cyclic antidepressant overdose. Am J Emerg Med 1993;11:336–41.
71. Smilkstein MJ. Reviewing cyclic antidepressant cardiotoxicity: wheat and chaff. J Emerg Med 1990;8:645–8.
72. Wason S, Lacouture PG, Lovejoy FH Jr. Single high-dose pyridoxine treatment for isoniazid overdose. JAMA 1981;246:1102–4.
73. Howland MA. Pyridoxine. In: Nelson LS, Howland MA, Lewin NA, et al, editors. Goldfrank's toxicologic emergencies. 11th edition. New York: McGraw-Hill Education; 2019. p. 2070.
74. Reade MC, Davies SR, Morley PT, et al. Review article: management of cyanide poisoning. Emerg Med Australas 2012;24:225–38.

Emerging Agents of Substance Use/Misuse

Avery E. Michienzi, DO*, Heather A. Borek, MD

KEYWORDS

- Novel psychoactive substances • Drugs of abuse • Kratom • Phenibut • Tianeptine
- Designer drugs

KEY POINTS

- The last decade has seen an emergence of numerous novel psychoactive substances (NPS) as well as the misuse of products marketed as "supplements."
- NPS are used specifically as agents of abuse or as unexpected adulterants in other substances, such as fentanyl analogs in heroin.
- Symptoms from NPS may be unpredictable due to varying potency.
- NPS are not detected on routine urine drug screen immunoassays.

INTRODUCTION

Over the last decade, the use of novel psychoactive substances (NPS) has been increasing. This is a broad category of substances often synthesized to mimic plants or existing drugs that includes substances such as synthetic cannabinoids, synthetic cathinones, kratom, phenibut, and designer opioids and benzodiazepines.[1] The production of these substances results from the diversion of new substances created for potential therapeutic use, the human desire to experiment, and the legal work-around to create unregulated substances once other substances of abuse become subject to regulatory scrutiny.[2] As new synthetic substances become popular, these substances often get banned or placed on the list of scheduled substances by the United States (U.S.) Drug Enforcement Administration (DEA) (**Table 1**)[3]. However, the legal regulation lags behind the substances that are being used, often for years.

Statistics on the use of NPS underrepresent their actual use due to underreporting, poor detection methods, and the prevalence of contaminants in many substances. Symptoms may mimic other drug classes such as opioids, benzodiazepines, or sympathomimetics. These substances may interact with multiple receptors or bind with

Department of Emergency Medicine, Division of Medical Toxicology, Medical Toxicology, University of Virginia School of Medicine, University of Virginia, PO Box 800774, Charlottesville, VA 22908, USA
* Corresponding author.
E-mail address: am6kf@virginia.edu

Emerg Med Clin N Am 40 (2022) 265–281
https://doi.org/10.1016/j.emc.2022.01.001 emed.theclinics.com
0733-8627/22/

Table 1 Drug Enforcement Administration (DEA) Scheduling definitions		
Schedule I	Substances, or chemicals are defined as drugs with no currently accepted medical use and a high potential for abuse	Heroin Ecstasy LSD Psilocybin Tetrahydrocannabinol
Schedule II	Substances, or chemicals are defined as drugs with a high potential for abuse, with use potentially leading to severe psychological or physical dependence. These drugs are also considered dangerous.	Oxycodone Cocaine Dextroamphetamine
Schedule III	Substances or chemicals are defined as drugs with a moderate to low potential for physical and psychological dependence. Schedule III drugs abuse potential is less than Schedule I and Schedule II drugs but more than Schedule IV.	Ketamine Buprenorphine/naloxone Acetaminophen with codeine
Schedule IV	Substances, or chemicals are defined as drugs with a low potential for abuse and low risk of dependence.	Lorazepam Barbital
Schedule V	Substances or chemicals are defined as drugs with lower potential for abuse than Schedule IV and consist of preparations containing limited quantities of certain narcotics. Schedule V drugs are generally used for antidiarrheal, antitussive, and analgesic purposes	Pregabalin Codeine preparations < 200 mg/100 mL

higher affinity than the traditional drugs of abuse, so symptoms can vary. Urine drug screens may detect the standard drugs of abuse such as cocaine, marijuana, phencyclidine, opiates, and amphetamines, but such standard drug screens do not routinely detect NPS due to the differences in chemical structure. It is, therefore, important to be aware of these ever-changing substances because diagnosis will largely be clinical. This article will review several of the novel substances that have emerged over the last two decades.

CANNABINOIDS

Background

Cannabis is the most widely used regulated drug worldwide.[4] The Cannabis plant contains over 100 different phytocannabinoids (plant-based cannabinoids) and is referred to colloquially as marijuana or hemp depending on the concentration of tetrahydrocannabinol (THC) it contains. Two of the most well-known phytocannabinoids are delta-9 THC and cannabidiol (CBD). Delta-9 THC is the primary psychoactive component of the cannabis plant while CBD may have anti-inflammatory and antiseizure properties.[5] In 2018, the Farm Bill defined hemp as the cannabis plant and any of its parts and extracts that contain no more than 0.3% THC on a dry weight basis. If the cannabis plant contains more than 0.3% THC, it is referred to as marijuana.[6,7] Over time, the delta-9 THC concentration contained in cannabis has increased such that it is more potent than it was in the past.[8–10] The percentage of THC in marijuana seized by the DEA in 2019 was about 15%, compared with about 4% in 1995.[11]

Marijuana and its cannabinoids are classified as Schedule I substances by the DEA with no approved medical use. Hemp, as it is defined by the Farm Bill, is not a controlled substance.[10] A synthetic form of THC (dronabinol) is approved by the Food and Drug Administration (FDA) for chemotherapy-induced nausea and vomiting and as an appetite stimulant for patients with acquired immune deficiency syndrome (AIDS). Dronabinol is classified as a Schedule III substance. An oral solution of CBD (brand name Epidiolex) is FDA approved for epilepsy from Dravet and Lennox–Gastaut syndromes and is classified as a Schedule V substance.[12,13] As of this writing, marijuana remains illegal at the federal level, but many states in the US have legalized it or decriminalized it at the state level.[14]

Cannabis is typically smoked, vaped, or eaten in the form of "edibles." Concentrated marijuana products with higher THC concentration are smoked in a process called "dabbing" using products referred to as wax, budder, or butane hash oil.[15]

Synthetic Cannabinoids

Synthetic cannabinoids were first developed in the 1960s for research, but it was not until 2004 that a synthetic cannabinoid called JWH-018 emerged as a substance of abuse.[5] Numerous variations have subsequently been introduced and are marketed as herbal incense and labeled "not for human consumption" to try to avoid regulation and potential legal ramifications. Herbal incense laced with synthetic cannabinoids is referred to by the brand names of the products such as K2, Spice, or Scooby Snax. These products are smoked by users much like marijuana but may also be brewed as tea or vaped in e-cigarettes. There are many synthetic cannabinoids currently listed as Schedule I Controlled substances in the US[13] The DEA has worked to ban many of these synthetic cannabinoids, but it is impossible to keep up with the rate at which new ones are created.

Delta-8 Tetrahydrocannabinol

Delta-8 THC emerged in 2021 as a new "legal" alternative to delta-9 THC.[16] Delta-8 THC has no current medical use, but because delta-8 THC is derived from the hemp plant, it is marketed as legal in many states under the 2018 Farm Bill.[17] It is sold for smoking or as edibles and labeled simply as "Delta 8" to eliminate the comparison between it and delta-9 THC. There has been a rise in calls to the U.S. Poison Centers in 2021 particularly regarding pediatric exposures to delta-8 THC.[18] Other cannabinoids such as delta-10 THC and THC-o have also emerged in 2021.

Mechanism of Action of Cannabinoids

Phytocannabinoids bind to cannabinoid 1 (CB1) and 2 (CB2) receptors which are located throughout the body. CB1 receptors are found predominantly in the central nervous system while CB2 receptors are found mainly in the immune system and hematopoietic cells. Synthetic cannabinoids also bind CB receptors but have a much higher potency than phytocannabinoids so they are known to cause unpredictable symptoms.[19,20]

Symptoms of Toxicity

Cannabis intoxication symptoms are generally associated with the psychoactive component, THC. Symptoms include altered mood, hallucinations, ataxia, central nervous system depression or excitation, tachycardia, and conjunctival injection.[21,22] Duration of symptoms tends to last longer with the ingestion of cannabinoids versus inhalation.

Peak plasma levels occur within minutes after smoking marijuana, but clinical impairment may be evident for 6 or more hours after use, which makes testing for impairment a challenge in marijuana users.[23] Cyclic vomiting syndrome has been associated with frequent cannabis use.[12] Psychosis is also a concern with marijuana use, especially in the setting of products with higher THC content. A recent meta-analysis showed an association with the dose of cannabis and the risk of psychosis.[24] There are not yet any published data on the symptoms associated with delta-8 THC, but based on the U.S. Poison Center experience, symptoms are similar to those seen with delta-9 THC intoxication with CNS depression, agitation, and tachycardia or bradycardia.[18]

Synthetic cannabinoids emerging in society are more potent than phytocannabinoids and can cause many different clinical effects depending on the product. Clinical effects reported from synthetic cannabinoid toxicity include tachycardia, agitation, mania, drowsiness, nausea, vomiting, hallucinations, and in rarer cases seizures, rhabdomyolysis, and acute kidney injury. Deaths have been reported but are uncommon.[5,25,26]

Treatment

There is no antidote for any of the cannabinoids and patients are treated with targeted supportive care based on their symptoms. Benzodiazepines are recommended for seizures and agitation. If psychosis or hallucinations are present with agitation, antipsychotics may be beneficial as well. Antiemetics, capsaicin topical cream, or haloperidol may be used for cyclic vomiting syndrome.[27]

SYNTHETIC CATHINONES

Background

Synthetic cathinones are psychoactive substances made to mimic plant-based cathinones derived from the shrub *Catha edulis.*[28] The leaves from this plant, also known as khat, are chewed or brewed as tea for their stimulant properties in the Middle East and East Africa.[28] The chemical structures of cathinones share a phenethylamine backbone with other stimulants such as cocaine, amphetamines, the 2-C series of designer drugs, 3,4-methylenedioxy methamphetamine, (MDMA) and the pharmaceutical drug bupropion. The first synthetic cathinone, methcathinone, was made in the 1920s as a homolog of ephedrine.[28–30] Methcathinone was listed as a Schedule I substance by the DEA in 1994 and it was not until the 2000s when other novel synthetic cathinones emerged as unscheduled alternatives to MDMA.[28,30] There are currently many synthetic cathinones listed as Schedule I substances by the DEA. However, as with other synthetic substances, new compounds are made faster than they are able to be regulated.[31]

Synthetic cathinones in their powdered or crystal forms have been falsely marketed as bath salts, stain removers, or jewelry cleaners and are labeled "not for human consumption" to attempt to avoid regulatory authorities. Some of the common synthetic cathinones and colloquial names are listed in **Table 2**.[28,32] Use of synthetic cathinones is reportedly high among those who frequent nightclubs and electronic dance music parties.[33–35] Data on the prevalence of use likely underestimate use due to people unknowingly consuming synthetic cathinones. This is either because they are unaware of the terminology for this class of substances or because synthetic cathinones are a common adulterant in the common club drug MDMA, also known as molly or ecstasy.[28,33]

Mechanism of Action

Synthetic cathinones work similarly to other stimulant drugs by altering the release and reuptake of neurotransmitters including dopamine, norepinephrine, and serotonin. The overall net effect is an increase in dopamine, norepinephrine, and serotonin.[30]

Table 2
Synthetic cathinones compounds and common names

Common Synthetic Cathinones	Colloquial Names for Synthetic Cathinones
• Eutylone • Butylone • Methylone • Mephedrone (MCAT) • Methylenedioxypyrovalerone (MDPV)	• Bath salts • Flakka • Zombie drug • Cloud nine • White lightning • Vanilla Sky • Lunar Wave • Bliss

Symptoms of Intoxication

Symptoms of intoxication with synthetic cathinones are similar to those seen with other stimulant and hallucinogenic substances. A sympathomimetic toxidrome would be expected, including tachycardia, diaphoresis, mydriasis, and hypertension. Desired effects from use include euphoria, increased empathy, increased libido, hallucinations, and increase sociability. Symptoms that may not be desired and can be harmful include paranoia, agitation, encephalopathy, self-mutilation, seizures, tachycardia, hypertension, hyperthermia, rhabdomyolysis, and acute renal failure.[30,32,36] In severe cases, patients may experience multisystem organ failure and even death.[30] In one case of psychosis made famous by the press, a man suspected to be intoxicated with cathinones was witnessed eating the face of another man.[37]

Treatment

There is no antidote for synthetic cathinone toxicity and treatment is tailored toward symptoms. Agitation, delirium, and sympathomimetic symptoms can be treated with benzodiazepines or antipsychotics. Targeted supportive care for end-organ damage, such as intravenous fluids for rhabdomyolysis, benzodiazepines for seizures, or cooling for hyperthermia can be considered.[30]

SYNTHETIC OPIOIDS

Background

Since the 1970s, illicitly manufactured opioids have been sold and abused. Illicit fentanyl and fentanyl analog production, in particular, has increased over the last decade and these substances have been implicated in numerous fatalities.[38] Starting in the mid-2000s, there was a rise in the use of fentanyl as an adulterant in other drugs such as heroin and cocaine. This has led to a serious risk in the use of other drugs as users may inadvertently overdose on opioids.[39] In the 2020 DEA Emerging Threat Report, fentanyl was the most common substance seized and analyzed in the DEA laboratory.[1] In addition to fentanyl and its analogs, many designer opioids have emerged including U-4770, AH-7921, and MT-45.

Much of the "heroin" being sold in the US currently contains fentanyl or a fentanyl analog.[40] Often times, this is not known to the person consuming the product, nor the dealer. Counterfeit pills have also been found to have fentanyl analogs, including oxycodone and alprazolam.[40,41]

Fentanyl and some of its analogs, such as remifentanil, do have medicinal uses and are classified by the DEA as Schedule II substances. Other fentanyl analogs and synthetic opioids are Schedule I substances and currently have no medical use (**Table 3**)[39,42].

Table 3
Synthetic opioids examples

Synthetic Opioid	DEA schedule
Fentanyl	II
Sufentanil	II
Alfentanil	II
Carfentanil	II
Remifentanil	II
Thiafentanil	I
U-4770	I
AH-7921	I
Thiafentanil	I
Acetylfentanyl	I
Butyryl fentanyl	I
Furanyl fentanyl	I

This list does not contain all synthetic opioids and some opioids are not yet scheduled.

Mechanism of Action

Fentanyl and its analogs are full μ-opioid receptor agonists and are known to be more potent than morphine and heroin. Carfentanil is the most dangerous analog with an analgesic potency 10,000 times that of morphine.[43] The designer opioids such as U-47700 are also μ-opioid receptor agonists but each has varied potency.[39]

Symptoms of Toxicity and Withdrawal

Symptoms of opioid intoxication include somnolence, respiratory depression, and miosis. Due to the high potency of many of the analogs, people can experience rapid and profound effects leading to death before having the chance to seek medical care. Both fentanyl and its analogs have been linked with chest wall rigidity syndrome.[44] Opioids have also been implicated in temporary hearing loss in overdose.[45] Symptoms of withdrawal include irritability, piloerection, nausea, vomiting, diarrhea, diaphoresis, and tachycardia. The Clinical Opioid Withdrawal Score can be used to help gauge severity of symptoms and indications for treatment.[46]

Treatment

Treatment of intoxication with designer opioids is with supportive care and the reversal agent, naloxone, if respiratory depression is present. Due to varied potency among the novel opioids, patients may require more than standard dosing of naloxone.[39] As it is not often known what agent the patient was exposed to at the time of presentation, naloxone should be titrated to effect to maintain adequate respiration. The authors recommend 0.04 mg naloxone every 10 to 20 seconds and titrate to the recovery of respiratory effort. Intubation can be performed if there is no response to naloxone or other concerns arise for airway compromise.

DESIGNER BENZODIAZEPINES

Background

Designer benzodiazepines are a class of substances that are derived from benzodiazepines and that work as gamma-aminobutyric acid (GABA)-A agonists (**Table 4**)[47,48].

Table 4
Categories and examples of designer benzodiazepines

	Benzodiazepines	Triazolobenzodiazepines	Thienotriazolobenzodiazepines	Thienodiazepines
FDA approved substances	Oxazepam Diazepam Clonazepam Lorazepam Midazolam	Alprazolam		
Designer benzodiazepines	Diclazepam Cloniprazepam Norflurazepam Flubromazepam Meclonazepam Phenazepam[a]	Clonazolam Bromazolam Pyrazolam Flubromazolam Flualprazolam Adinazolam	Etizolam[a] Brotizolam Deschloroetizolam Metizolam Fluclotizolam	Clotiazepam

[a] Etizolam is available for prescription in Japan, Italy, and India. Phenazepam is available for prescription in Russia, Estonia, Latvia, Lithuania, and Belarus.

Some designer benzodiazepines are approved for prescription use in countries outside of the US Common indications for use are anxiety and alcohol withdrawal.[48] Designer benzodiazepine misuse emerged in the US in the 2010s with an increase in exposures reported to the U.S. Poison Control Centers from 2014 to 2017.[47] Etizolam and clonazolam were the most frequently identified substances being used.[47] These substances tend to be ingested orally in pill or capsule form and may be obtained from the internet and/or as counterfeit prescription benzodiazepines, such as alprazolam made via a pill press.[48,49] Prescription benzodiazepines are listed as Schedule IV substances by the DEA, but most designer benzodiazepines are not yet classified.[13]

Symptoms of Toxicity and Withdrawal

Designer benzodiazepine intoxication causes sedative/hypotonic toxidrome. Symptoms include drowsiness, slurred speech, confusion, agitation, ataxia, hypotension, tachy/bradycardia, and coma. Rarely they can also cause respiratory depression and cardiac arrest though that is seen more commonly in cases with co-ingestions.[47,48] Symptoms of withdrawal are similar to withdrawal from other GABA agents and can cause delirium, agitation, seizures, tachycardia, and hyperthermia.

Treatment

Treatment is supportive and specific to symptoms present. Intravenous fluids and supplemental oxygen may be used for hypotension and hypoxia. For severe respiratory compromise especially in the setting of co-ingestants, intubation and mechanical ventilation may be necessary. Flumazenil, the reversal agent for benzodiazepines, is generally used with caution in acute overdoses due to the risk of inducing seizures, but could be considered in select cases (eg, difficult intubation). For withdrawal symptoms, treatment is with GABA agonists such as benzodiazepines or barbiturates.

KRATOM (MITRAGYNINE)

Background

Mitragyna speciosa, commonly known as kratom, is a plant native to Southeast Asia. Kratom contains multiple psychoactive alkaloids including mitragynine and it is known to have both stimulant and opioid-like effects. Kratom has long been used in Southeast Asia, but due to its high abuse potential, it has now been banned in several countries. It is used to treat pain, fatigue and as an alternative to medication-assisted therapy for opioid withdrawal but is also used as a recreational drug in its own right.[50–52] Kratom leaves may be smoked, chewed, or brewed as tea. It is sold as a concentrated powder or as capsules. In the last decade, there has been a notable rise in reported kratom use in the US with a significant increase in calls made to the poison centers for kratom use starting in 2015.[50] Kratom is not FDA approved for any medicinal use and the DEA has listed it as Drug and Chemical of Concern. It is not, however, listed as a controlled substance and is currently available to purchase in all states in the US except for Alabama, Arkansas, Indiana, Wisconsin, Rhode Island, and Vermont. Other states have various regulations such as minimum age requirements for purchase.[53] Due to the lack of regulations, kratom has been known to contain many contaminants such as synthetic opioids, o-desmethyltramadol, Salmonella, and toxic metals.[54–56]

Mechanism of Action

Kratom contains several psychogenic alkaloids. Only mitragynine, 7-hydroxymitragynine, speciociliatine, and corynantheidine are currently known to be pharmacologically active. Mitragynine and 7-hydroxymitragynine function as partial agonists at the μ-opioid receptors and antagonists at the δ-opioid receptors.[50] These alkaloids are referred to as atypical opioids because while they do bind the opioid receptors, they do not activate the β-arrestin pathway which is the pathway responsible for the respiratory depression, constipation and sedation seen in other opioids.[50,57] The mechanism of the stimulant effects is not entirely understood and may be the result of the synergistic effects of the various alkaloids present. Mitragynine is proposed to also work as a neuronal calcium channel blocker and as a COX-2 inhibitor which contributes to its analgesic properties.[50]

Symptoms of Toxicity and Withdrawal

At low doses, kratom has stimulant properties and at higher doses, it has euphoric and analgesic effects similar to opioids. Clinical effects reported with kratom toxicity include agitation, tachycardia, drowsiness, confusion, hallucinations, seizures, and coma.[58] Transaminitis, acute kidney injury, cardiac arrhythmia, and acute respiratory distress syndrome have all been reported.[50] Respiratory depression is reported only rarely and this is thought to be due to the fact that kratom does not activate the β-arrestin pathway.[50,51] Deaths have occurred with kratom use, though these are often in the setting of multiple substance intoxications.

Kratom does have addictive properties and patients can develop withdrawal symptoms with the cessation of use. Symptoms of kratom withdrawal mimic those seen in opioid withdrawal with nausea, vomiting, chills, diarrhea, rhinorrhea, body aches, irritability, and restlessness. Withdrawal is not known to cause altered mental status.[50]

Treatment

Treatment is largely supportive and tailored to symptoms as they are variable. If respiratory depression is present, naloxone may be of benefit according to case reports though there are no clinical studies on its efficacy for reversing kratom toxicity.[59] Symptoms of kratom withdrawal can be treated with clonidine or buprenorphine-naloxone.[50]

PHENIBUT

Background

Phenibut (4-amino-3-phenyl-butyric acid) is a GABA analog first synthesized in the former Soviet Union in the 1960s.[60] In Russia, phenibut is prescribed for anxiety, post-traumatic stress disorder, stuttering, and vestibular disorders.[61] In the US, it is not currently available for prescription use but phenibut can be purchased online where it is marketed for stress relief and cognitive enhancement. Phenibut is classified as a dietary supplement in the US and is, therefore, not subject to the same regulations as FDA-approved medications. With increased use since 2015, people most commonly ingest phenibut in its powdered or tablet form for its euphoric and anxiolytic properties.[62,63]

Mechanism of Action

Phenibut works primarily as a GABA-B receptor agonist but also acts as a GABA-A agonist, B-phenethylamine receptor antagonist, and activator of dopamine metabolism.[60,61,63,64] Other commonly known GABA-B agonists are baclofen and gamma-hydroxybutyrate (GHB) (**Fig. 1**). Most other GABA agonists work at the GABA-A receptor such as benzodiazepines, barbiturates, alcohol, propofol, and etomidate.

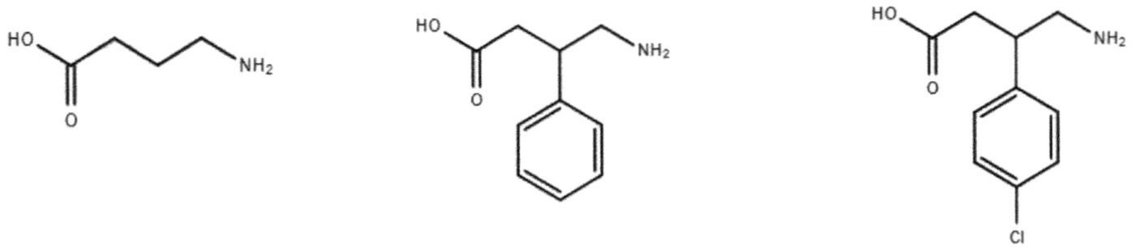

GABA Phenibut Baclofen

Fig. 1. Chemical structures of gamma aminobutyric acid (GABA), phenibut, and baclofen. Phenibut and baclofen both work primarily as agonists at the GABA-B receptors.

Symptoms of Toxicity and Withdrawal

Phenibut toxicity will cause a sedative/hypnotic toxidrome and lead to clinical effects such as decreased consciousness, stupor, and depressed respiratory drive. It may paradoxically also cause agitation, hallucinations, seizures, and delirium. Seizures are thought to be related to the feedback inhibition of GABA-B on GABA-A receptors. Treatment is supportive with monitoring and GABA agonist agents if seizures occur. Withdrawal from phenibut causes symptoms similar to withdrawal from other GABA agonist agents and may include hallucinations, psychosis, agitation, tachycardia, hyperthermia, seizures, and myoclonus.

Treatment

The mainstay of treatment of withdrawal is with other GABA agonists such as benzodiazepines or barbiturates. However, withdrawal symptoms from phenibut can be severe and may not respond to GABA-A agonists. In severe withdrawal cases, treatment with the GABA-B agonist baclofen should be considered. There is no approved regimen for the dose of baclofen for phenibut withdrawal and dosing should be titrated to symptom control.[60,64–66]

TIANEPTINE

Background

Tianeptine is an atypical tricyclic drug used as an antidepressant in Europe, Asia, and Latin America.[67] Tianeptine is not approved by the FDA and is it listed as a Schedule II controlled substance by Michigan and Alabama due to its opioid effects.[68] It is often used to self-treat opioid withdrawal, but can cause dependence and withdrawal with prolonged use. Since 2015, there has been a significant rise in calls to the poison centers regarding tianeptine use.[67,69] In the US, tianeptine was previously sold as a dietary supplement under the names “ZaZa” and “Tianaa,” both of which are available for purchase online and at gas stations.[69,70] According to the FDA, however, tianeptine does not meet criteria for a dietary ingredient and thus products marketed as dietary supplements are considered adulterated under the Federal Food, Drug and Cosmetic Act.[71] In 2018, the FDA issued warning letters to 2 companies who sold products marketed as dietary supplements but were labeled as containing tianeptine. Tianeptine-containing products continue to be sold but may be marketed as nootropics or may not be labeled as tianeptine to circumvent these warnings by the FDA.

Mechanism

Tianeptine is structurally similar to tricyclic antidepressants but has a different mechanism of action. It is known to increase serotonin reuptake, increase dopamine concentrations, and works as a mu-opioid receptor agonist.[69]

Symptoms of Toxicity and Withdrawal

Tianeptine products claim to help calm anxiety and depression. Due to the opioid effects, users report a feeling of euphoria with use and can develop dependence. The most commonly reported symptoms of tianeptine toxicity are lethargy or agitation, and hypertension. There are also reports of myoclonic jerking and tachycardia. Symptoms of withdrawal mimic that of opioid withdrawal and can include agitation, anxiety, gastrointestinal distress, and myoclonic jerking.[67,69]

Treatment

Treatment of both tianeptine toxicity and withdrawal is with symptomatic and supportive care. For lethargy or respiratory depression from toxicity, naloxone has been reported to work to reverse opioid effects.[69,72,73] Agitation due to toxicity or withdrawal can be treated with benzodiazepines, alpha 2 agonists, antipsychotics, or barbiturates. There is limited information on the use of buprenorphine-naloxone for tianeptine use disorder but it has been reported as a possible treatment.[74]

DETECTION OF NOVEL PSYCHOACTIVE SUBSTANCES

Diagnosis of NPS use is based on history and the presenting clinical signs and symptoms. Testing to detect these substances is not widely available. Urine drug screens (UDSs) use immunoassay techniques to screen for some of the more "classic" drugs of abuse such as cocaine, marijuana, and opiates, but do not reliably detect the substances discussed in this article. Liquid or gas chromatography-mass spectrometry (LC/GC-MS) can be used to identify specific substances but the equipment is not available at most hospitals. There are forensic labotatories that can run standard tests on urine samples to detect some of the known substances, such as clonazolam, kratom, acrylfentanyl; however, the results and not typically available for several days and will subsequently not help in the acute management of a toxic patient presenting to the emergency department.[75] Specific testing for these substances is useful for epidemiologic and forensic purposes.

Synthetic Cannabinoids and Delta-8 Tetrahydrocannabinol

UDS immunoassays for marijuana screen for delta-9 THC. Anecdotal experience suggests that delta-8 THC may turn the typical urine hospital drug screen positive. Products containing CBD or synthetic cannabinoids do not reliably trigger a positive screen.

Synthetic Cathinones

Synthetic cathinones are not routinely detected by a routine UDS. While the structure of synthetic cathinones is related to amphetamines, these substances are often not detected by the typical urine amphetamine screening tests. However, depending on the agent, amount consumed, and lab cut-off values, cathinones may trigger positive amphetamine screens.

Designer Opioids

Routine urine drug screens test for opiates (eg, morphine, codeine, heroin) and not opioids (synthetic and semisynthetic opioid receptor agonists) and will be negative in patients using the designer opioids, including fentanyl and its analogs.[76]

Designer Benzodiazepines

The typical UDS used to detect benzodiazepines will detect agents related to diazepam and its metabolites.[77] These immunoassays will routinely miss other benzodiazepines including the designer substances. A negative UDS for benzodiazepines should not be taken as evidence that no benzodiazepine designer substances are present.

Kratom, Phenibut, and Tianeptine

These substances will not show up on routine typical UDS.

SUMMARY

In the last decade, there has been a rise in the use of NPS for recreational purposes. Many of these synthetic psychoactive substances are derived or based on older substances of abuse, but because of their novel structures, they are not easily detectable by routine immunoassay urine drug screens. Clinical effects encountered in patients using these substances depend on the substance's structure, but can be unpredictable due to the effects on various receptors at varying doses. It is important for clinicians to be aware that these novel substances exist because the diagnosis is often clinical and not based on UDS. Treatment for these substances is generally supportive and aimed at the presenting signs and symptoms.

CLINICS CARE POINTS

- There are a variety of NPS, most of which do not turn a typical urine drug screen positive.
- Treatment is mainly supportive and directed at controlling the airway for sedating agents and managing agitation for stimulating agents.
- There is poor regulatory control of supplements and agents that can be ordered over the internet. Clinicians should rely on physical examination to guide management, as history is often lacking and the content of the supplements is usually not known at the time of presentation.
- Synthetic versions of common substances of abuse (opiates, benzodiazepines) are on the rise.

DISCLOSURE

The authors have nothing to disclose.

REFERENCES

1. Drug Enforcement Administration. DEA Emerging Threat Report: Annual 2020 | CESAR I Center for Substance Abuse Research I University of Maryland. Available at: https://cesar.umd.edu/publicationprofile/236. Accessed June 30, 2021.
2. Hassan Z, Bosch OG, Singh D, et al. Novel Psychoactive Substances-Recent Progress on Neuropharmacological Mechanisms of Action for Selected Drugs. Front Psychiatry 2017;8:152.
3. Drug Enforcement Administration. Drug Scheduling. Available at: https://www.dea.gov/drug-information/drug-scheduling. Accessed June 30, 2021.
4. United Nations Office on Drugs and Crime, United Nations. World Drug Report. 2014. Available at: https://www.unodc.org/documents/wdr2014/World_Drug_Report_2014_web.pdf. Accessed June 30, 2021.

5. Lapoint J. Cannabinoids McGraw Hill Medical. In: Goldfrank's Toxicologic Emergencies. 11th ed. McGraw Hill Medical; 2019. p. 1111–23. Available at: https://accesspharmacy.mhmedical.com/Content.aspx?bookid=1163§ionid=65097986. Accessed June 30, 2021.
6. Johnson R, Monke J. What Is the Farm Bill? Congr Res Serv 2019;17.
7. Mead A. Legal and Regulatory Issues Governing Cannabis and Cannabis-Derived Products in the United States. Front Plant Sci 2019;10:697.
8. Chandra S, Radwan MM, Majumdar CG, et al. New trends in cannabis potency in USA and Europe during the last decade (2008-2017). Eur Arch Psychiatry Clin Neurosci 2019;269(1):5–15.
9. Pijlman FTA, Rigter SM, Hoek J, et al. Strong increase in total delta-THC in cannabis preparations sold in Dutch coffee shops. Addict Biol 2005;10(2):171–80.
10. Mehmedic Z, Chandra S, Slade D, et al. Potency trends of Δ9-THC and other cannabinoids in confiscated cannabis preparations from 1993 to 2008. J Forensic Sci 2010;55(5):1209–17.
11. National Institute on Drug. Marijuana potency. National Institute on Drug Abuse; 2021. Available at: https://www.drugabuse.gov/drug-topics/marijuana/marijuana-potency. Accessed June 30, 2021.
12. Drug Enforcement Administration. Marijuana Drug Fact Sheet. Available at: https://www.dea.gov/factsheets/marijuana. Accessed June 30, 2021.
13. Drug Enforcement Administration. Controlled Substance Schedules. Available at: https://www.deadiversion.usdoj.gov/schedules/. Accessed June 30, 2021.
14. National Conference of State Legislatures. State Medical Marijuana Laws. 2021. Available at: https://www.ncsl.org/research/health/state-medical-marijuana-laws.aspx. Accessed June 30, 2021.
15. National Institute on Drug. Marijuana Concentrates DrugFacts. National Institute on Drug Abuse. 2020. Available at: https://www.drugabuse.gov/publications/drugfacts/marijuana-concentrates. Accessed June 30, 2021.
16. Ritchel M. What Is Delta-8-THC?: The Hemp Derivative That's a Hot Seller - The New York Times. Available at: https://web.archive.org/web/20210227182840/https://www.nytimes.com/2021/02/27/health/marijuana-hemp-delta-8-thc.html. Accessed June 30, 2021.
17. Sullivan K. Delta-8 THC is legal in many states, but some want to ban it. 2021. Available at: https://www.nbcnews.com/health/health-news/delta-8-thc-legal-many-states-some-want-ban-it-n1272270. Accessed July 1, 2021.
18. McKenzie B. Area poison center sees hike in crisis calls from hemp-derived THC | Local News | dailyprogress.com. 2021. Available at: https://dailyprogress.com/news/local/area-poison-center-sees-hike-in-crisis-calls-from-hemp-derived-thc/article_12ad7caa-d53d-11eb-bddd-dfa221278399.html#utm_source=dailyprogress.com&utm_campaign=%2Fnewsletter-templates%2Fnews-alert&utm_medium=PostUp&utm_content=aa8b1fa27e8bfb7c66e847308886fd08794cf64b. Accessed June 30, 2021.
19. Debruyne D, Le Boisselier R. Emerging drugs of abuse: current perspectives on synthetic cannabinoids. Subst Abuse Rehabil 2015;6:113–29.
20. Le Boisselier R, Alexandre J, Lelong-Boulouard V, et al. Focus on cannabinoids and synthetic cannabinoids. Clin Pharmacol Ther 2017;101(2):220–9.
21. Noble MJ, Hedberg K, Hendrickson RG. Acute cannabis toxicity. Clin Toxicol Phila Pa 2019;57(8):735–42.

22. Turner AR, Spurling BC, Agrawal S. Marijuana Toxicity. In: StatPearls. StatPearls Publishing; 2021. Available at: http://www.ncbi.nlm.nih.gov/books/NBK430823/. Accessed June 30, 2021.
23. Crean RD, Crane NA, Mason BJ. An Evidence Based Review of Acute and Long-Term Effects of Cannabis Use on Executive Cognitive Functions. J Addict Med 2011;5(1):1–8.
24. Marconi A, Di Forti M, Lewis CM, et al. Meta-analysis of the Association Between the Level of Cannabis Use and Risk of Psychosis. Schizophr Bull 2016;42(5): 1262–9.
25. Courts J, Maskill V, Gray A, et al. Signs and symptoms associated with synthetic cannabinoid toxicity: systematic review. Australas Psychiatry Bull R Aust N Z Coll Psychiatr 2016;24(6):598–601.
26. Kourouni I, Mourad B, Khouli H, et al. Critical Illness Secondary to Synthetic Cannabinoid Ingestion. JAMA Netw Open 2020;3(7):e208516.
27. Ruberto AJ, Sivilotti MLA, Forrester S, et al. Intravenous Haloperidol Versus Ondansetron for Cannabis Hyperemesis Syndrome (HaVOC): A Randomized, Controlled Trial. Ann Emerg Med 2021;77(6):613–9.
28. Oliver CF, Palamar JJ, Salomone A, et al. Synthetic cathinone adulteration of illegal drugs. Psychopharmacology (Berl) 2019;236(3):869–79.
29. Hyde JF, Browning E, Adams R. Sythetic Homologs of d,l-Ephedrirne. J Am Chem Soc 1928;50(8):2287–92.
30. Karila L, Megarbane B, Cottencin O, et al. Synthetic cathinones: a new public health problem. Curr Neuropharmacol 2015;13(1):12–20.
31. National Archives and Records Administration. Schedules of Controlled Substances: Temporary Placement of 10 Synthetic Cathinones into Schedule I. Federal Register. 2014. Available at: https://www.federalregister.gov/documents/2014/01/28/2014-01172/schedules-of-controlled-substances-temporary-placement-of-10-synthetic-cathinones-into-schedule-i. Accessed June 30, 2021.
32. National Institute on Drug. Synthetic cathinones ("Bath salts") DrugFacts. National Institute on Drug Abuse; 2020. Available at: https://www.drugabuse.gov/publications/drugfacts/synthetic-cathinones-bath-salts. Accessed June 30, 2021.
33. Palamar JJ, Salomone A, Vincenti M, et al. Detection of "bath salts" and other novel psychoactive substances in hair samples of ecstasy/MDMA/"Molly" users. Drug Alcohol Depend 2016;161:200–5.
34. Palamar JJ, Salomone A, Gerace E, et al. Hair testing to assess both known and unknown use of drugs amongst ecstasy users in the electronic dance music scene. Int J Drug Policy 2017;48:91–8.
35. Palamar JJ, Martins SS, Su MK, et al. Self-reported use of novel psychoactive substances in a US nationally representative survey: Prevalence, correlates, and a call for new survey methods to prevent underreporting. Drug Alcohol Depend 2015;156:112–9.
36. Borek HA, Holstege CP. Hyperthermia and multiorgan failure after abuse of "bath salts" containing 3,4-methylenedioxypyrovalerone. Ann Emerg Med 2012;60(1): 103–5.
37. Memmott M. Bath Salts" Drug Suspected In Miami Face-Eating Attack. NPR.org. Available at: https://www.npr.org/sections/thetwo-way/2012/05/30/153989768/bath-salts-drug-suspected-in-miami-face-eating-attack. Accessed June 30, 2021.

38. Centers for Disease Control. Nonpharmaceutical Fentanyl-Related Deaths Multiple States, April 2005 to March 2007. Available at: https://www.cdc.gov/mmwr/preview/mmwrhtml/mm5729a1.htm. Accessed June 30, 2021.
39. Armenian P, Vo KT, Barr-Walker J, et al. Fentanyl, fentanyl analogs and novel synthetic opioids: A comprehensive review. Neuropharmacology 2018;134(Pt A):121–32.
40. National Institute on Drug NI on D. The True, Deadly Scope of America's Fentanyl Problem. National Institute on Drug Abuse. 2018. Available at: https://www.drugabuse.gov/about-nida/noras-blog/2018/05/true-deadly-scope-americas-fentanyl-problem. Accessed July 1, 2021.
41. Drug Enforcement Administration. 2019 National Drug Threat Assessment. Available at: https://www.dea.gov/documents/2020/2020-01/2020-01-30/2019-national-drug-threat-assessment. Accessed July 1, 2021.
42. Drug Enforcement Administration. Drugs of Abuse. 2017. Available at: https://www.dea.gov/documents/2017/2017-06/2017-06-15/drugs-abuse. Accessed June 30, 2021.
43. Leen JLS, Juurlink DN. Carfentanil: a narrative review of its pharmacology and public health concerns. Can J Anaesth J Can Anesth 2019;66(4):414–21.
44. Torralva R, Janowsky A. Noradrenergic Mechanisms in Fentanyl-Mediated Rapid Death Explain Failure of Naloxone in the Opioid Crisis. J Pharmacol Exp Ther 2019;371(2):453–75.
45. Mozeika AM, Ruck BE, Nelson LS, et al. Opioid-Associated Hearing Loss: A 20-Year Review from the New Jersey Poison Center. J Med Toxicol Off J Am Coll Med Toxicol 2020;16(4):416–22.
46. Wesson DR, Ling W. The Clinical Opiate Withdrawal Scale (COWS). J Psychoactive Drugs 2003;35(2):253–9.
47. Carpenter JE, Murray BP, Dunkley C, et al. Designer benzodiazepines: a report of exposures recorded in the National Poison Data System, 2014-2017. Clin Toxicol Phila Pa 2019;57(4):282–6.
48. Zawilska JB, Wojcieszak J. An expanding world of new psychoactive substances—designer benzodiazepines. NeuroToxicol 2019;73:8–16.
49. Arens AM, van Wijk XMR, Vo KT, et al. Adverse Effects From Counterfeit Alprazolam Tablets. JAMA Intern Med 2016;176(10):1554–5.
50. Eastlack SC, Cornett EM, Kaye AD. Kratom-Pharmacology, Clinical Implications, and Outlook: A Comprehensive Review. Pain Ther 2020;9(1):55–69.
51. Prozialeck WC, Avery BA, Boyer EW, et al. Kratom policy: The challenge of balancing therapeutic potential with public safety. Int J Drug Policy 2019;70:70–7.
52. Sethi R, Hoang N, Ravishankar DA, et al. Kratom (Mitragyna speciosa): Friend or Foe? Prim Care Companion CNS Disord 2020;22(1):19nr02507.
53. Olsen EO. Notes from the Field: Unintentional Drug Overdose Deaths with Kratom Detected — 27 States, July 2016–December 2017. MMWR Morb Mortal Wkly Rep 2019;68. https://doi.org/10.15585/mmwr.mm6814a2.
54. FDA. FDA In Brief: FDA releases test results identifying dangerous levels of heavy metals in certain kratom products. FDA 2019. Available at: https://www.fda.gov/news-events/fda-brief/fda-brief-fda-releases-test-results-identifying-dangerous-levels-heavy-metals-certain-kratom. Accessed July 1, 2021.
55. FDA. Statement from FDA Commissioner Scott Gottlieb, M.D. and FDA Deputy Commissioner for Foods and Veterinary Medicine Stephen Ostroff, M.D., on the ongoing risk of salmonella in kratom products. FDA 2020. Available at: https://www.fda.gov/news-events/press-announcements/statement-fda-commissioner-scott-gottlieb-md-and-fda-deputy-commissioner-foods-and-veterinary. Accessed June 30, 2021.

56. Kronstrand R, Roman M, Thelander G, et al. Unintentional fatal intoxications with mitragynine and O-desmethyltramadol from the herbal blend Krypton. J Anal Toxicol 2011;35(4):242–7.
57. Váradi A, Marrone GF, Palmer TC, et al. Mitragynine/Corynantheidine Pseudoindoxyls As Opioid Analgesics with Mu Agonism and Delta Antagonism, Which Do Not Recruit β-Arrestin-2. J Med Chem 2016;59(18):8381–97.
58. Eggleston W, Stoppacher R, Suen K, et al. Kratom Use and Toxicities in the United States. Pharmacotherapy 2019;39(7):775–7.
59. Overbeek DL, Abraham J, Munzer BW. Kratom (Mitragynine) Ingestion Requiring Naloxone Reversal. Clin Pract Cases Emerg Med 2019;3(1):24–6.
60. Jouney EA. Phenibut (β-Phenyl-γ-Aminobutyric Acid): an Easily Obtainable "Dietary Supplement" With Propensities for Physical Dependence and Addiction. Curr Psychiatry Rep 2019;21(4):23.
61. Lapin I. Phenibut (beta-phenyl-GABA): a tranquilizer and nootropic drug. CNS Drug Rev 2001;7(4):471–81.
62. Graves JM, Dilley J, Kubsad S, et al. Notes from the Field: Phenibut Exposures Reported to Poison Centers - United States, 2009-2019. MMWR Morb Mortal Wkly Rep 2020;69(35):1227–8.
63. Owen DR, Wood DM, Archer JRH, et al. Phenibut (4-amino-3-phenyl-butyric acid): Availability, prevalence of use, desired effects and acute toxicity. Drug Alcohol Rev 2016;35(5):591–6.
64. Hardman MI, Sprung J, Weingarten TN. Acute phenibut withdrawal: A comprehensive literature review and illustrative case report. Bosn J Basic Med Sci 2019;19(2):125–9.
65. Coenen NCB, Dijkstra BAG, Batalla A, et al. Detoxification of a Patient With Comorbid Dependence on Phenibut and Benzodiazepines by Tapering With Baclofen: Case Report. J Clin Psychopharmacol 2019;39(5):511–4.
66. Samokhvalov AV, Paton-Gay CL, Balchand K, et al. Phenibut dependence. BMJ Case Rep 2013;2013:bcr2012008381. https://doi.org/10.1136/bcr-2012-008381.
67. Zahran T, Schier J, Glidden E. Characteristics of Tianeptine Exposures Reported to the National Poison Data System — United States, 2000–2017 | MMWR. Available at: https://www.cdc.gov/mmwr/volumes/67/wr/mm6730a2.htm. Accessed June 30, 2021.
68. Tianeptine is Now a Schedule II Controlled Substance | DTPM. Available at: https://dtpm.com/articles/tianeptine-is-now-a-schedule-ii-controlled-substance/. Accessed July 1, 2021.
69. Rushton W, Whitworth B, Brown J, et al. Characteristics of tianeptine effects reported to a poison control center: a growing threat to public health. Clin Toxicol Phila Pa 2021;59(2):152–7.
70. Glenn J. Gas station dope:" The legal and personal battles over Tianeptine. 2020. Available at: https://www.alreporter.com/2020/12/16/gas-station-dope-the-legal-and-personal-battles-over-tianeptine/. Accessed June 30, 2021.
71. Nutrition C for FS and A. Tianeptine in Dietary Supplements. FDA 2020. Available at: https://www.fda.gov/food/dietary-supplement-products-ingredients/tianeptine-dietary-supplements. Accessed June 30, 2021.
72. Lauhan R, Hsu A, Alam A, et al. Tianeptine Abuse and Dependence: Case Report and Literature Review. Psychosomatics 2018;59(6):547–53.
73. Pillai AG, Anilkumar S, Chattarji S. The same antidepressant elicits contrasting patterns of synaptic changes in the amygdala vs hippocampus. Neuropsychopharmacol Off Publ Am Coll Neuropsychopharmacol 2012;37(12):2702–11.

74. Trowbridge P, Walley AY. Use of Buprenorphine-Naloxone in the Treatment of Tianeptine Use Disorder. J Addict Med 2019;13(4):331–3.
75. Novel Psychoactive Substances. NMS Labs. Available at: https://www.nmslabs.com/forensic-testing/novel-psychoactive-substances. Accessed July 1, 2021.
76. Mayo Clinic. Urine Drug Screening: Practical Guide for Clinicians - Mayo Clinic Proceedings. Available at: https://www.mayoclinicproceedings.org/article/S0025-6196(11)61120-8/fulltext. Accessed June 30, 2021.
77. Craven C, S M, Fileger M, et al. Demystifying Benzodiazepine Urine Drug Screen Results. Practical Pain Management. 2014. Available at: https://www.practicalpainmanagement.com/treatments/addiction-medicine/drug-monitoring-screening/demystifying-benzodiazepine-urine-drug. Accessed July 1, 2021.

Carbon Monoxide Toxicity

Kristine A. Nañagas, MD[a,*], Shannon J. Penfound, MPH[b,1], Louise W. Kao, MD[c,1]

KEYWORDS

- Carbon monoxide • Normobaric oxygen • Hyperbaric oxygen
- Neuropsychometric testing • Poisoning • Toxicity • Carboxyhemoglobin
- Delayed neurologic sequelae

KEY POINTS

- When carbon monoxide (CO) toxicity is diagnosed, consider others that may be at risk at the scene of exposure.
- A mechanism of toxicity is oxidative stress and impaired mitochondrial activity.
- A high degree of suspicion for CO toxicity must be maintained because the symptoms are similar to other benign disease processes.
- The mainstay of therapy is high-flow oxygen for 6 hours.
- Hyperbaric oxygen remains controversial, and no one standard treatment regimen has been established.

INTRODUCTION

Carbon monoxide (CO) is an insidious poison that mimics a great number of other disease processes. The clinical presentations associated with CO toxicity may be diverse and nonspecific and may include syncope, new-onset seizure, flulike illness, headache, or chest pain. Unrecognized CO exposure can lead to significant morbidity and mortality. Given that the exposure is sometimes unrecognized by the patient, vigilance is required on behalf of the provider to detect occult poisoning.

Epidemiology and Sources

CO is a colorless, odorless, nonirritating gas produced primarily owing to incomplete combustion of any carbonaceous fossil fuel. CO poisoning is a leading cause of

[a] Department of Emergency Medicine, Medical Toxicology, Indiana University School of Medicine, Indiana Poison Center, 1701 North Senate Boulevard, B412b, Indianapolis, IN 46202, USA; [b] Indiana Poison Center, Epidemiologist, 1701 North Senate Boulevard, B418, Indianapolis, IN 46202, USA; [c] Department of Emergency Medicine, Medical Toxicology, Indiana University School of Medicine, Indiana Poison Center, 1701 North Senate Boulevard, B412a, Indianapolis, IN 46202, USA
[1] Co-authors.
* Corresponding author.
E-mail address: knanagas@iuhealth.org

Emerg Med Clin N Am 40 (2022) 283–312
https://doi.org/10.1016/j.emc.2022.01.005

poisoning in the United States, accounting for an estimated 1555 annual deaths[1] and an estimated 50,000 annual emergency department (ED) visits.[2] CO poisoning may be responsible for more than half of all fatal poisonings worldwide.[3,4] Most accidental deaths are due to house fires, faulty furnaces, and automobile exhaust.[5–7] Unintentional deaths are more common in men and the elderly and peak in the winter months with the use of indoor heating.[8–10] Annual rates of all deaths from CO poisoning in the United States have declined in recent years, perhaps related to increased use of residential CO detectors as well as improved control of motor vehicle emissions.[1,9,11,12]

Environmental CO exposure is typically less than 0.001%, or 10 parts per million (ppm)[13] but may be higher in urban areas.[14] The amount of CO absorbed by the body is dependent on minute ventilation, duration of exposure, and air concentrations of CO and O_2.[15–20] A cigarette smoker is exposed to 400 to 500 ppm of CO while actively smoking.[3] After cooking with a gas stove, indoor air concentrations of CO may reach 100 ppm.[14] In an enclosed garage, a gasoline-powered generator can produce air concentrations of CO exceeding 1000 ppm in under 15 minutes.[11] Automobile exhaust may contain up to 10% (100,000 ppm) CO, although a functioning catalytic converter should reduce this to less than 1000 ppm.[11,21] After 4 hours, exposure to 70 ppm may produce CO-Hgb levels of 10%, and exposure to 350 ppm may produce CO-Hgb levels of 40%.[3,22] The current OSHA (Occupational Safety and Health Administration) permissible exposure limit for CO exposure in workers is 50 ppm averaged over an 8-hour workday.[23]

In addition to the above sources (**Box 1**), CO poisoning has been reported in children riding in the back of pickup trucks,[24] recreational boaters,[25] workers operating propane-powered forklifts,[26–28] campers using gas-powered stoves,[29] and persons in an ice-skating rink using resurfacing machines.[30–32] Methylene chloride, a solvent found in paint remover and aerosol propellants, is converted by the liver to CO after exposure.[20,33–35]

Endogenous production of CO occurs during heme catabolism by heme oxygenase and generates CO-Hgb levels of about 1%, which may increase to 3% to 4% with hemolytic anemia.[21,36,37] Sepsis and severe respiratory illness have also been shown to elevate endogenous CO production.[38]

Box 1
Sources of carbon monoxide

Endogenous
- Normal heme catabolism by heme oxygenase
- Increased in hemolytic anemia, sepsis, severe respiratory illness

Exogenous
- Incomplete combustion of carbonaceous fossil fuel
  - House fires
  - Automobile exhaust
  - Propane-powered vehicles (forklifts, ice-skating rink resurfacers)
  - Gas-powered furnaces, ovens, and fireplaces
  - Heaters
  - Indoor grills
  - Camp stoves
  - Boat exhaust
  - Cigarette smoke
- Methylene chloride
  - A solvent found primarily in paint remover
  - Endogenously converted to CO after inhalation exposure

A patient who presents from a house fire or after a suicide attempt with automobile exhaust may not represent a diagnostic dilemma. However, a family presenting with flulike symptoms or a patient with headache can be easily misdiagnosed and discharged back to the dangerous environment.

Pathophysiology

Hemoglobin binding

The pathophysiology of CO poisoning was initially thought to be only due to the cellular hypoxia imposed by replacing oxyhemoglobin by (CO-Hgb.[39] CO binds to hemoglobin with a 200-fold affinity over oxygen.[15,40,41] It causes a leftward shift in the oxygen-hemoglobin dissociation curve, decreasing oxygen delivery to the tissues and resulting in tissue hypoxia.[41]

Direct Cellular Toxicity

CO poisoning is much more complex than initially presumed and clearly has mechanisms of toxicity beyond the formation of CO-Hgb. In a classic study, Goldbaum and colleagues[42] demonstrated that dogs breathing 13% CO died within one hour after achieving CO-Hgb levels from 54% to 90%. However, exchange transfusion with blood containing 80% CO-Hgb to otherwise healthy dogs resulted in no toxic effects, despite resultant CO-Hgb levels of 57% to 64%. This suggests that CO toxicity is not dependent on CO-Hgb formation, a finding confirmed in subsequent investigations.[43–46]

The current understanding of the pathophysiology of CO poisoning relates its clinical effects to a combination of hypoxia/ischemia as well as direct CO toxicity at the cellular level via a host of interrelated mechanisms. CO exposure intensity and duration are also important factors determining the extent of injury. This helps to explain why CO-Hgb levels do not correlate well with the severity of clinical effects.[47–49] An outline of some proposed mechanisms is presented in **Fig. 1**.

Protein binding (cytochromes, myoglobin, guanylyl cyclase)

CO binds to heme-containing proteins, including cytochromes, myoglobin, and guanylyl cyclase. CO binding to cytochrome a3[50,51] and cytochrome C oxidase[52,53] disrupts oxidative metabolism and leads to the generation of reactive oxygen species (ROS), resulting in oxidative stress.[54,55] Cellular respiration may also be inhibited via inactivation of mitochondrial enzymes and impaired electron transport.[20,56–58] Cellular energy metabolism is inhibited even after normalization of CO-Hgb levels,[47,59] which may explain the prolonged clinical effects after CO-Hgb levels decrease.[16] Binding to cardiac myoglobin may contribute to arrhythmias and cardiac dysfunction,[16,20,60–62] and binding to skeletal muscle myoglobin may result in rhabdomyolysis.[63–65] CO also stimulates guanylyl cyclase, which increases cyclic guanylyl monophosphate, resulting in cerebral vasodilation, which has been associated with loss of consciousness in animal models.[66,67]

Nitric oxide and reactive oxygen species

The role of nitric oxide (NO) and other ROS has been extensively researched in the setting of CO poisoning. Exogenous CO is thought to compete with NO for protein targets, leading to increased NO levels.[20] NO affects the function of platelets and neutrophils, resulting in oxidative stress on the vascular endothelium.[57,68] CO-induced cerebral vasodilation has been associated with increased NO levels,[69–74] as well as activation of vascular calcium channels.[73] NO is a peripheral vasodilator,[75] and increased NO activity may result in systemic hypotension.[76] Clinically, the presence of systemic hypotension in CO poisoning is correlated with the severity of cerebral

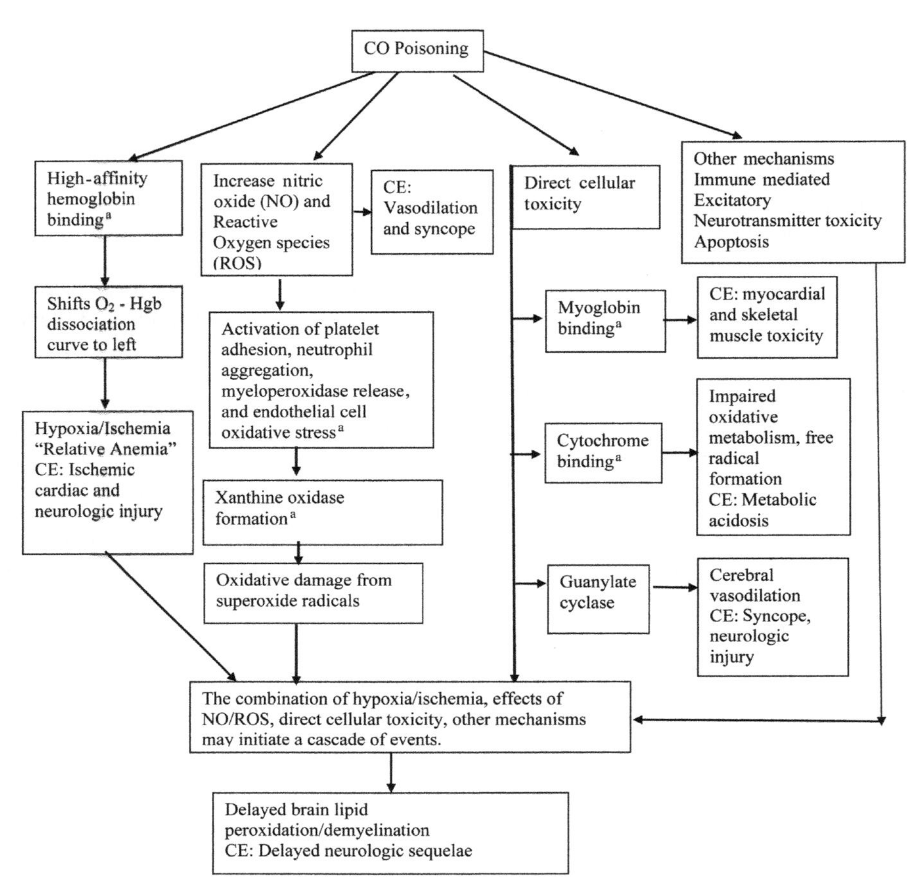

Fig. 1. Pathophysiology of CO poisoning. [a] Potential HBOT target. CE, clinical effect.

lesions, particularly in watershed areas of perfusion (ie, basal ganglia, white matter, hippocampus).[16,77–81]

CO is thought to increase ROS via several mechanisms, including inducing intracellular ROS formation, inhibiting cytochrome C resulting in superoxide excess in mitochondria, and production of peroxynitrite. The widespread effects of excessive ROS contribute to the diverse physiology and neuropathology of CO poisoning.[20,76,82,83]

NO and ROS appear to play a pivotal role in a cascade of events culminating in oxidative damage to the brain, resulting in brain lipid peroxidation and demyelination. These are thought to be the underlying processes responsible for the clinical syndrome of delayed neurologic sequelae (DNS).[68,76,82–86] Neuropathologic changes after CO exposure appear to be mediated by alterations in cerebral blood flow, as well as oxidative free radical damage, and are distinct from changes induced by hypoxia alone.[56,72,82,86–91] A period of hypotension and unconsciousness may be required for lipid peroxidation to occur.[76,83,85]

Immune Mediated

An immune-mediated mechanism of DNS has been postulated. CO induced structural and antigenic changes in myelin basic protein (MBP) interacting with products of lipid peroxidation and promoting an immunologic cascade. Rats made immunologically tolerant to MBP before CO poisoning did not suffer the cognitive and neuropathologic deficits displayed by nonimmunologically tolerant rats.[54] The utility of MBP as a diagnostic or prognostic marker for DNS remains to be elucidated.[92–94]

Other Mechanisms

Other potential mechanisms of CO toxicity include catecholamine or glutamate-mediated neuronal injury,[82,95–98] increased atherogenesis,[99,100] involvement with cytochrome p450,[16,101] actions on neuronal and cardiac ion channels,[76,102–104] and apoptosis.[95] Recent investigations discuss the role of CO as an endogenous signaling molecule with possible therapeutic effects.[76,105–108] Further research is likely to continue to elucidate the complex pathophysiology of CO poisoning.

Clinical Effects: Acute

The clinical effects of CO poisoning are diverse and easily confused with other illnesses, such as viral syndromes. The most common symptom following CO exposure is headache.[109] As exposure increases, patients develop more pronounced and severe symptoms, with oxygen-dependent organs (the brain and the heart) showing the earliest signs of injury. **Table 1** lists commonly reported signs and symptoms.[7,83,110]

Neurologic symptoms with increasing exposure include altered mental status, confusion, syncope, seizure, acute strokelike syndromes, and coma. Neuroimaging abnormalities, particularly bilateral globus pallidus lesions, are often

Table 1
Clinical signs and symptoms associated with carbon monoxide poisoning

Severity	Signs and Symptoms
Mild	Headache Nausea Vomiting Dizziness Blurred vision
Moderate	Confusion Syncope Chest pain Dyspnea Weakness Tachycardia Tachypnea Rhabdomyolysis
Severe	Palpitations Dysrhythmias Hypotension Myocardial ischemia Cardiac arrest Respiratory arrest Noncardiogenic pulmonary edema Seizures Coma

Adapted from Refs.[7,83,110]

seen.[62,83,85,111,112] The presence of systemic hypotension in CO poisoning is correlated with the severity of central nervous system structural damage.[16,77–81]

Cardiovascular effects of CO poisoning include tachycardia, hypotension, dysrhythmia, ischemia, infarction, and, in extreme cases, cardiac arrest.[113] Hypotension may result from myocardial injury owing to hypoxia/ischemia, direct myocardial depressant activity, effects on cardiac ion channels, peripheral vasodilation, or a combination of these effects.[114,115]

CO poisoning may also result in rhabdomyolysis and acute renal failure, potentially as a direct toxic effect of CO on skeletal muscle.[63,64,116,117] Cutaneous blisters[118] and noncardiogenic pulmonary edema[119–122] have been reported in patients with severe CO poisoning. The "cherry red" skin color often discussed in textbooks is not commonly seen in practice.[13,56,119]

CO binds more tightly to fetal hemoglobin than adult hemoglobin, making infants particularly vulnerable.[123] Occult CO poisoning may present as an acute life-threatening event in the infant.[124] Older pediatric patients are more susceptible to CO poisoning owing to higher metabolic rate and oxygen uptake.[125–127] Symptoms in pediatric patients are often nonspecific and can be easily misdiagnosed.[124,125,128,129]

CO exposure in the pregnant patient presents a unique scenario. Adverse fetal outcomes, such as stillbirth, anatomic malformations, and neurologic disability, are clearly associated with more severe maternal exposure.[130–134] However, even in mildly symptomatic mothers, the effects on the fetus can be severe, including anatomic malformations and fetal demise.[131,135] Earlier gestational age of the fetus during CO exposure has been associated with anatomic malformations, while functional disturbances and poor neurologic development are reported after CO exposure at any gestational age.[130,131,136–138]

Clinical Effects: Delayed

The effects of CO are not confined to the period immediately after exposure. Most concerning is a syndrome of apparent recovery from acute CO poisoning followed by behavioral and neurologic deterioration after a latency period of 2 to 40 days. This syndrome, often referred to as DNS, may manifest as almost any conceivable neurologic and psychiatric symptom, including memory loss, confusion, ataxia, seizures, urinary and fecal incontinence, emotional lability, disorientation, hallucinations, parkinsonism, mutism, cortical blindness, psychosis, and gait and other motor disturbances.[139–144] Neuroimaging is often abnormal and may correlate with the development of DNS,[145] although DNS is also reported in patients with normal neuroimaging.[146]

The true incidence of DNS is difficult to determine with estimates ranging from less than 1% up to 47% of patients after CO poisoning.[120,141–143,146–150] The large variability in incidence is at least partially explained by a lack of consistency in defining DNS using either clinical, subclinical (ie, neuropsychometric testing results), self-reported, or combination criteria. The 2 largest case series are from Korea, where CO poisoning is common owing to the use of coal stoves for cooking and heating.[141,142] Of 2360 victims of acute CO poisoning, DNS were diagnosed in 2.75% of all CO-poisoned patients and 11.8% of hospitalized patients. Symptoms included mental deterioration, memory impairment, gait disturbance, urinary and fecal incontinence, and mutism. The lucid interval between recovery from the initial exposure and the development of DNS was 2 to 40 days (mean, 22.4 days). Of those followed, 75% recovered within 1 year. The incidence of DNS increased in accordance with the duration of unconsciousness and with age greater than 30 years.[142] Another large series reporting 2967 patients with CO poisoning had findings almost identical to the above cohort. More than 90% of patients who developed DNS in this series were unconscious during the acute intoxication, and the incidence of DNS was higher in patients over 50 years of age.[141]

In general, patients who present with a more symptomatic initial clinical picture are the most likely to develop DNS. DNS occurs most frequently in patients who present comatose, in older patients, and in those with a prolonged exposure.[27,141,142,147,148,150–154] Neuropsychometric testing abnormalities have been associated with decreased level of consciousness at presentation.[147,152]

Variable definitions of DNS are used by different investigators and may refer to clinical symptoms, abnormal physical examination findings, neuropsychometric test abnormalities, or a combination. Although using gross neurologic abnormalities to define DNS may underestimate subtle cognitive dysfunction, neuropsychometric testing may reveal subclinical and perhaps temporary cognitive dysfunction with unknown clinical and prognostic significance. These results may also be confounded by mental health issues or coingestion of intoxicants.[155–158] In addition, CO-poisoned patients generally do not have a baseline for comparison.[16,159] Despite these limitations, neuropsychometric testing provides an objective measure of cognitive function that can be used to screen and follow CO-poisoned patients.[160]

Diagnosis

A high index of suspicion must be maintained in order to avoid missing CO-poisoned patients. In prospective observational studies, patients presenting to the ED with nonspecific symptoms have had elevated CO-Hgb levels without a known history of exposure.[161–164] Conventional pulse oximetry may falsely overestimate the percentage of oxyhemoglobin in CO poisoning, as CO-Hgb is difficult to distinguish from oxyhemoglobin by wavelength.[165] Fingertip pulse oximeters capable of measuring CO-Hgb are available, but as these devices are less accurate than blood co-oximetry, they have been most commonly used as a screening tool.[165–169]

Assessment of Acutely Poisoned Patient

Carboxyhemoglobin levels

In patients with suspected exposure, blood CO-Hgb levels should be measured via a co-oximeter.[165] Co-oximetry measures total, oxygenated, and deoxygenated hemoglobin concentrations, and hemoglobins such as CO-Hgb and methemoglobin.[21] Routine blood gas analyzers without co-oximeters do not recognize the contribution of abnormal hemoglobins. Arterial sampling is not necessary, as prospective comparison of arterial and venous CO-Hgb levels in poisoned patients have shown a high degree of correlation.[170,171]

Interpretation of the CO-Hgb level can be challenging. CO-Hgb levels decline with time and with oxygen therapy, so a result drawn after a considerable delay after exposure will not accurately predict the magnitude of a patient's exposure. A nonsmoker would be expected to have a baseline level of less than 1% to 3%, whereas patients who have smoked may have levels from less than 5% to 38% depending on the timing of levels and the substance used.[172,173] The severity of CO poisoning symptoms do not correlate well to CO-Hgb levels.[48,174–176] Serial CO-Hgb levels are generally not necessary during the patient's course of treatment.[177]

Other diagnostic testing

Other diagnostic testing in the CO-poisoned patient is dependent on the clinical scenario and may include complete blood count with differential, arterial blood gas monitoring, electrolytes, blood urea nitrogen, cardiac markers, creatinine, creatine phosphokinase, lactate, chest radiography, electrocardiography (ECG), and neuroimaging studies (**Box 2**). The presence of metabolic acidosis has been found to correlate with severity of clinical symptoms and/or adverse sequelae after CO poisoning.[48,178] Lactate has been found to be a marker for severe poisoning and may be a better estimate of severity than CO-Hgb levels.[179–184] An elevated neutrophil count has also been found to be a marker of severity.[176,185–187] In the setting of smoke inhalation, concomitant cyanide toxicity may occur with CO poisoning.[188–190] Fetal monitoring may be helpful to detect fetal compromise in the CO-poisoned pregnant patient.[191] Other biochemical markers of brain damage (neuron specific enolase, S-100 beta) after CO poisoning have been investigated,[192–194] but are not commonly used.

Given that the myocardium is very oxygen dependent, it is particularly vulnerable to injury via CO. Manifestations of cardiac involvement include cardiomyopathy, arrhythmia, infarction, and cardiogenic shock[110,181,195,196] and can occur in the absence of coronary artery disease.[122] Troponin concentrations can be elevated and may correlate better with severity of exposure than CO-Hgb levels[127,180,181,185,197,198]; therefore, the provider should have a low threshold to obtain an ECG and cardiac markers in a CO-poisoned patient.[169] Cardiac injury is associated with worse long-term mortality in CO-poisoned patients.[199]

A computed tomographic (CT) scan of the brain in patients with severe CO exposure may show signs of cerebral infarction. Bilateral globus pallidus lesions are frequently reported (**Fig. 2**).[200–202] Concomitant white matter lesions may also be seen.[203] Globus pallidus lesions are not pathognomonic for CO poisoning and may be seen in other intoxications, such as methanol or hydrogen sulfide poisoning.[204,205] MRI may also show globus palladi lesions[110,200] and diffuse white matter lesions.[206,207] MRI findings present in patients who have been diagnosed with DNS include demyelinating lesions in diffuse areas of white matter as well as the globus pallidus and other structures.[85,201,207,208]

Neuropsychometric Testing

A battery of neuropsychometric tests has been developed specifically to screen for cognitive dysfunction as a result of CO poisoning. The Carbon Monoxide

Box 2
Clinical care points

Acute evaluation of the CO-poisoned patient
- Basic metabolic panel
- Complete blood count with differential
- Liver function tests
- Blood carboxyhemogobin level
- Troponin
- Creatine phosphokinase
- Lactate
- Chest radiograph
- ECG
- CT scan of the head

Evaluation for delayed neurologic sequelae
- Neuropsychometric testing
- MRI of the brain

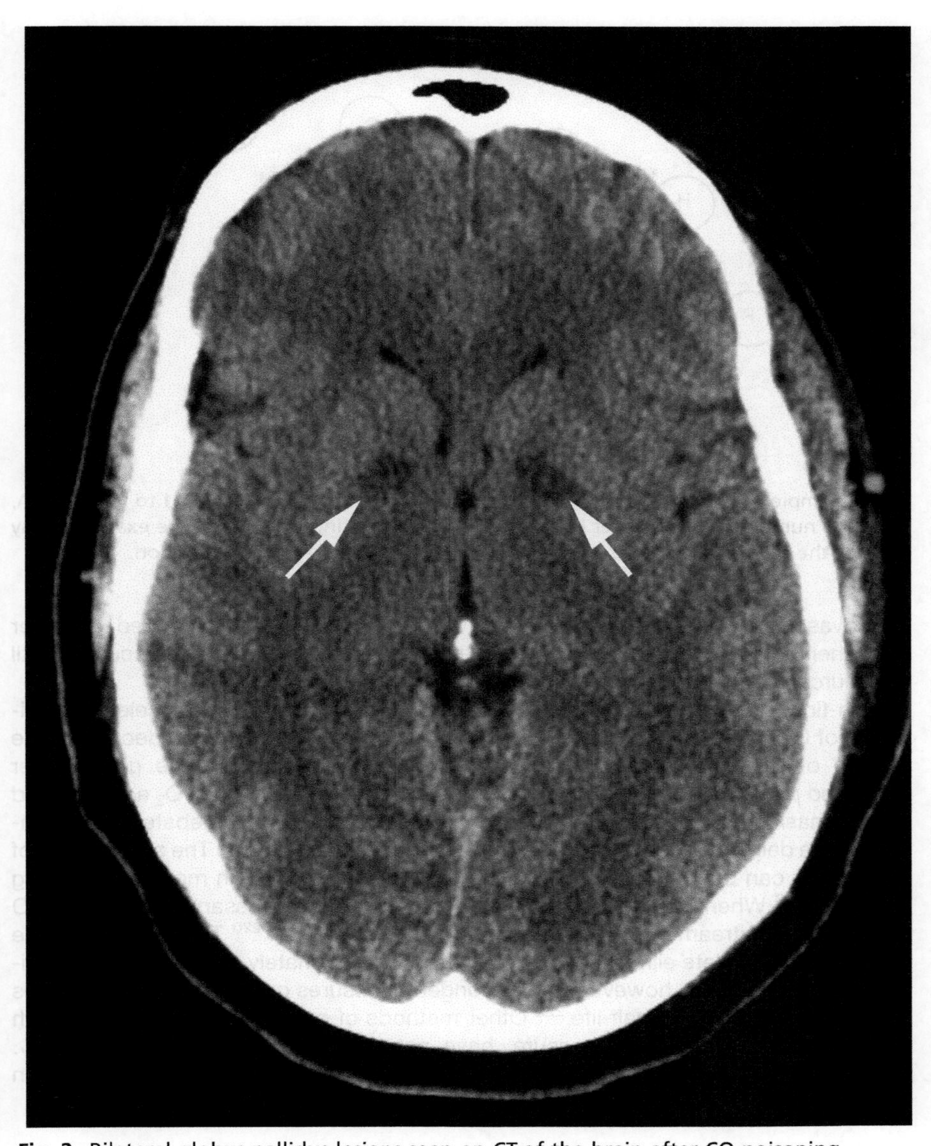

Fig. 2. Bilateral globus pallidus lesions seen on CT of the brain after CO poisoning.

Neuropsychological Screening Battery consists of 6 subtests assessing general orientation, digit span, trail making, digit symbol, aphasia, and block design (**Fig. 3**).[209] The utility of neuropsychometric testing in CO poisoning in the ED setting has yet to be determined,[210] and the practice is not widespread. Neuropsychometric testing is generally used to assess patients for DNS rather than in the acute phase of toxicity.

Treatment

Treatment of the CO-poisoned patient begins with supplemental oxygen and aggressive supportive care, including airway management, and stabilization of the

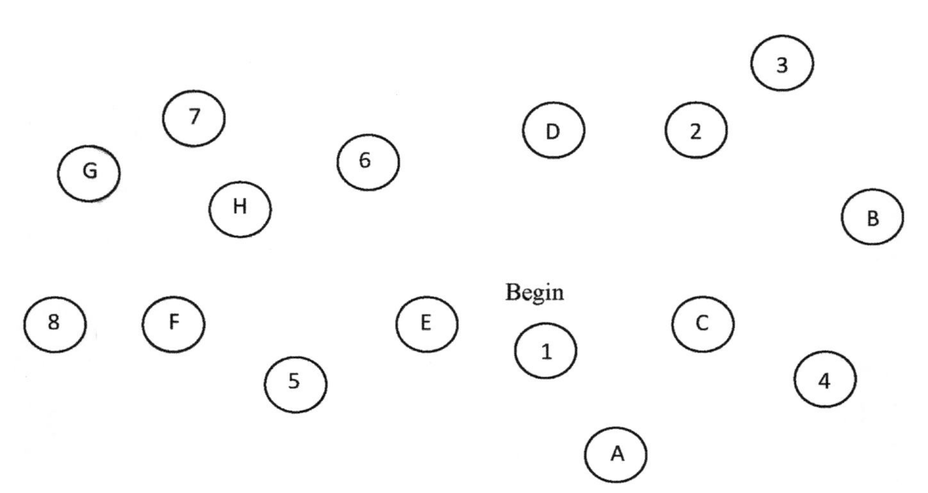

Fig. 3. Sample trail making test. Instructions: Draw a line from the number 1 to the letter A, from the number 2 to the letter B, and so on without lifting the pencil. The examiner may prompt the patient. The score is the total time in seconds for task completion.

cardiovascular and respiratory systems. When CO poisoning is discovered, consider that other patients may remain at the scene and should be warned and evacuated until the source is identified and the environment is safe.

High-flow oxygen therapy should be administered immediately to accelerate elimination of CO from the body. Increasing the partial pressure of oxygen decreases the half-life of CO-Hgb (**Table 2**).[175,210–216] Whether oxygen should be given under increased pressure with hyperbaric oxygen therapy (HBOT) or 100% O_2 administered via facemask under ambient pressures (NBO) is a subject of much debate. HBOT consists of the delivery of 100% oxygen within a pressurized chamber. The acute phase of CO toxicity can be managed by NBO, as there is no decrease in mortality by giving HBOT.[217,218] When using NBO, continue for as long as necessary to eliminate CO from the bloodstream[219] and until symptoms have resolved.[220] The amount of time required for complete elimination (5 half-lives) is approximately 6 hours.[221] Wide individual variation exists, however, and prolonged exposures or high CO concentrations may result in prolonged half-life.[222] Other methods of oxygen delivery, such as with continuous positive airway pressure, have not been studied for clinical efficacy. Some patients poisoned with CO will subsequently develop DNS. HBOT has been

Table 2
Half-life of carboxyhemoglobin

Oxygen delivery	CO-Hgb t½ (in minutes)
Normobaric oxygen[213]	74 ± 25 (26–148)
High-flow nasal cannula[214]	36.8 ± 9.26
High-flow nasal cannula[216]	48.5 ± 12.4
Continuous positive airway pressure[215]	45(30–120)
Continuous positive airway pressure[177]	36.20 ± 4.58
100% HBOT at 2.5–3.0 ATA[218,219]	20 min

theorized to prevent DNS, and several trials have attempted to address this question. HBOT is not universally available and is not entirely risk-free. Furthermore, most HBO chambers in the United States are not equipped to treat high-acuity patients,[223] and only about 75 centers are available on an emergency basis at all times.[224]

HBOT was thought beneficial merely by accelerating the dissociation of CO from hemoglobin. However, it appears that HBOT may have other mechanisms. HBOT has been shown in CO-poisoned animals to not only reduce CO binding to hemoglobin[215,225] but also reduce CO binding to other heme-containing proteins, such as cytochrome a3.[226,227] Animal studies that evaluate the role of HBOT in reducing oxidative damage or preventing neurologic impairment have had mixed results, with some showing benefit and some showing no difference.[90,226,228–233]

Six prospective, randomized, controlled trials compared HBOT to NBO for CO poisoning (**Table 3**).[149,234–238] Another trial has been conducted, but results have only been published in abstract form.[239] The data and conclusions drawn from these studies are conflicting and highlight the controversy surrounding the utility of HBOT. All trials have been criticized for flaws and other issues that may compromise the strength of the conclusions shown by each.

Various meta-analyses have been performed to determine if the preponderance of evidence favors HBOT for the treatment of CO toxicity.[218,240,241] They have each drawn somewhat different conclusions regarding the efficacy of HBO. Buckley and colleagues[240] summarized their findings as "[t]here is insufficient evidence to support the use of hyperbaric oxygen for treatment of patients with carbon monoxide poisoning", with the explanation that "the review of published trials found conflicting, potentially biased, and generally weak evidence regarding the usefulness of hyperbaric oxygen for the prevention of neurological injury." They excluded the trial by Ducasse and colleagues[234] because of methodologic flaws and the lack of clinically significant endpoints. Wang and colleagues[218] found that almost all endpoints (moderate/severe sequelae, death, headache, concentration/behavioral impairment, resumption of activity) were not different for NBO versus HBOT, with some exceptions. They determined that 1 session of HBO appears to reduce the risk of memory impairment, but 2 sessions increase the risk, and that those receiving HBOT scored better on 2 specific neuropsychometric subtests (block design and trail making) but not on others (digit span and digit symbol). They included all 7 published randomized controlled trials, including Mathieu[239] and Ducasse[234], in their analysis. Lin and colleagues[241] found that there was a trend toward a decreased proportion of patients treated with HBOT compared with NBO that developed neuropsychological sequelae that did not reach statistical significance. They also found that 2 treatments of HBO were associated with worse memory impairment and difficulty concentrating compared with 1 treatment of HBO. They excluded the abstract published by Mathieu and colleagues[244] from their analysis. Because of significant variations in study design, HBOT and NBO protocols used, and outcomes measured, no firm recommendations can be made based on the weight of the evidence.

No widespread agreement exists regarding selection criteria of patients for HBOT in the setting of CO poisoning. The American College of Emergency Physicians Clinical Policy states that "Emergency physicians should use HBO_2 therapy or high-flow normobaric therapy for acute CO-poisoned patients. It remains unclear whether HBO_2 therapy is superior to normobaric oxygen therapy for improving long-term neurocognitive outcomes." The Undersea and Hyperbaric Medical Society has recommended HBOT for patients who demonstrate transient or prolonged unconsciousness, an abnormal neurologic examination, cardiovascular dysfunction, or severe acidosis, are greater than 36 years old, who were exposed constantly or intermittently for

Table 3
Prospective trials of hyperbaric oxygen treatment for carbon monoxide poisoning

Author Year	Description	Treatment Protocols	Outcomes Measured	HBO Benefit?	Results
Raphael[149] 1989	Randomized Single blind N = 649	*Group A: (−) LOC* 6 h 100% NBO vs 2 h HBO @ 2 ATA & 4 h 100% NBO *Group B: (+) LOC* 2 h HBO @ 2 ATA & 4 h 100% NBO vs 2 h HBO @ 2 ATA * 2 & 4 h 100% NBO	Self-assessment questionnaire and PE @ 1 mo	No	(−) LOC group, no benefit shown for HBO (+) LOC group, no benefit to 2 sessions compared with 1
Ducasse[234] 1995	Randomized Nonblinded N = 26	6 h 100% NBO & 6 h 50% NBO vs 2 h HBO @ 2.5 ATA & 4 h 100% NBO & 6 h 50% NBO	PE CO-Hgb @ arrival, 2 h & 12 h EEG @ 1 & 21 d	Yes	At 2 & 12 h more NBO patients were symptomatic HBO better CO-Hgb level and PE at 2 h, but no differences by discharge More abnormal EEGs in NBO group at 21 d
Thom[235] 1995	Randomized Nonblinded N = 65	100% NBO until symptom resolution vs 30 min HBO @ 2.8 ATA then 90 min @ 2 ATA	NPT & PE after HBO NPT @ 3–4 wk Telephone follow-up @ 3 mo	Yes	Terminated early More in NBO group had DNS
Scheinkestel[236] 1999	Randomized Double blind N = 191	*Group A: Normal PE and NPT* 100 min 100% NBO @ 1.0 ATA QD × 3 d vs 60 min HBO @ 2.8 ATA QD × 3 d *Group B: Abnormal PE or NPT* NBO QD × 6 d, with 100% O_2 in between treatments vs HBO QD × 6 d, with 100% O_2 between treatments	NPT & PE after HBO and @ 1 mo	No	More DNS in HBO group No benefit of HBO demonstrated

Weaver[237] 2002	Randomized Double blind N = 152	*3 sessions NBO @ intervals of 6–12 h* Session 1: 150 min 100% NBO @ 1 ATA Sessions 2 & 3: 2 h 100% NBO @ 1 ATA vs *3 sessions of HBO at intervals of 6–12 h* Session 1: 1 h @ 3 ATA & 1 h @ 2 ATA Sessions 2 & 3: 2 h @ 2 ATA	NPT after 1st and 3rd tx, 2 wk, 6 wk, 6 mo, and 1 y PE before 1st tx after 3rd tx Questionnaire @ 2 wk and 6 wk	Yes	Terminated early Cognitive sequelae less frequent in the HBO group @ 6 wk (OR, 0.39; 95% CI, 0.2–0.78; *P* = .007)
Annane[238] 2011	Randomized Single blind N = 385	*Group A: patients with syncope* 6 h 100% NBO vs 4 h 100% NBO & 2 h HBO @ 2 ATA *Group B: patients with coma* 4 h 100% NBO & 2 h HBO @ 2 ATA vs 4 h 100% NBO & 2 h HBO @ 2 ATA * 2	Self-assessment questionnaire and PE @ 1 mo	No	Terminated early Group A: No benefit of HBO Group B: Complete recovery rate lower in arm with 2 sessions of HBO

Abbreviations: CI, confidence interval; EEG, electroencephalography; HBO, hyperbaric oxygen; LOC, loss of consciousness; NPT, neuropsychometric testing; OR, odds ratio; PE, physical examination; tx, treatment.

24 hours or more, or for a CO-Hgb level of 25% or higher.[219] Surveys of practice patterns show a wide variability in the criteria used to determine if HBOT should be used for patients exposed to CO.[242–244] Variables that must be considered when deciding whether to use HBOT include distance of available facility, length of delay of treatment, cost of treatment, need for specialized treatment of comorbidities (such as burn care or interventional cardiology), and risk of complications of HBOT. A risk-benefit analysis should be considered for each patient.

There is no current evidence that supports a specific HBOT treatment protocol over another. A survey showed 19 different treatment protocols used among centers queried.[243] Another survey showed Japanese centers use a range of regimens from 2.0 to 2.8 atmospheres absolute (ATA).[244] Randomized trials used 2 to 3 ATA for 60 to 120 minutes. Seizures occur more frequently at higher pressures.[245] Given the lack of an established protocol, the exact regimen should be left to the treating physician.[221]

A maternal CO-Hgb level greater than 15% to 20%, evidence of fetal distress, or other standard criteria for HBOT in CO poisoning are often cited as indications for HBOT in the pregnant CO-poisoned patient.[246–249] Because fetal CO-Hgb levels increase and diminish more slowly than maternal CO-Hgb, and at equilibrium are higher than maternal levels,[250,251] maternal CO-Hgb levels do not reflect fetal levels.[191] The safety of HBOT in pregnancy has been questioned,[252] but many investigators recommend it because of the potential benefit to both mother and fetus and the difficulty of assessing intrauterine hypoxia.[132,135,137,188,191,220,249,253,254] Some case series have evaluated the safety of HBOT in pregnancy and did not identify any obvious harm from HBOT to the fetus.[132,137,255] The value of transferring an unstable pregnant patient, especially one with evidence of fetal distress, is questionable. If a CO-poisoned pregnant patient is at a viable fetal gestational age, the risks and benefits of delivery should be considered.[256] Pregnant women may require longer treatment with oxygen than the nonpregnant patient[133,138,250,251,253,255,257,258]; however, there are no established protocols to suggest the ideal duration.

HBOT is not entirely risk free. Most commonly, patients complain of painful barotrauma affecting the ears and sinuses, and patients with claustrophobia are often unable to tolerate the close confines of a monoplace (sized for a single individual) hyperbaric chamber. Other less common risks include oxygen toxicity seizures, pulmonary edema and hemorrhage, decompression sickness including pneumothorax and nitrogen emboli, and fire hazard.[148,245,259–263] Potentially, hyperoxygenation injuries, such as radical formation or DNA damage, could occur.[264] The only absolute contraindication to HBOT is an untreated pneumothorax.[248] Relative contraindications include claustrophobia, otosclerosis or other scarring of middle ear, bowel obstruction, significant chronic obstructive pulmonary disease particularly with bullae formation, difficulty lying flat, and requirement of care beyond what can be provided in a monoplace chamber. In addition, if the patient requires an emergency intervention while undergoing HBOT, several minutes are required to decompress the patient safely before interventions can proceed.[229]

Ongoing research is being performed to delineate the possible role of free radical scavengers,[82,265] CO binding compounds,[165,266] *n*-acetylcyesteine,[267] and hydroxocobalamin.[268] Various means of oxygen delivery[212,214,269,270] are being researched as well.

Disposition

Patients with mild symptoms can often be treated and released from an ambulatory setting. Mild poisoning is defined by some investigators as a CO-Hgb level less than 25% with mild gastrointestinal symptoms (nausea, vomiting) and/or mild neurologic symptoms (headache, dizziness, blurry vision).[15,247] The source of CO poisoning may require investigation, and discharging a patient may depend on determining safety of the living environment. There are no well-defined mandatory admission criteria, but hospitalization is recommended by many investigators for patients experiencing persistent symptoms after initial treatment, signs of end-organ damage, refractory acidosis, seizures, rhabdomyolysis, pregnancy, or persistent symptoms suggesting an exacerbation of a comorbidity.[248,257,271] As arrhythmia is sometimes precipitated by CO exposure, telemetry is advisable.[272]

The disposition of a CO-poisoned patient may present a dilemma, particularly when intrahospital transfer is required for HBOT. Therefore, the decision to transfer becomes complicated by further questions regarding where to transfer, which of the patient's medical needs takes precedence, and if the receiving facility has a multiplace or monoplace chamber.[221,248,271,273] The Divers Alert Network can provide information on the location and use of hyperbaric oxygen facilities (1-800-446-2671 or www.diversalertnetwork.org). The treating physician may also contact the local poison center, medical toxicologist, or local hyperbaric unit for assistance.

Prevention

Prevention of high indoor concentrations of CO can be accomplished by maintenance and proper use of furnaces and fireplaces, and avoidance of indoor unvented combustion sources, such as generators and running cars.[274,275] CO detectors prevent unintentional exposure in both the workplace and residential areas.[276–278] Furthermore, CO detectors are cost-effective compared with the economic burden of unintentional non-fire-related poisoning.[279] There are disparities in the implementation of CO detector use, however, with lower use among Hispanic/Latinx and African American/black households[280] and residences with low income.[281]

SUMMARY

CO is a ubiquitous poison with many sources of exposure. CO poisoning produces diverse signs and symptoms, which are often subtle and can be easily misdiagnosed. Failure to diagnose CO poisoning may result in significant morbidity and mortality and allows for continued exposure to a dangerous environment.

Treatment of CO poisoning begins with inhalation of supplemental oxygen and aggressive supportive care. Securing the scene of exposure is critical, as this can prevent additional exposures. HBOT accelerates dissociation of CO from hemoglobin, but its ability to prevent DNS remains uncertain, given the weaknesses and limitations of existing randomized trials. Hyperbaric chambers are not ubiquitously available and may require long transport times or may not be able to provide for all the specialized needs of the patient. The ideal regimen of oxygen therapy has yet to be determined, and significant controversy exists regarding HBOT treatment protocols. Often the local medical toxicologist, poison control center, or hyperbaric unit can assist the treating physician with decisions regarding therapy.

DISCLOSURE

No authors have any financial disclosures, and none received compensation to write the article.

REFERENCES

1. Hampson NB. U.S. mortality due to carbon monoxide poisoning, 1999-2014. Accidental and intentional deaths. Ann Am Thorac Soc 2016;13(10):1768–74.
2. Hampson NB, Weaver LK. Carbon monoxide poisoning: a new incidence for an old disease. Undersea Hyperb Med 2007;34(3):163–8.
3. Raub JA, Mathieu-Nolf M, Hampson NB, et al. Carbon monoxide poisoning–a public health perspective. Toxicology 2000;145(1):1–14.
4. Mattiuzzi C, Lippi G. Worldwide epidemiology of carbon monoxide poisoning. Hum Exp Toxicol 2020;39(4):387–92.
5. Mah JC. Non-fire carbon monoxide deaths and injuries associated with the use of consumer produces: annual estimates -1998 annual estimates. Bethesda, (MD): US Consumer Product Safety Commission; 2003. http://www.cpsc.gov/library/data.html.
6. CfDCa Prevention. Unintentional non-fire-related carbon monoxide exposures–United States, 2001-2003. MMWR Morb Mortal Wkly Rep 2005;54(2):36–9.
7. Tomaszewski C. Carbon monoxide. In: Nelson L, Howland MA, Lewin NA, et al, editors. Goldfrank's toxicologic Emergencies. 11th edition. McGraw Hill; 2019.
8. Cobb N, Etzel RA. Unintentional carbon monoxide-related deaths in the United States, 1979 through 1988. JAMA 1991;266(5):659–63.
9. Sircar K, Clower J, Shin MK, et al. Carbon monoxide poisoning deaths in the United States, 1999 to 2012. Am J Emerg Med 2015;33(9):1140–5.
10. Prevention CfDCa. QuickStats: number of deaths resulting from unintentional carbon monoxide poisoning,* by month and year—National Vital Statistics System, United States, 2010–2015. MMWR Morb Mortal Wkly Rep 2017;66:234.
11. Hampson NB, Holm JR, Courtney TG. Garage carbon monoxide levels from sources commonly used in intentional poisoning. Undersea Hyperb Med 2017;44(1):11–5.
12. Hampson NB, Holm JR. Suicidal carbon monoxide poisoning has decreased with controls on automobile emissions. Undersea Hyperb Med 2015;42(2):159–64.
13. Ernst A, Zibrak JD. Carbon monoxide poisoning. New Engl J Med 1998;339(22):1603–8.
14. Abelsohn A, Sanborn MD, Jessiman BJ, et al. Identifying and managing adverse environmental health effects: 6. Carbon monoxide poisoning. CMAJ Can Med Assoc J 2002;166(13):1685–90.
15. Ilano AL, Raffin TA. Management of carbon monoxide poisoning. Chest 1990;97(1):165–9.
16. Olson KR. Carbon monoxide poisoning: mechanisms, presentation, and controversies in management. J Emerg Med 1984;1(3):233–43.
17. Forbes WH, Sargent F, Roughton FJW. The rate of carbon monoxide uptake by normal men. Am J Physiol 1945;143(4):594–608.
18. Roughton FJW. The kinetics of the reaction CO+O2Hb <-> O2 + COHb in human blood at body temperature. Am J Physiolgy 1945;143(4):609–20.
19. Coburn RF. Carbon monoxide uptake and excretion: testing assumptions made in deriving the Coburn-Forster-Kane equation. Respir Physiol Neurobiol 2013;187(3):224–33.
20. Thom SR. Carbon monoxide transport and actions in blood and tissues. Compr Physiol 2011;1(1):421–46.
21. Widdop B. Analysis of carbon monoxide. Ann Clin Biochem 2002;39(Pt 4):378–91.

22. Raub JA, Benignus VA. Carbon monoxide and the nervous system. Neurosci Biobehavioral Rev 2002;26(8):925–40.
23. Carbon Monoxide Fact Sheet. Occupational Safety and Health Administration. Available at: https://www.osha.gov/sites/default/files/publications/carbonmonoxide-factsheet.pdf.
24. Hampson NB, Norkool DM. Carbon monoxide poisoning in children riding in the back of pickup trucks. JAMA 1992;267(4):538–40.
25. LaSala G, McKeever R, Okaneku J, et al. The epidemiology and characteristics of carbon monoxide poisoning among recreational boaters. Clin Toxicol (Phila) 2015;53(2):127–30.
26. Anonymous. From the Centers for Disease Control and Prevention. Carbon monoxide poisoning associated with use of LPG-powered (propane) forklifts in industrial settings–Iowa, 1998. Jama 2000;283(3):331–2.
27. Ely EW, Moorehead B, Haponik EF. Warehouse workers' headache: emergency evaluation and management of 30 patients with carbon monoxide poisoning. Am J Med 1995;98(2):145–55.
28. Fawcett TA, Moon RE, Fracica PJ, et al. Warehouse workers' headache. Carbon monoxide poisoning from propane-fueled forklifts [comment]. J Occup Med 1992;34(1):12–5.
29. Leigh-Smith S. Carbon monoxide poisoning in tents–a review. *Wilderness Environ Med* Fall 2004;15(3):157–63.
30. Pelham TW, Holt LE, Moss MA. Exposure to carbon monoxide and nitrogen dioxide in enclosed ice arenas. Occup Environ Med 2002;59(4):224–33.
31. Anonymous. Carbon monoxide poisoning at an indoor ice arena and bingo hall–Seattle, 1996. From the Centers for Disease Control and Prevention. Jama 1996; 275(19):1468–9.
32. Cox A, Sleeth D, Handy R, et al. Characterization of CO and NO(2) exposures of ice skating rink maintenance workers. *J Occup Environ Hyg* Feb 2019;16(2): 101–8.
33. Rioux JP, Myers RA. Hyperbaric oxygen for methylene chloride poisoning: report on two cases. Ann Emerg Med 1989;18(6):691–5.
34. Nager EC, O'Connor RE. Carbon monoxide poisoning from spray paint inhalation. Acad Emerg Med 1998;5(1):84–6.
35. Langehennig PL, Seeler RA, Berman E. Paint removers and carboxyhemoglobin. New Engl J Med 1976;295(20):1137.
36. Piantadosi CA. Diagnosis and treatment of carbon monoxide poisoning. Respir Care Clin North America 1999;5(2):183–202.
37. Naik JS, O'Donaughy TL, Walker BR. Endogenous carbon monoxide is an endothelial-derived vasodilator factor in the mesenteric circulation. Am J Physiol - Heart Circulatory Physiol 2003;284(3):H838–45.
38. Zegdi R, Perrin D, Burdin M, et al. Increased endogenous carbon monoxide production in severe sepsis. Intensive Care Med 2002;28(6):793–6.
39. Haldane J. Medicolegal contributions of historical interest. The action of carbonic oxide on man. Forensic Sci 1972;1(4):451–83.
40. Sendroy J, Liu SH, Van Slyke DO. The gasometric estimation of the relative affinity constant for carbon monoxide and oxygen in whole blood at 38C. Am J Physiol 1929;90:511–2.
41. Roughton FJW, Darling RC. The effect of carbon monoxide on the oxyhemoglobin dissociation curve. Am J Physiolgy 1944;141:17–31.
42. Goldbaum LR, Ramirez RG, Absalon KB. What is the mechanism of carbon monoxide toxicity? Aviation Space Environ Med 1975;46(10):1289–91.

43. Goldbaum LR, Orellano T, Dergal E. Mechanism of the toxic action of carbon monoxide. Ann Clin Lab Sci 1976;6(4):372–6.
44. Ramirez RG, Albert SN, Agostin JC, et al. Lack of toxicity of transfused carboxyhemoglobin. Surg Forum 1974;25:165–8.
45. Meilin S, Rogatsky GG, Thom SR, et al. Effects of carbon monoxide on the brain may be mediated by nitric oxide. J Appl Physiol 1996;81(3):1078–83.
46. Mendelman A, Zarchin N, Meilin S, et al. Blood flow and ionic responses in the awake brain due to carbon monoxide. Neurol Res 2002;24(8):765–72.
47. Brown SD, Piantadosi CA. Recovery of energy metabolism in rat brain after carbon monoxide hypoxia. J Clin Invest 1992;89(2):666–72.
48. Clower JH, Hampson NB, Iqbal S, et al. Recipients of hyperbaric oxygen treatment for carbon monoxide poisoning and exposure circumstances. Am J Emerg Med 2012;30(6):846–51.
49. Rottman SJ. Carbon monoxide screening in the ED [comment]. Am J Emerg Med 1991;9(2):204–5.
50. Hill BC. The pathway of CO binding to cytochrome c oxidase. Can the gateway be closed? FEBS Lett 1994;354(3):284–8.
51. Chance B, Erecinska M, Wagner M. Mitochondrial responses to carbon monoxide toxicity. Ann New York Acad Sci 1970;174(1):193–204.
52. Taskiran D, Nesil T, Alkan K. Mitochondrial oxidative stress in female and male rat brain after ex vivo carbon monoxide treatment. Hum Exp Toxicol 2007; 26(8):645–51.
53. Piantadosi CA. Carbon monoxide, reactive oxygen signaling, and oxidative stress. Free Radic Biol Med 2008;45(5):562–9.
54. Thom SR, Bhopale VM, Fisher D, et al. Delayed neuropathology after carbon monoxide poisoning is immune-mediated. Proc Natl Acad Sci U S A 2004; 101(37):13660–5.
55. Cheng Y, Mitchell-Flack MJ, Wang A, et al. Carbon monoxide modulates cytochrome oxidase activity and oxidative stress in the developing murine brain during isoflurane exposure. Free Radic Biol Med 2015;86:191–9.
56. Hardy KR, Thom SR. Pathophysiology and treatment of carbon monoxide poisoning. J Toxicol - Clin Toxicol 1994;32(6):613–29.
57. Thom SR, Ohnishi ST, Ischiropoulos H. Nitric oxide released by platelets inhibits neutrophil B2 integrin function following acute carbon monoxide poisoning. Toxicol Appl Pharmacol 1994;128(1):105–10.
58. Radi R, Rodriguez M, Castro L, et al. Inhibition of mitochondrial electron transport by peroxynitrite. Arch Biochem Biophys 1994;308(1):89–95.
59. Piantadosi CA, Tatro L, Zhang J. Hydroxyl radical production in the brain after CO hypoxia in rats. Free Radic Biol Med 1995;18(3):603–9.
60. DeBias DA, Banerjee CM, Birkhead NC, et al. Effects of carbon monoxide inhalation on ventricular fibrillation. Arch Environ Health 1976;31(1):42–6.
61. Sangalli BC, Bidanset JH. A review of carboxymyoglobin formation: a major mechanism of carbon monoxide toxicity. Vet Hum Toxicol 1990;32(5):449–53.
62. Prockop LD, Chichkova RI. Carbon monoxide intoxication: an updated review. J Neurol Sci 2007;262(1–2):122–30.
63. Florkowski CM, Rossi ML, Carey MP, et al. Rhabdomyolysis and acute renal failure following carbon monoxide poisoning: two case reports with muscle histopathology and enzyme activities. J Toxicol - Clin Toxicol 1992;30(3):443–54.
64. Herman GD, Shapiro AB, Leikin J. Myonecrosis in carbon monoxide poisoning. Vet Hum Toxicol 1988;30(1):28–30.

65. Richardson RS, Noyszewski EA, Saltin B, et al. Effect of mild carboxyhemoglobin on exercising skeletal muscle: intravascular and intracellular evidence. Am J Physiol 2002;283(5):R1131–9.
66. Barinaga M. Carbon monoxide: killer to brain messenger in one step [comment]. Science 1993;259(5093):309.
67. Verma A, Hirsch DJ, Glatt CE, et al. Carbon monoxide: a putative neural messenger [comment] [erratum appears in Science 1994 Jan 7;263(5143):15]. Science 1993;259(5093):381–4.
68. Thom SR, Kang M, Fisher D, et al. Release of glutathione from erythrocytes and other markers of oxidative stress in carbon monoxide poisoning. J Appl Physiol 1997;82(5):1424–32.
69. Meyer-Witting M, Helps S, Gorman DF. Acute carbon monoxide exposure and cerebral blood flow in rabbits. Anaesth Intensive Care 1991;19(3):373–7.
70. Sinha AK, Klein J, Schultze P, et al. Cerebral regional capillary perfusion and blood flow after carbon monoxide exposure. J Appl Physiol 1991;71(4):1196–200.
71. Jiang J, Tyssebotn I. Cerebrospinal fluid pressure changes after acute carbon monoxide poisoning and therapeutic effects of normobaric and hyperbaric oxygen in conscious rats. Undersea Hyperb Med 1997;24(4):245–54.
72. Ischiropoulos H, Beers MF, Ohnishi ST, et al. Nitric oxide production and perivascular tyrosine nitration in brain after carbon monoxide poisoning in the rat [comment]. J Clin Invest 1996;97(10):2260–7.
73. Leffler CW, Parfenova H, Jaggar JH. Carbon monoxide as an endogenous vascular modulator. Am J Physiol Heart Circ Physiol 2011;301(1):H1–11.
74. Koehler RC, Traystman RJ. Cerebrovascular effects of carbon monoxide. Antioxid Redox Signal 2002;4(2):279–90.
75. Landry DW, Oliver JA. The pathogenesis of vasodilatory shock. New Engl J Med 2001;345(8):588–95.
76. Roderique JD, Josef CS, Feldman MJ, et al. A modern literature review of carbon monoxide poisoning theories, therapies, and potential targets for therapy advancement. Toxicology 2015;334:45–58.
77. Ginsberg MD, Myers RE, McDonagh BF. Experimental carbon monoxide encephalopathy in the primate. II. Clinical aspects, neuropathology, and physiologic correlation. Arch Neurol 1974;30(3):209–16.
78. Koehler RC, Jones MD Jr, Traystman RJ. Cerebral circulatory response to carbon monoxide and hypoxic hypoxia in the lamb. Am J Physiol 1982;243(1):H27–32.
79. Okeda R, Funata N, Song SJ, et al. Comparative study on pathogenesis of selective cerebral lesions in carbon monoxide poisoning and nitrogen hypoxia in cats. Acta Neuropathologica 1982;56(4):265–72.
80. Okeda R, Funata N, Takano T, et al. The pathogenesis of carbon monoxide encephalopathy in the acute phase–physiological and morphological correlation. Acta Neuropathologica 1981;54(1):1–10.
81. Song SY, Okeda R, Funata N, et al. An experimental study of the pathogenesis of the selective lesion of the globus pallidus in acute carbon monoxide poisoning in cats. Acta Neuropathol (Berl) 1983;61:232–8.
82. Akyol S, Erdogan S, Idiz N, et al. The role of reactive oxygen species and oxidative stress in carbon monoxide toxicity: an in-depth analysis. Redox Rep 2014;19(5):180–9.
83. Betterman K, Patel S. Neurologic complications of carbon monoxide intoxication. Handb Clin Neurol 2014;120:971–9.

84. Sönmez BM, İşcanlı MD, Parlak S, et al. Delayed neurologic sequelae of carbon monoxide intoxication. Turk J Emerg Med 2018;18(4):167–9.
85. Tormoehlen LM. Toxic leukoencephalopathies. Neurol Clin 2011;29(3):591–605.
86. Sekiya K, Nishihara T, Abe N, et al. Carbon monoxide poisoning-induced delayed encephalopathy accompanies decreased microglial cell numbers: distinctive pathophysiological features from hypoxemia-induced brain damage. Brain Res 2019;1710:22–32.
87. Thom SR. Leukocytes in carbon monoxide-mediated brain oxidative injury. Toxicol Appl Pharmacol 1993;123(2):234–47.
88. Thom SR. Dehydrogenase conversion to oxidase and lipid peroxidation in brain after carbon monoxide poisoning. J Appl Physiol 1992;73(4):1584–9.
89. Thom SR. Carbon monoxide-mediated brain lipid peroxidation in the rat. J Appl Physiol 1990;68(3):997–1003.
90. Zhang J, Piantadosi CA. Mitochondrial oxidative stress after carbon monoxide hypoxia in the rat brain. J Clin Invest 1992;90(4):1193–9.
91. Penney DG. Acute carbon monoxide poisoning: animal models: a review. Toxicology 1990;62(2):123–60.
92. Ide T, Kamijo Y. Myelin basic protein in cerebrospinal fluid: a predictive marker of delayed encephalopathy from carbon monoxide poisoning. Am J Emerg Med 2008;26(8):908–12.
93. Kamijo Y, Soma K, Ide T. Recurrent myelin basic protein elevation in cerebrospinal fluid as a predictive marker of delayed encephalopathy after carbon monoxide poisoning. Am J Emerg Med 2007;25(4):483–5.
94. Kuroda H, Fujihara K, Kushimoto S, et al. Novel clinical grading of delayed neurologic sequelae after carbon monoxide poisoning and factors associated with outcome. Neurotoxicology 2015;48:35–43.
95. Piantadosi CA, Zhang J, Levin ED, et al. Apoptosis and delayed neuronal damage after carbon monoxide poisoning in the rat. Exp Neurol 1997;147(1):103–14.
96. Penney DG, Chen K. NMDA receptor-blocker ketamine protects during acute carbon monoxide poisoning, while calcium channel-blocker verapamil does not. J Appl Toxicol 1996;16(4):297–304.
97. Ishimaru H, Katoh A, Suzuki H, et al. Effects of N-methyl-D-aspartate receptor antagonists on carbon monoxide-induced brain damage in mice. J Pharmacol Exp Ther 1992;261(1):349–52.
98. Park EJ, Min YG, Kim GW, et al. Pathophysiology of brain injuries in acute carbon monoxide poisoning: a novel hypothesis. Med Hypotheses 2014;83(2):186–9.
99. Lightfoot NF. Chronic carbon monoxide exposure. Proc R Soc Med 1972;65(9):798–9.
100. Thom SR, Fisher D, Xu YA, et al. Role of nitric oxide-derived oxidants in vascular injury from carbon monoxide in the rat. Am J Physiol 1999;276(3 Pt 2):H984–92.
101. Estabrook RW, Franklin MR, Hildebrandt AG. Factors influencing the inhibitory effect of carbon monoxide on cytochrome P-450-catalyzed mixed function oxidation reactions. Ann New York Acad Sci 1970;174(1):218–32.
102. Chamberland DL, Wilson BD, Weaver LK. Transient cardiac dysfunction in acute carbon monoxide poisoning. Am J Med 2004;117(8):623–5.
103. Peers C, Steele DS. Carbon monoxide: a vital signalling molecule and potent toxin in the myocardium. J Mol Cell Cardiol 2012;52(2):359–65.

104. Dallas ML, Yang Z, Boyle JP, et al. Carbon monoxide induces cardiac arrhythmia via induction of the late Na+ current. Am J Respir Crit Care Med 2012;186(7): 648–56.
105. Ryter SW, Choi AM. Carbon monoxide in exhaled breath testing and therapeutics. J Breath Res 2013;7(1):017111.
106. Ryter SW, Ma KC, Choi AMK. Carbon monoxide in lung cell physiology and disease. Am J Physiol Cell Physiol 2018;314(2):C211–27.
107. Schallner N, Romão CC, Biermann J, et al. Carbon monoxide abrogates ischemic insult to neuronal cells via the soluble guanylate cyclase-cGMP pathway. PLoS One 2013;8(4):e60672.
108. Stucki D, Stahl W. Carbon monoxide - beyond toxicity? Toxicol Lett 2020;333: 251–60.
109. Hampson NB, Hampson LA. Characteristics of headache associated with acute carbon monoxide poisoning. Headache 2002;42(3):220–3.
110. Bleecker ML. Carbon monoxide intoxication. Handb Clin Neurol 2015;131: 191–203.
111. Silver DA, Cross M, Fox B, et al. Computed tomography of the brain in acute carbon monoxide poisoning. Clin Radiol 1996;51(7):480–3.
112. Jones JS, Lagasse J, Zimmerman G. Computed tomographic findings after acute carbon monoxide poisoning. Am J Emerg Med 1994;12(4):448–51.
113. Lippi G, Rastelli G, Meschi T, et al. Pathophysiology, clinics, diagnosis and treatment of heart involvement in carbon monoxide poisoning. Clin Biochem 2012; 45(16–17):1278–85.
114. Yanir Y, Shupak A, Abramovich A, et al. Cardiogenic shock complicating acute carbon monoxide poisoning despite neurologic and metabolic recovery. Ann Emerg Med 2002;40(4):420–4.
115. Lee KK, Spath N, Miller MR, et al. Short-term exposure to carbon monoxide and myocardial infarction: a systematic review and meta-analysis. Environ Int 2020; 143:105901.
116. Wolff E. Carbon monoxide poisoning with severe myonecrosis and acute renal failure. Am J Emerg Med 1994;12(3):347–9.
117. Lee HD, Lee SY, Cho YS, et al. Sciatic neuropathy and rhabdomyolysis after carbon monoxide intoxication: a case report. Medicine (Baltimore) 2018;97(23): e11051.
118. Myers RA, Snyder SK, Majerus TC. Cutaneous blisters and carbon monoxide poisoning. Ann Emerg Med 1985;14(6):603–6.
119. Thom SR. Smoke inhalation. Emerg Med Clin North America 1989;7(2):371–87.
120. Goulon M, Barois A, Rapin M, et al. Carbon monoxide poisoning and acute anoxia due to breathing coal tar gas and hydrocarbons. J Hyperb Med 1986; 1(1):23–41.
121. Krantz T, Thisted B, Strom J, et al. Acute carbon monoxide poisoning. Acta Anaesthesiologica Scand 1988;32(4):278–82.
122. Kalay N, Ozdogru I, Cetinkaya Y, et al. Cardiovascular effects of carbon monoxide poisoning. Am J Cardiol 2007;99(3):322–4.
123. Vreman HJ, Mahoney JJ, Stevenson DK. Carbon monoxide and carboxyhemoglobin. Adv Pediatr 1995;42:303–34.
124. Foster M, Goodwin SR, Williams C, et al. Recurrent acute life-threatening events and lactic acidosis caused by chronic carbon monoxide poisoning in an infant. Pediatrics 1999;104(3):e34.
125. Crocker PJ, Walker JS. Pediatric carbon monoxide toxicity. J Emerg Med 1985; 3(6):443–8.

126. Liebelt EL. Hyperbaric oxygen therapy in childhood carbon monoxide poisoning. Curr Opin Pediatr 1999;11(3):259–64.
127. Akcan Yildiz L, Gultekingil A, Kesici S, et al. Predictors of severe clinical course in children with carbon monoxide poisoning. Pediatr Emerg Care 2021;37(6): 308–11.
128. Baker MD, Henretig FM, Ludwig S. Carboxyhemoglobin levels in children with nonspecific flu-like symptoms. J Pediatr 1988;113(3):501–4.
129. Kurt F, Bektaş Ö, Kalkan G, et al. Does age affect presenting symptoms in children with carbon monoxide poisoning? Pediatr Emerg Care 2013;29(8):916–21.
130. Norman CA, Halton DM. Is carbon monoxide a workplace teratogen. Ann Occup Hyg 1990;34(4):335–47.
131. Caravati EM, Adams CJ, Joyce SM, et al. Fetal toxicity associated with maternal carbon monoxide poisoning [erratum appears in Ann Emerg Med 1988 Oct;17(10):1097]. Ann Emerg Med 1988;17(7):714–7.
132. Koren G, Sharav T, Pastuszak A, et al. A multicenter, prospective study of fetal outcome following accidental carbon monoxide poisoning in pregnancy. Reprod Toxicol 1991;5(5):397–403.
133. Farrow JR, Davis GJ, Roy TM, et al. Fetal death due to nonlethal maternal carbon monoxide poisoning. J Forensic Sci 1990;35(6):1448–52.
134. Yildiz H, Aldemir E, Altuncu E, et al. A rare cause of perinatal asphyxia: maternal carbon monoxide poisoning. Arch Gynecol Obstet 2010;281(2):251–4.
135. Cramer CR. Fetal death due to accidental maternal carbon monoxide poisoning. J Toxicol - Clin Toxicol 1982;19(3):297–301.
136. Woody RC, Brewster MA. Telencephalic dysgenesis associated with presumptive maternal carbon monoxide intoxication in the first trimester of pregnancy. J Toxicol - Clin Toxicol 1990;28(4):467–75.
137. Elkharrat D, Raphael JC, Korach JM, et al. Acute carbon monoxide intoxication and hyperbaric oxygen in pregnancy. Intensive Care Med 1991;17(5):289–92.
138. Friedman P, Guo XM, Stiller RJ, et al. Carbon monoxide exposure during pregnancy. Obstet Gynecol Surv 2015;70(11):705–12.
139. Thom SR, Keim LW. Carbon monoxide poisoning: a review. Epidemiology, pathophysiology, clinical findings, and treatment options including hyperbaric oxygen therapy. J Toxicol - Clin Toxicol 1989;27(3):141–56.
140. Garland H, Pearce J. Neurological complications of carbon monoxide poisoning. Q J Med 1967;36(144):445–55.
141. Min SK. A brain syndrome associated with delayed neuropsychiatric sequelae following acute carbon monoxide intoxication. Acta Psychiatrica Scand 1986; 73(1):80–6.
142. Choi IS. Delayed neurologic sequelae in carbon monoxide intoxication. Arch Neurol 1983;40(7):433–5.
143. Myers RA, Snyder SK, Emhoff TA. Subacute sequelae of carbon monoxide poisoning. Ann Emerg Med 1985;14(12):1163–7.
144. Lee MS, Marsden CD. Neurological sequelae following carbon monoxide poisoning clinical course and outcome according to the clinical types and brain computed tomography scan findings. Movement Disord 1994;9(5):550–8.
145. Jeon SB, Sohn CH, Seo DW, et al. Acute brain lesions on magnetic resonance imaging and delayed neurological sequelae in carbon monoxide poisoning. JAMA Neurol 2018;75(4):436–43.
146. Nah S, Choi S, Kim HB, et al. Cerebral white matter lesions on diffusion-weighted images and delayed neurological sequelae after carbon monoxide

poisoning: a prospective observational study. Diagnostics (Basel) 2020;(9):10. https://doi.org/10.3390/diagnostics10090698.
147. Smith JS, Brandon S. Morbidity from acute carbon monoxide poisoning at three-year follow-up. Br Med J 1973;1(5849):318–21.
148. Norkool DM, Kirkpatrick JN. Treatment of acute carbon monoxide poisoning with hyperbaric oxygen: a review of 115 cases. Ann Emerg Med 1985;14(12): 1168–71.
149. Raphael JC, Elkharrat D, Jars-Guincestre MC, et al. Trial of normobaric and hyperbaric oxygen for acute carbon monoxide intoxication [comment]. Lancet 1989;2(8660):414–9.
150. Shillito FH, Drinker CK, Shaugnessy TJ. The problem of nervous and mental sequelae in carbon monoxide poisoning. JAMA 1936;106(9):669–74.
151. Kim JK, Coe CJ. Clinical study on carbon monoxide intoxication in children. Yonsei Med J 1987;28(4):266–73.
152. Parkinson RB, Hopkins RO, Cleavinger HB, et al. White matter hyperintensities and neuropsychological outcome following carbon monoxide poisoning. Neurology 2002;58(10):1525–32.
153. Mathieu D, Nolf M, Durocher A, et al. Acute carbon monoxide poisoning. Risk of late sequelae and treatment by hyperbaric oxygen. J Toxicol - Clin Toxicol 1985; 23(4–6):315–24.
154. Weaver LK, Valentine KJ, Hopkins RO. Carbon monoxide poisoning: risk factors for cognitive sequelae and the role of hyperbaric oxygen. Am J Respir Crit Care Med 2007;176(5):491–7.
155. Schiltz KL. Failure to assess motivation, need to consider psychiatric variables, and absence of comprehensive examination: a skeptical review of neuropsychologic assessment in carbon monoxide research [comment]. Undersea Hyperb Med 2000;27(1):48–50.
156. Seger D, Welch L. Carbon monoxide controversies: neuropsychologic testing, mechanism of toxicity, and hyperbaric oxygen [comment]. Ann Emerg Med 1994;24(2):242–8.
157. Hampson NB, Mathieu D, Piantadosi CA, et al. Carbon monoxide poisoning: interpretation of randomized clinical trials and unresolved treatment issues. Undersea Hyperb Med 2001;28(3):157–64.
158. Deschamps D, Geraud C, Julien H, et al. Memory one month after acute carbon monoxide intoxication: a prospective study. Occup Environ Med 2003;60(3): 212–6.
159. Gorman D, Drewry A, Huang YL, et al. The clinical toxicology of carbon monoxide. Toxicology 2003;187(1):25–38.
160. Katirci Y, Kandis H, Aslan S, et al. Neuropsychiatric disorders and risk factors in carbon monoxide intoxication. Toxicol Ind Health 2011;27(5):397–406.
161. Clarke S, Keshishian C, Murray V, et al. Screening for carbon monoxide exposure in selected patient groups attending rural and urban emergency departments in England: a prospective observational study. BMJ Open 2012;2(6). https://doi.org/10.1136/bmjopen-2012-000877.
162. Dolan MC, Haltom TL, Barrows GH, et al. Carboxyhemoglobin levels in patients with flu-like symptoms. Ann Emerg Med 1987;16(7):782–6.
163. Deniz T, Kandis H, Eroglu O, et al. Carbon monoxide poisoning cases presenting with non-specific symptoms. Toxicol Ind Health 2017;33(1):53–60.
164. Chee KJ, Nilson D, Partridge R, et al. Finding needles in a haystack: a case series of carbon monoxide poisoning detected using new technology in the emergency department. Clin Toxicol (Phila) 2008;46(5):461–9.

165. Rose JJ, Wang L, Xu Q, et al. Carbon monoxide poisoning: pathogenesis, management, and future directions of therapy. Am J Respir Crit Care Med 2017;195(5):596–606.
166. Sanders RW, Katz KD, Suyama J, et al. Seizure during hyperbaric oxygen therapy for carbon monoxide toxicity: a case series and five-year experience. J Emerg Med 2012;42(4):e69–72.
167. Villalba N, Osborn ZT, Derickson PR, et al. Diagnostic performance of carbon monoxide testing by pulse oximetry in the emergency department. Respir Care 2019;64(11):1351–7.
168. Roth D, Bayer A, Schrattenbacher G, et al. Exposure to carbon monoxide for patients and providers in an urban emergency medical service. Prehosp Emerg Care 2013;17(3):354–60.
169. Wolf SJ, Maloney GE, Shih RD, et al. Clinical policy: critical issues in the evaluation and management of adult patients presenting to the emergency department with acute carbon monoxide poisoning. Ann Emerg Med 2017;69(1):98–107.e6.
170. Touger M, Gallagher EJ, Tyrell J. Relationship between venous and arterial carboxyhemoglobin levels in patients with suspected carbon monoxide poisoning. Ann Emerg Med 1995;25(4):481–3.
171. Lopez DM, Weingarten-Arams JS, Singer LP, et al. Relationship between arterial, mixed venous, and internal jugular carboxyhemoglobin concentrations at low, medium, and high concentrations in a piglet model of carbon monoxide toxicity. Crit Care Med 2000;28(6):1998–2001.
172. Dorey A, Scheerlinck P, Nguyen H, et al. Acute and chronic carbon monoxide toxicity from tobacco smoking. Mil Med 2020;185(1–2):e61–7.
173. Schimmel J, George N, Schwarz J, et al. Carboxyhemoglobin levels induced by cigarette smoking outdoors in smokers. J Med Toxicol 2018;14(1):68–73.
174. Hampson NB. Myth busting in carbon monoxide poisoning. Am J Emerg Med 2016;34(2):295–7.
175. Bal U, Sönmez BM, Inan S, et al. The efficiency of continuous positive airway pressure therapy in carbon monoxide poisoining in the emergency department. Eur J Emerg Med 2020;27(3).
176. Grieb G, Simons D, Schmitz L, et al. Glasgow Coma Scale and laboratory markers are superior to COHb in predicting CO intoxication severity. Burns 2011;37(4):610–5.
177. Thornton SL, Gallagher R, Gallagher D, et al. Trends and characteristics of cases when serial carboxyhemoglobins are obtained. Undersea Hyperb Med 2019;46(5):655–8. Sep - Dec - Fourth Quarter.
178. Myers RA, Britten JS. Are arterial blood gases of value in treatment decisions for carbon monoxide poisoning? Crit Care Med 1989;17(2):139–42.
179. Doğruyol S, Akbaş I, Tekin E, et al. Carbon monoxide intoxication in geriatric patients: how important are lactate values at admission? Hum Exp Toxicol 2020;39(6):848–54.
180. Güzel M, Atay E, Ö Terzi, et al. The role of lactate and troponin-I levels in predicting length of hospital stay in patients with carbon monoxide poisoning. Clin Lab 2019;65(5).
181. Cervellin G, Comelli I, Rastelli G, et al. Initial blood lactate correlates with carboxyhemoglobin and clinical severity in carbon monoxide poisoned patients. Clin Biochem 2014;47(18):298–301.

182. Damlapinar R, Arikan FI, Sahin S, et al. Lactate level is more significant than carboxihemoglobin level in determining prognosis of carbon monoxide intoxication of childhood. Pediatr Emerg Care 2016;32(6):377–83.
183. Huang CC, Ho CH, Chen YC, et al. Effects of hyperbaric oxygen therapy on acute myocardial infarction following carbon monoxide poisoning. Cardiovasc Toxicol 2020;20(3):291–300.
184. Jeong Mi M, Min Ho S, Byeong Jo C. The value of initial lactate in patients with carbon monoxide intoxication: in the emergency department. Hum Exp Toxicol 2010;30(8):836–43.
185. Coşkun A, Eren FA, Eren Ş H, et al. Predicting of neuropsychosis in carbon monoxide poisoning according to the plasma troponin, COHb, RDW and MPV levels: neuropsychoses in carbon monoxide poisoning. Am J Emerg Med 2019;37(7): 1254–9.
186. Moon JM, Chun BJ, Cho YS. The predictive value of scores based on peripheral complete blood cell count for long-term neurological outcome in acute carbon monoxide intoxication. Basic Clin Pharmacol Toxicol 2019;124(4):500–10.
187. Gao H, Sun L, Wu H, et al. The predictive value of neutrophil-lymphocyte ratio at presentation for delayed neurological sequelae in carbon monoxide poisoning. Inhal Toxicol 2021;1–13.
188. Culnan DM, Craft-Coffman B, Bitz GH, et al. Carbon monoxide and cyanide poisoning in the burned pregnant patient: an indication for hyperbaric oxygen therapy. Ann Plast Surg 2018;80(3 Suppl 2):S106–12.
189. Huzar TF, George T, Cross JM. Carbon monoxide and cyanide toxicity: etiology, pathophysiology and treatment in inhalation injury. Expert Rev Respir Med 2013; 7(2):159–70.
190. Lawson-Smith P, Jansen EC, Hilsted L, et al. Effect of hyperbaric oxygen therapy on whole blood cyanide concentrations in carbon monoxide intoxicated patients from fire accidents. Scand J Trauma Resusc Emerg Med 2010;18:32.
191. Roderique EJ, Gebre-Giorgis AA, Stewart DH, et al. Smoke inhalation injury in a pregnant patient: a literature review of the evidence and current best practices in the setting of a classic case. J Burn Care Res 2012;33(5):624–33.
192. Akdemir HU, Yardan T, Kati C, et al. The role of S100B protein, neuron-specific enolase, and glial fibrillary acidic protein in the evaluation of hypoxic brain injury in acute carbon monoxide poisoning. Hum Exp Toxicol 2014;33(11):1113–20.
193. Akelma AZ, Celik A, Ozdemir O, et al. Neuron-specific enolase and S100B protein in children with carbon monoxide poisoning: children are not just small adults. Am J Emerg Med 2013;31(3):524–8.
194. Hafez AS, El-Sarnagawy GN. S-100β in predicting the need of hyperbaric oxygen in CO-induced delayed neurological sequels. Hum Exp Toxicol 2020;39(5): 614–23.
195. Garg J, Krishnamoorthy P, Palaniswamy C, et al. Cardiovascular abnormalities in carbon monoxide poisoning. Am J Ther 2018;25(3):e339–48.
196. Satran D, Henry CR, Adkinson C, et al. Cardiovascular manifestations of moderate to severe carbon monoxide poisoning. J Am Coll Cardiol 2005;45(9): 1513–6.
197. Ozyurt A, Karpuz D, Yucel A, et al. Effects of acute carbon monoxide poisoning on ECG and echocardiographic parameters in children. *Cardiovasc Toxicol* Jul 2017;17(3):326–34.
198. Holstege CP, Baer AB, Eldridge DL, et al. Case series of elevated troponin I following carbon monoxide poisoning. J Toxicol - Clin Toxicol 2004;42(5):742–3.

199. Henry CR. Myocardial injury and long-term mortality following moderate to severe carbon monoxide poisoning. JAMA 2006;295(4):398.
200. Chawla A, Ray S, Matettore A, et al. Arterial carboxyhaemoglobin levels in children admitted to PICU: a retrospective observational study. PLoS One 2019;14(3):e0209452.
201. Beppu T. The role of MR imaging in assessment of brain damage from carbon monoxide poisoning: a review of the literature. AJNR Am J Neuroradiol 2014;35(4):625–31.
202. Açıkalın A, Satar S, Sebe A, et al. H-FABP in cases of carbon monoxide intoxication admitted to the emergency room. Hum Exp Toxicol 2010;30(6):443–7.
203. Ozcan N, Ozcam G, Kosar P, et al. Correlation of computed tomography, magnetic resonance imaging and clinical outcome in acute carbon monoxide poisoning. Braz J Anesthesiol 2016;66(5):529–32.
204. Hegde AN, Mohan S, Lath N, et al. Differential diagnosis for bilateral abnormalities of the basal ganglia and thalamus. Radiographics 2011;31(1):5–30.
205. Alquist CR, McGoey R, Bastian F, et al. Bilateral globus pallidus lesions. J La State Med Soc 2012;164(3):145–6.
206. O'donnell P, Buxton P, Pitkin A, et al. The magnetic resonance imaging appearances of the brain in acute carbon monoxide poisoning. Clin Radiol 2000;55(4):273–80.
207. Wang X, Li Z, Berglass J, et al. MRI and clinical manifestations of delayed encephalopathy after carbon monoxide poisoning. Pak J Pharm Sci 2016;29(6 Suppl):2317–20.
208. Lin YT, Chen SY, Lo CP, et al. Utilizing cerebral perfusion scan and diffusion-tensor MR imaging to evaluate the effect of hyperbaric oxygen therapy in carbon monoxide-induced delayed neuropsychiatric seqeulae- a case report and literature review. Acta Neurol Taiwan 2015;24(2):57–62.
209. Messier LD, Myers RA. A neuropsychological screening battery for emergency assessment of carbon-monoxide-poisoned patients. J Clin Psychol 1991;47(5):675–84.
210. Weaver LK, Howe S, Hopkins R, et al. Carboxyhemoglobin half-life in carbon monoxide-poisoned patients treated with 100% oxygen at atmospheric pressure. Chest 2000;117(3):801–8.
211. Ozturan IU, Yaka E, Suner S, et al. Determination of carboxyhemoglobin half-life in patients with carbon monoxide toxicity treated with high flow nasal cannula oxygen therapy. Clin Toxicol (Phila) 2019;57(7):617–23.
212. Turgut K, Yavuz E. Comparison of non-invasive CPAP with mask use in carbon monoxide poisoning. Am J Emerg Med 2020;38(7):1454–7.
213. Kim Y-M, Shin H-J, Choi D-w, et al. Comparison of high-flow nasal cannula oxygen therapy and conventional reserve-bag oxygen therapy in carbon monoxide intoxication: a pilot study. The Am J Emerg Med 2020;38(8):1621–6. https://doi.org/10.1016/j.ajem.2019.158451.
214. Caglar B, Serin S, Yilmaz G, et al. The impact of treatment with continuous positive airway pressure on acute carbon monoxide poisoning. Prehosp Disaster Med 2019;34(6):588–91.
215. Pace N, Stajman E, Walker EL. Acceleration of carbon monoxide elimination in man by high pressure oxygen. Science 1950;111:652–4.
216. Jay GD, McKindley DS. Alterations in pharmacokinetics of carboxyhemoglobin produced by oxygen under pressure. Undersea Hyperb Med 1997;24(3):165–73.

217. Simonsen C, Thorsteinsson K, Mortensen RN, et al. Carbon monoxide poisoning in Denmark with focus on mortality and factors contributing to mortality. PLoS One 2019;14(1):e0210767.
218. Wang W, Cheng J, Zhang J, et al. Effect of hyperbaric oxygen on neurologic sequelae and all-cause mortality in patients with carbon monoxide poisoning: a meta-analysis of randomized controlled trials. Med Sci Monit 2019;25: 7684–93.
219. Weaver LK. Clinical practice. Carbon monoxide poisoning. N Engl J Med 2009; 360(12):1217–25.
220. Eichhorn L, Thudium M, Jüttner B. The diagnosis and treatment of carbon monoxide poisoning. Dtsch Arztebl Int 2018;115(51–52):863–70.
221. Hampson NB, Piantadosi CA, Thom SR, et al. Practice recommendations in the diagnosis, management, and prevention of carbon monoxide poisoning. Am J Respir Crit Care Med 2012;186(11):1095–101.
222. Pan KT, Leonardi GS, Croxford B. Factors contributing to CO uptake and elimination in the body: a critical review. Int J Environ Res Public Health 2020;17(2). https://doi.org/10.3390/ijerph17020528.
223. Chin W, Jacoby L, Simon O, et al. Hyperbaric programs in the United States: locations and capabilities of treating decompression sickness, arterial gas embolisms, and acute carbon monoxide poisoning: survey results. *Undersea Hyperb Med* Jan-feb 2016;43(1):29–43.
224. Shea S. In: Kris Nanagas M, editor. 24 HBO chamber availability, according to Divers Alert Network. 2021.
225. End E, Long CW. Oxygen under pressure in carbon monoxide poisoning. J Ind Hyg Toxicol 1942;24(10):302–6.
226. Thom SR. Antagonism of carbon monoxide-mediated brain lipid peroxidation by hyperbaric oxygen. Toxicol Appl Pharmacol 1990;105(2):340–4.
227. Brown SD, Piantadosi CA. Reversal of carbon monoxide-cytochrome c oxidase binding by hyperbaric oxygen in vivo. Adv Exp Med Biol 1989;248:747–54.
228. Thom SR. Functional inhibition of leukocyte B2 integrins by hyperbaric oxygen in carbon monoxide-mediated brain injury in rats. Toxicol Appl Pharmacol 1993; 123(2):248–56.
229. Thom SR. Antidotes in depth: hyperbaric oxygen. In: Goldfrank LR, Flomenbaum NE, Lewin NA, et al, editors. Goldfrank's toxicologic emergencies. 7 ed. McGraw-Hill; 2002. p. 1492–7.
230. Thom SR, Bhopale VM, Fisher D. Hyperbaric oxygen reduces delayed immune-mediated neuropathology in experimental carbon monoxide toxicity. Toxicol Appl Pharmacol 2006;213(2):152–9.
231. Tomaszewski C, Rosenberg N, Wanthen J, et al. Prevention of neurological sequelae from carbon monoxide by hyperbaric oxygen in rats. *Neurology.* April 1992;42(Suppl 3):196.
232. Gilmer B, Kilkenny J, Tomaszewski C, et al. Hyperbaric oxygen does not prevent neurologic sequelae after carbon monoxide poisoning. Acad Emerg Med 2002; 9(1):1–8.
233. Carstairs SD, Miller AD, Minns AB, et al. Single versus multiple hyperbaric sessions for carbon monoxide poisoning in a murine model. J Med Toxicol 2016; 12(4):386–90.
234. Ducasse JL, Celsis P, Marc-Vergnes JP. Non-comatose patients with acute carbon monoxide poisoning: hyperbaric or normobaric oxygenation? Undersea Hyperb Med 1995;22(1):9–15.

235. Thom SR, Taber RL, Mendiguren II, et al. Delayed neuropsychologic sequelae after carbon monoxide poisoning: prevention by treatment with hyperbaric oxygen [comment]. Ann Emerg Med 1995;25(4):474–80.
236. Scheinkestel CD, Bailey M, Myles PS, et al. Hyperbaric or normobaric oxygen for acute carbon monoxide poisoning: a randomised controlled clinical trial [comment]. Med J Aust 1999;170(5):203–10.
237. Weaver LK, Hopkins RO, Chan KJ, et al. Hyperbaric oxygen for acute carbon monoxide poisoning [comment]. N Engl J Med 2002;347(14):1057–67.
238. Annane D, Chadda K, Gajdos P, et al. Hyperbaric oxygen therapy for acute domestic carbon monoxide poisoning: two randomized controlled trials. *Intensive Care Med* Mar 2011;37(3):486–92. https://doi.org/10.1007/s00134-010-2093-0.
239. Mathieu D, Wattel F, Mathieu-Nolf M, et al. Randomized prospective study comparing the effect of HBO versus 12 hours NBO in noncomatose CO poisoned patients: results of the interim analysis. Undersea Hyperb Med 1996;23:7–8.
240. Buckley NA, Juurlink DN, Isbister G, et al. Hyperbaric oxygen for carbon monoxide poisoning. Cochrane Database Syst Rev 2011;(4):CD002041.
241. Lin CH, Su WH, Chen YC, et al. Treatment with normobaric or hyperbaric oxygen and its effect on neuropsychometric dysfunction after carbon monoxide poisoning: a systematic review and meta-analysis of randomized controlled trials. Medicine (Baltimore) 2018;97(39):e12456.
242. Hampson NB, Dunford RG, Kramer CC, et al. Selection criteria utilized for hyperbaric oxygen treatment of carbon monoxide poisoning. J Emerg Med 1995; 13(2):227–31.
243. Byrne BT, Lu JJ, Valento M, et al. Variability in hyperbaric oxygen treatment for acute carbon monoxide poisoning. *Undersea Hyperb Med* Mar-apr 2012;39(2): 627–38.
244. Fujita M, Oda Y, Kaneda K, et al. Variability in treatment for carbon monoxide poisoning in Japan: a multicenter retrospective survey. Emerg Med Int 2018; 2018:2159147.
245. Hampson NB, Simonson SG, Kramer CC, et al. Central nervous system oxygen toxicity during hyperbaric treatment of patients with carbon monoxide poisoning. Undersea Hyperb Med 1996;23(4):215–9.
246. Aubard Y, Magne I. Carbon monoxide poisoning in pregnancy. BJOG: An Int J Obstet Gynaecol 2000;107(7):833–8.
247. Tomaszewski C. Carbon monoxide. In: Goldfrank LR, Flomenbaum NE, Lewin NA, et al, editors. Goldfrank's toxicologic Emergencies. 7 ed. McGraw-Hill; 2002.
248. Tomaszewski CA, Thom SR. Use of hyperbaric oxygen in toxicology. Emerg Med Clin North America 1994;12(2):437–59.
249. Van Hoesen KB, Camporesi EM, Moon RE, et al. Should hyperbaric oxygen be used to treat the pregnant patient for acute carbon monoxide poisoning? A case report and literature review. JAMA 1989;261(7):1039–43.
250. Longo LD, Hill EP. Carbon monoxide uptake and elimination in fetal and maternal sheep. Am J Physiol 1977;232(3):H324–30.
251. Hill EP, Hill JR, Power GG, et al. Carbon monoxide exchanges between the human fetus and mother: a mathematical model. Am J Physiol 1977;232(3): H311–23.
252. Greingor J, Tosi J, Ruhlmann S, et al. Acute carbon monoxide intoxication during pregnancy. One case report and review of the literature. Emerg Med J 2001; 18(5):399–401.

253. Margulies JL. Acute carbon monoxide poisoning during pregnancy. Am J Emerg Med 1986;4(6):516–9.
254. Brown DB, Mueller GL, Golich FC. Hyperbaric oxygen treatment for carbon monoxide poisoning in pregnancy: a case report. Aviation Space Environ Med 1992;63(11):1011–4.
255. Arslan A. Hyperbaric oxygen therapy in carbon monoxide poisoning in pregnancy: maternal and fetal outcome. Am J Emerg Med 2021;43:41–5.
256. Ullmann Y, Blumenfeld Z, Hakim M, et al. Urgent delivery, the treatment of choice in term pregnant women with extended burn injury. Burns 1997;23(2): 157–9.
257. Gozubuyuk AA, Dag H, Kacar A, et al. Epidemiology, pathophysiology, clinical evaluation, and treatment of carbon monoxide poisoning in child, infant, and fetus. North Clin Istanb 2017;4(1):100–7.
258. Longo LD. Carbon monoxide in the pregnant mother and fetus and its exchange across the placenta. Ann New York Acad Sci 1970;174(1):312–41.
259. Camporesi EM. Side effects of hyperbaric oxygen therapy. Undersea Hyperb Med J Undersea Hyperb Med Soc Inc. 2014;41(3):253–7.
260. Gabb G, Robin ED. Hyperbaric oxygen. A therapy in search of diseases. Chest 1987;92(6):1074–82.
261. Weaver LK, Hopkins RO, Elliott G. Carbon monoxide poisoning [comment]. New Engl J Med 1999;340(16):1290 ; author reply 1292.
262. Chen W, Liang X, Nong Z, et al. The multiple applications and possible mechanisms of the hyperbaric oxygenation therapy. Med Chem 2019;15(5):459–71.
263. Lee CH, Choi JG, Lee JS, et al. Seizure during hyperbaric oxygen therapy: experience at a single academic hospital in Korea. Undersea Hyperb Med 2021;48(1):43–51.
264. Mannaioni PF, Vannacci A, Masini E. Carbon monoxide: the bad and the good side of the coin, from neuronal death to anti-inflammatory activity. Inflamm Res : official J Eur Histamine Res Soc [et al] 2006;55(7):261–73.
265. Akyol S, Gulec MA, Erdemli HK, et al. A new therapeutic approach for carbon monoxide poisoning: antioxidants. Toxicology 2015;336:34–5.
266. Rose JJ, Bocian KA, Xu Q, et al. A neuroglobin-based high-affinity ligand trap reverses carbon monoxide-induced mitochondrial poisoning. J Biol Chem 2020;295(19):6357–71.
267. Kekec Z, Seydaoglul G, Sever H, et al. The effect of antioxidants (N-acetylcysteine and melatonin) on hypoxia due to carbonmonoxide poisoning. Bratisl Lek Listy 2010;111(4):189–93.
268. Roderique JD, Josef CS, Newcomb AH, et al. Preclinical evaluation of injectable reduced hydroxocobalamin as an antidote to acute carbon monoxide poisoning. The J Trauma acute Care Surg 2015;79(4 Suppl 2):S116–20. https://doi.org/10.1097/TA.0000000000000740.
269. Sein Anand J, Schetz D, Waldman W, et al. Hyperventilation with maintenance of isocapnia. An "old new" method in carbon monoxide intoxication. PLoS One 2017;12(1):e0170621.
270. Fisher JA, Iscoe S, Fedorko L, et al. Rapid elimination of CO through the lungs: coming full circle 100 years on. Exp Physiol 2011;96(12):1262–9.
271. Haddad LM. Carbon monoxide poisoning: to transfer or not to transfer? Ann Emerg Med 1986;15(11):1375.
272. Lee FY, Chen WK, Lin CL, et al. Carbon monoxide poisoning and subsequent cardiovascular disease risk: a nationwide population-based cohort study. Medicine (Baltimore) 2015;94(10):e624.

273. Olson KR, Seger D. Hyperbaric oxygen for carbon monoxide poisoning: does it really work? [comment]. Ann Emerg Med 1995;25(4):535–7.
274. Johnson-Arbor KK, Quental AS, Li D. A comparison of carbon monoxide exposures after snowstorms and power outages. Am J Prev Med 2014;46(5):481–6. https://doi.org/10.1016/j.amepre.2014.01.006.
275. CfDCa Prevention. Carbon monoxide poisoning prevention guidance. https://www.cdc.gov/co/guidelines.htm. Accessed May 30, 2021.
276. Iqbal S, Clower JH, Saha S, et al. Residential carbon monoxide alarm prevalence and ordinance awareness. J Public Health Manag Pract 2012;18(3):272–8.
277. Christensen GM, Creswell PD, Theobald J, et al. Carbon monoxide detector effectiveness in reducing poisoning, Wisconsin 2016. Clin Toxicol 2020;58(12):1335–41.
278. Hammond S, Phillips JA. Carbon monoxide poisoning. *Workplace Health Saf* Jan 2019;67(1):47–8.
279. Cho K, Minami T, Okuno Y, et al. Convulsive seizure and pulmonary edema during hyperbaric oxygen therapy: a case report. J Med Invest 2018;65(34):286–8.
280. Hampson N. Racial and ethnic trends in unintentional carbon monoxide poisoning deaths. Undersea Hyperb Med : J Undersea Hyperb Med Soc Inc. 2019;46 4:495–501.
281. Johnson-Arbor K, Liebman DL, Carter EM. A survey of residential carbon monoxide detector utilization among Connecticut Emergency Department patients. Clin Toxicol 2012;50(5):384–9.

North American Envenomation Syndromes

George P. Warpinski, MD[a,b,*], Anne-Michelle Ruha, MD[a,b]

KEYWORDS

- North American envenomations • Pit viper envenomation • Scorpion envenomation
- Black widow envenomation • Brown recluse envenomation
- Envenomation management

KEY POINTS

- Envenomation from the Crotalinae subfamily produces a clinical syndrome that ranges from local tissue effects and coagulopathy to circulatory collapse and anaphylactoid reactions.
- Envenomation from coral snake species produces neurotoxicity; the incidence coral snake envenomation is low.
- Loxosceles envenomation can produce cutaneous lesions as well as systemic toxicity involving hemolysis and end-organ damage.
- Latrodectus species envenomation produces musculoskeletal pain as well as autonomic dysfunction through dysregulation of acetylcholine release.
- Symptoms of Centruroides sculpturatus envenomation can range from pain at the site of envenomation to musculoskeletal symptoms and cranial nerve dysfunction.

INTRODUCTION

The purpose of this review is to acquaint readers with the variety of envenomation syndromes caused by snakes, scorpions, and spiders of North America. Although the venomous species discussed here are endemic to specific geographic regions of North America, there are opportunities for envenomations to occur outside of their natural range. Therefore, the medical management of these envenomation syndromes is an essential skill set for physicians no matter where they practice.

[a] Department of Medical Toxicology, Banner University Medical Center Phoenix, 1012 East Willetta Street, Fl 2, Phoenix, AZ 85006, USA; [b] University of Arizona College of Medicine, Phoenix, AZ, USA
* Corresponding author.
E-mail address: george.warpinski@bannerhealth.com

Emerg Med Clin N Am 40 (2022) 313–326
https://doi.org/10.1016/j.emc.2022.01.006

DISCUSSION

North American Venomous Snakes

Epidemiology

Approximately 5000 venomous snake bites are reported to US poison centers each year.[1] Venomous North American snakes come from 2 families. These are the families Elapidae and Viperidae, the latter of which can be divided into 2 subfamilies: Crotalinae and Viperinae. Snakes from the Crotalinae subfamily are those that are found in North America, whereas snakes from Viperinae are found in Europe, Asia, and Africa. There are 3 genera within the Crotalinae subfamily found in North America: *Crotalus*, *Sistrurus*, and *Agkistrodon*. *Agkistrodon* includes both copperheads and cottonmouths, whereas *Crotalus* and *Sistrurus* comprise the rattlesnakes.

Common to all snakes within the Crotalinae subfamily are the presence of heat-detecting "pits" near the nostril that help snakes detect prey. Other distinguishing features of these snakes are a triangular head and elliptical pupil. Pit vipers are responsible for most of the snake envenomations reported to North American poison centers.[1]

The minority of snake envenomations in North America are from snakes belonging to the Elapidae family, specifically the genus *Micrurus*. These are the coral snakes. The geographic range of coral snakes extends from Southeastern to the Southwestern states. There are 3 known species: *Micrurus fulvius* (Eastern coral snake), *Micrurus tener* (Texas coral snake), and *Micruroides euryxanthus* (Arizona coral snake). Of the 3, the Eastern and Texas coral snakes do produce significant human envenomation, whereas the Arizona coral snake does not.

Taken as a group, snakes from the Crotalinae subfamily produce an envenomation syndrome that is distinct from those in the Elapidae family; this review delineates the clinical presentation, assessment, and management of each separately.

Pit Vipers

Clinical presentation

The clinical effects of pit viper bite range from so-called dry bites, where no venom is injected, to severe envenomation with circulatory collapse and death. The venom responsible for these effects is composed of different proteins including serine proteases, phospholipases, and metalloproteases; the relative proportion of these proteins in the venom varies between species and even individual snakes.[2]

Rattlesnakes are responsible for the most severe envenomations reported among the pit vipers and copperheads the least severe. Severity occurs along a spectrum however, and a given rattlesnake envenomation may be minor, whereas the rare copperhead envenomation has been fatal in part depending on the amount of venom injected and the exact site of the envenomation.

Most pit viper envenomations are associated with swelling, which can be severe and extend from the bite site as the envenomation progresses. Without treatment, and occasionally despite treatment, swelling can continue to progress. Swelling at bite sites on a distal extremity can even progress to involve the torso. After swelling, ecchymosis, erythema, and superficial necrosis are the next most common local tissue effects.[3] Erythema in the immediate hours to days after envenomation is due to venom-induced inflammation rather than infection. Location of the bite site is clinically important as well. In one study, bites to digits of the hand were more likely to result in local tissue necrosis compared with bites at other locations[4]; airway obstruction can result as a consequence of bites to the face and neck, as demonstrated in several case reports.[5–7] Clinical signs of copperhead envenomation are most often limited to tissue swelling.

Hematologic toxicity is a frequent finding in rattlesnake envenomations. Patients may develop thrombocytopenia or coagulopathy or a combination of the two. Coagulopathy primarily results from the effect of thrombinlike enzymes in venom on fibrinogen and fibrin; other coagulation factors are not directly affected. As fibrinogen levels decrease, prothrombin time may also increase. Hemotoxicity typically occurs early in the course of the envenomation, but late-onset or delayed hemotoxicity can occur for up to 2 weeks following antivenom treatment.[8]

Less commonly, envenomation results in systemic toxicity. Findings may include gastrointestinal symptoms such as diarrhea and vomiting; cardiopulmonary symptoms such as hypotension, tachycardia, and respiratory failure; rhabdomyolysis; and bleeding.[3] Major bleeding is rare after rattlesnake envenomation.[9]

Perhaps the most severe manifestation of systemic toxicity is circulatory shock, which may be caused by an anaphylactoid reaction to venom. Patients can develop symptoms of angioedema and upper airway obstruction as well as hypotension, tachycardia, and gastrointestinal symptoms such as nausea, vomiting, and diarrhea. Anaphylaxis to venom may also occur in patients with presensitization to venom proteins.

Neurotoxicity is also sometimes seen after rattlesnake envenomation. Some populations of the Mohave rattlesnake, *Crotalus scutulatus*, and the Timber rattlesnake, *Crotalus horridus*, have caused severe muscular weakness and respiratory failure. A more common effect of neurotoxicity is myokymia or fasciculations. These have been associated with bites by several rattlesnake species. One poison center review suggested that patients with fasciculations near the upper torso were more likely to develop weakness necessitating mechanical ventilation.[10] Patients exhibiting neurotoxicity are much more likely to also have rhabdomyolysis than patients without neurotoxic findings.

Compartment syndrome can develop as a consequence of pit viper envenomation, although this is an extremely rare event.[11]

Assessment

Initially, patients who present following a pit viper envenomation need their airway, breathing, and circulation assessed. Historical information should be sought, such as circumstances surrounding the bite, history of previous snake envenomations and antivenom treatment, concomitant medical problems such as hypertension or cardiac disease, and use of medications such as β-blockers, which can blunt innate systemic responses to envenomation, or anticoagulants, which may predispose to bleeding.[9]

Approximately 20% of patients who sustain a pit viper bite will not receive any venom.[12] Any patient suspected of having a “dry bite” from a rattlesnake should be monitored for at least 8 hours for development of local tissue effects, hemotoxicity, or systemic symptoms. An initial complete blood count, prothrombin time, and fibrinogen should be checked, and in the case of rattlesnake bites, these laboratory tests should be repeated toward the end of the observation period.

Most patients who are bitten will be envenomated. The physical examination should initially focus on the bite site. Local tissue findings are carefully documented and monitored throughout the duration of the emergency department course. Frequent reassessment, up to every 15 minutes while determining need for treatment, is recommended, with attention paid to progression of swelling and neurovascular integrity. The circumference should be measured at 3 different sites along the involved extremity. Mark the sites to be measured by outlining the tape measure location in ink on the skin so that measurements can be repeated in a consistent fashion.

If compartment syndrome is suspected, measure intracompartmental pressures. Compartment syndrome cannot be diagnosed clinically following a snakebite, given that both can result in grossly swollen, tight, and painful extremities.

All patients with pit viper bite need an initial complete blood count to assess the platelet count as well as a baseline hemoglobin and hematocrit. Presence of coagulopathy is determined with a prothrombin time and fibrinogen level. In patients with rattlesnake bites these values should be repeated at least 4 hours later, as venom-induced thrombocytopenia and coagulopathy may not be immediately apparent. Any trend toward abnormal should prompt further monitoring. Most patients with pit viper bite do not develop rhabdomyolysis but a CPK should be obtained if there is any concern for neuro or myotoxicity. Patients presenting with systemic toxicity should have electrolytes, acid-base status, and liver and renal function assessed. Negative inspiratory force can be monitored to determine respiratory muscle strength in patients with neurotoxicity.

Management

Prehospital management involves ensuring rapid transport to a nearby health care facility. Tourniquets should never be applied in the setting of pit viper bite, and the bite site should not be manipulated. Applying suction or incising the wound can be harmful and worsen tissue damage rather than alleviate it.

The patient's airway, breathing, and circulation are addressed first. All patients should have prompt intravenous access and be placed on a cardiac monitor. Those with bites to the face or neck should be monitored closely for upper airway swelling and at onset of symptoms intubated immediately. Progression of envenomation in such cases can lead to rapid complete airway obstruction.

Patients with hypotension should receive crystalloid boluses followed by an epinephrine infusion if not immediately responsive to fluids. If there is suspicion for an anaphylactoid or anaphylactic reaction to venom, epinephrine, antihistamines, and corticosteroids are administered.

There are no studies to evaluate the effect of limb position on progression of envenomation or pain. It is the investigator's experience that elevation of the bitten extremity helps to ameliorate pain and lessen distal edema. The authors apply a posterior splint to keep the extremity in full extension and then apply a noncompressive stocking net around the splinted extremity. They then suspend affected upper extremities from an intravenous (IV) pole at the bedside and raise affected lower extremities on several pillows above the level of the heart. When opioid analgesia is used, fentanyl is preferred to avoid histamine-releasing effects of other opioids that may lead to confusion as to the cause of an allergic reaction when antivenom is administered. There is no indication for prophylactic antibiotics; however, the patient's tetanus status should be ascertained and updated as needed.

If physical examination findings raise concern for compartment syndrome, compartment pressures are obtained. If elevated, fasciotomy may be considered. In one review, it was suggested that antivenom alone can improve intracompartmental pressures and tissue perfusion rather than fasciotomy or dermotomy.[11] There is no evidence that fasciotomy decreases myonecrosis in the setting of venom-induced compartment syndrome. However, it is the investigator's practice to proceed with fasciotomy when intracompartmental pressures are extremely elevated (eg, >75 mm Hg).

Antivenom is indicated for treatment of patients with progressive swelling, hemotoxicity, systemic envenomation, and neurotoxicity.[13,14] There are currently 2 Food and Drug Administration (FDA)-approved antivenoms available. The first is an ovine-derived Fab antivenom, crotalidae polyvalent immune Fab, sold as Crofab. The second newer product is equine-derived crotalidae immune F(ab')2, sold as Anavip. All antivenoms have the potential to cause life-threatening hypersensitivity reactions and should be administered in a monitored setting.

Dosing of Crofab starts with a recommended initial dose of 4 to 6 vials for any signs of local tissue injury, coagulopathy, or systemic signs of envenomation. An additional 4 to 6 vials after a 1-hour period of observation can be given to achieve control of the patient's symptoms, if necessary. This includes cessation of progression of swelling, stabilization of coagulation parameters, and resolution of systemic signs of envenomation. After control is achieved, some patients may benefit from maintenance doses of antivenom given as 2 vials every 6 hours for 18 hours. Consultation with a regional medical toxicologist is recommended.

The dosing strategy for Anavip begins with 10 vials given for signs of local tissue injury, coagulopathy, and systemic signs of envenomation. An additional 10 vials can be given if needed to obtain control of swelling, coagulopathy, and any further symptoms of systemic envenomation. Once control has been achieved, any reemergence of findings is treated with 4 vials of Anavip. After completion of antivenom, the patient is monitored for an additional 18 hours for further progression or recurrence of venom effects.

Acute adverse reactions to both crotalidae polyvalent immune Fab and crotalidae immune F(ab')2 include hypersensitivity reactions. These reactions can either be an anaphylactoid response that is related to the infusion rate or true anaphylaxis if the patient previously received the product or if they have an allergy. Symptoms of hypersensitivity include urticaria and pruritic rash, angioedema, dyspnea and wheezing, and hypotension. In patients with only mild symptoms such as urticaria, symptomatic management with antihistamines can be provided. Depending on the degree of symptom severity, the patient's infusion rate can be decreased or the antivenom stopped in addition to providing supportive care.

A risk-to-benefit assessment should be undertaken when deciding whether to give antivenom to a patient with a previous allergy to it. In cases of severe systemic toxicity, for example, where antivenom is strongly indicated, the patient can be given corticosteroids and antihistamines before antivenom administration and have an epinephrine infusion at the bedside. If hypersensitivity symptoms develop, the antivenom is held and epinephrine infused at a low rate. When symptoms abate, the antivenom can be restarted with rates of both antivenom and epinephrine titrated to facilitate completion of antivenom.

Serum sickness, a late hypersensitivity reaction, is a risk with any antivenom product. Urticaria, rash, myalgias, arthralgias, and/or fever may develop between 3 days and 3 weeks from the time of antivenom treatment. Serum sickness is treated with steroids and antihistamines.

After patients have completed treatment with antivenom, they must be monitored for late onset of hemotoxicity. Platelets and fibrinogen are measured 2 to 3 days and again 5 to 7 days after the last antivenom administration.[8] Late hemotoxicity is more commonly seen with Fab antivenom compared with F(ab')2 antivenom. **Table 1** points out other differences between the 2 antivenom products.

Coral Snakes

Epidemiology

The Eastern coral snake, *M fulvius*, and the Texas coral snake, *M tener*, are responsible for a small number of snake bites in the United States annually. There were 72 cases of coral snake bites reported to North American Poison Centers in 2018.[16]

Table 1
Comparison of available antivenoms for Crotalinae envenomation

	Fab	F(ab')2
Brand name	Crofab	Anavip
Source	Ovine	Equine
Loading dose	4–6 vials[a]	10 vials[b]
Maintenance dose	2 vials every 6 h	None
Experienced late coagulopathy [15]	29.7%	10.3%

[a] CroFab package insert.
[b] Anavip package insert.
Data from Bush, Sean P, Ruha, Anne-Michelle, Seifert, Steven A, Morgan, David L, Lewis, Brandon J, Arnold, Thomas C, Clark, Richard F, Meggs, William J, Toschlog, Eric A, Borron, Stephen W, Figge, Gary R, Sollee, Dawn R, Shirazi, Farshad M, Wolk, Robert, De Chazal, Ives, Quan, Dan, García-Ubbelohde, Walter, Alagón, Alejandro, Gerkin, Richard D, and Boyer, Leslie V. "Comparison of F(ab')2 versus Fab Antivenom for Pit Viper Envenomation: A Prospective, Blinded, Multicenter, Randomized Clinical Trial." *Clinical Toxicology (Philadelphia, Pa.)* 53.1 (2015): 37-45.

Clinical presentation

Bites from *Micrurus* species can produce very mild local tissue swelling; however, the main feature of envenomation is neurotoxicity, and this can present with muscle fasciculations and paresthesias. Patients can also develop bulbar symptoms such as slurred speech, ptosis, and dysphagia.[17] Patients with these symptoms are at risk for respiratory depression due to paralysis of the diaphragm and intercostal muscles.

Assessment and management

Prehospital management of patients with suspected coral snake envenomation involves transport to a health care facility and airway support if there is evidence of respiratory failure. If transport is delayed or prolonged after the bite occurs, there is some evidence in an animal model that pressure immobilization bandages may delay onset of neurotoxicity without exacerbating local tissue effects.[18]

Patients who present to health care following a potential coral snake bite require admission to monitor for development of muscle weakness. Patients are at risk for respiratory depression and some require mechanical ventilation. Onset of neurotoxicity has been delayed up to 13 hours,[17] and it is important that patients be admitted to a monitored setting regardless of symptoms at the time of presentation.

An equine-derived antivenom is commercially available. North American coral snake antivenin (equine) should be administered if there are symptoms of neurotoxicity including motor weakness and paresthesias; patients exhibiting respiratory depression should also receive the antivenom with close monitoring of the airway; intubation may be required. As a practice, providers should obtain the antivenom but withhold giving it unless there is evidence of neurotoxicity.

The recommended dose of antivenom is 3 to 5 vials. As with any equine-derived product, there is potential for this treatment to cause anaphylaxis and serum sickness. Patients with previous hypersensitivity to horse serum should not receive the antivenom unless the benefits of receiving outweigh the risks.[19]

In the event that antivenom is not immediately available, the acetylcholinesterase inhibitor neostigmine can be administered in an attempt to overcome venom-induced neuromuscular blockade. Although it has been inconsistently effective in improving venom-induced neurotoxicity, it has been shown in some case reports of nonnative coral snake envenomation to delay progression of symptoms until antivenom can be acquired.[20]

North American Spiders

All spiders are venomous by definition, that is, they contain fangs that inject venom following a bite. However, only 2 venomous genera—the *Latrodectus* and *Loxosceles*—are responsible for clinically significant envenomation symptoms in humans in North America. Approximately 1800 spider envenomations from these 2 genera were reported to poison centers in 2018.[16]

Brown Recluse

Epidemiology

The most well-known species within the genus *Loxosceles* is the *reclusa*, the brown recluse spider. Data from the National Poison Data System database cite an estimated 734 brown recluse bites in the United States in 2018.[16] Unlike the black widow spider, the brown recluse has a much more limited geographic range within the United States, from the southern Atlantic states through Texas and the Southern Plains.

The main constituent of Loxosceles venom is sphingomyelinase D; however, there are many other components of the venom. Sphingomyelinase D is cytotoxic and has the ultimate effect of producing local tissue necrosis secondary to inflammation and microvascular occlusion through vessel thrombosis by inflammatory cells.[21]

Clinical presentation

Cutaneous loxoscelism. The bite from the brown recluse spider is sometimes painless. Patients can develop skin erythema around the bite site several hours afterward. A firm papule can form and there may be associated pruritus.[22] In the days afterward, this papule can progress to a blue-violet plaque that eventually evolves into a necrotic eschar that spreads gravitationally. In some cases, this can evolve to ulceration and necrosis.

Viscerocutaneous loxoscelism. In addition to developing the skin lesion described earlier, patients can develop viscerocutaneous—systemic—loxoscelism, and hemotoxicity. Patients can exhibit hemolysis and in severe cases disseminated intravascular coagulopathy, with complications including acute kidney injury, hematuria, and shock.

In cases of both cutaneous and viscerocutaneous loxoscelism, patients can exhibit fever, chills, arthralgias, headache, nausea, and vomiting.

Assessment and management

The patient's airway, breathing, and circulation need to be assessed first, as patients with systemic loxoscelism can present in shock. Intravenous access should be secured, given that patients may require crystalloid infusions or in some cases, blood products depending on the degree of anemia secondary to hemolysis.

The only manner to definitively diagnose brown recluse spider envenomation is to identify the spider in question. In the absence of this, clinicians should use their knowledge of the spider's endemic range coupled with history and physical examination findings to arrive at a tentative diagnosis.

Laboratory workup should be undertaken if viscerocutaneous envenomation is suspected; this includes a complete blood count with a differential to assess for the degree of anemia and serum haptoglobin, lactate dehydrogenase, and indirect bilirubin to determine whether hemolysis is present. Urine analysis may show hemoglobinuria.

Other than initial resuscitation and supportive care, no definitive treatment exists for viscerocutaneous loxoscelism. For this and for isolated cutaneous lesions, there has been no convincing evidence to support the use of dapsone, corticosteroids, antibiotics, or hyperbaric oxygen, although these have all been proposed. The patient's tetanus status should be assessed and updated if needed.

Lesions from Loxosceles envenomation can progress in size for several days. Surgical debridement and skin grafting in cases of skin necrosis may ultimately be required. Patients presenting with cutaneous loxoscelism should have follow-up with either dermatology or plastic surgery.

Black Widow

Epidemiology

There are 5 species of spiders within the genus *Latrodectus* found in North America. In 2018, 1015 cases were reported in the Annual Report of the American Association of Poison Control Centers.[16] As a group, spiders from this genus produce envenomation, resulting in a syndrome termed "latrodectism." The venom of *Latrodectus* consists of 7 active components, with alpha-latrotoxin being the mediator of toxicity in vertebrates. Latrotoxin is a neurotoxin capable of producing musculoskeletal pain as well as pain in the abdomen and thorax through a mechanism ultimately involving acetylcholine release at the neuromuscular junction as well as other neurotransmitters such as dopamine and norepinephrine within the central nervous system.

This pain has been variously described as cramping, pressurelike, or tight. It can also give rise to a myopathic syndrome where the patient experiences muscle hypertonicity, fibrillations, tonic contractions, and tremor. Muscle symptoms can involve both the affected extremity as well as muscles of the face. Latrotoxin can also produce autonomic disturbances such as hypertension, tachycardia, and diaphoresis.

Clinical presentation

Patients can present with a visible sign of envenomation such as a target lesion; in one retrospective study this amounted to 48% of patients; however the most common complaint among those presenting after *Latrodectus* envenomation is muscle pain about the abdomen, back, and legs.

This pain has been variously described as cramping, pressurelike, or tight. It can also give rise to a myopathic syndrome where the patient experiences muscle hypertonicity, fibrillations, tonic contractions, and tremor. Muscle symptoms can involve both the affected extremity as well as muscles of the face. Latrotoxin can also produce autonomic disturbances such as hypertension, tachycardia, and diaphoresis. The diaphoresis can be localized to the area of the bite site early following the envenomation. Symptom onset can range from immediate pain to a delay of 1 hour after the bite, with the average time of onset being about 1 hour in one retrospective review.[23] Symptoms gradually resolve over several days, with the symptoms at their worst usually 12 to 24 hours after the bite with a waxing and waning course during this time.

Assessment and management

There is no specific laboratory marker that can be used to diagnose or risk-stratify patients who have sustained a bite from *Latrodectus* species. In the review cited earlier by Clark and colleagues, the most common laboratory abnormalities included leukocytosis and elevated creatine phosphokinase.

Treatment following *Latrodectus* envenomation involves supportive care, with both parenteral opioids and benzodiazepines used to manage pain and muscle spasms, respectively. Patients who remain in distress despite oral analgesics should be admitted for pain control.

Antivenom does exist for *Latrodectus* envenomations. Currently in the United States, there is whole immunoglobulin G antivenom that is available and can produce rapid and irreversible symptom improvement for patients experiencing symptoms. As with any immunoglobulin-based therapy, there is risk for hypersensitivity reaction. Although one retrospective study by Nordt and colleagues[24] did report a low incidence of adverse reactions to the antivenom, severe anaphylaxis resulting in death has been reported.[25] Given the self-resolving nature of latrodectism over the course of 24 to 48 hours, its treatment with a potentially life-threatening intervention would need to be preceded by a risk-benefit calculation individual to each patient's circumstances (**Table 2**).

North American Scorpions

Epidemiology

There are approximately 1700 known species of scorpion across the world; within North America there is only a single species capable of producing a systemic envenomation syndrome—*Centruroides sculpturatus*—the Arizona bark scorpion. Within the United States, there were approximately 9700 cases of scorpion sting reported to poison centers in 2018.[16] It is suspected that this number underrepresents the actual number of scorpion stings, as these often go unreported by adults who have mild symptoms.

Clinical presentation

Scorpion venom is a constituent of proteins, lipids, proteases, and other compounds. One of the main consequences of scorpion envenomation on a physiologic level is the binding of sodium channels by α-toxins and β-toxins; this leads to delayed sodium channel inactivation, prolongs depolarization, and leads to increased neuronal excitation.[26] The immediate clinical effect of scorpion envenomation is pain at the sting site. Pain is the most common clinical presentation following a bark scorpion sting based on a review by Kang and Brooks,[27] although paresthesias can also be present. It should be noted that pain occurs in the absence of any local tissue effects. In fact, the presence of local tissue signs such as edema or erythema can be used to rule out bark scorpion envenomation.

Aside from local pain or paresthesias, patients can also experience systemic symptoms of toxicity, which includes manifestations of cranial nerve dysfunction such as roving eye movements, hypersalivation, slurred speech, and dysconjugate gaze; musculoskeletal dysfunction in the form of fasciculations and myoclonic jerking, which may be mistaken for seizure activity, can also occur.

In 1984, Curry and colleagues published a review article on bark scorpion envenomations, which introduced the grading system frequently used today. The grades of envenomation, which are included in **Table 3**, categorize the medically important envenomation findings as grade III and for the most severe grade IV. There is a large spectrum of severity even within grade IV classification however, ranging from patients with mild oculomotor and neuromuscular findings to patients with severe neuromuscular agitation and inability to handle secretions and protect their airway. Potential complications of severe scorpion envenomation are also described in **Table 3**.

Table 2
Comparison of US native Arachnid envenomation syndromes

	Loxosceles sp.	Latrodectus sp.
Primary venom component	Sphingomyelinase D	Alpha-latrotoxin
Mechanism of toxicity	Cytotoxicity	Acetylcholine release
Clinical presentation	Skin lesion, hemolysis	Musculoskeletal pain, autonomic dysfunction
Treatment	Supportive	Supportive, antivenom can be considered

Table 3
Envenomation grades and other clinical findings associated with Centruroides sculpturatus envenomation

Envenomation Grade	Clinical Findings
I	Pain and/or paresthesias at the envenomation site
II	Pain and/or paresthesias remote from the envenomation site, in addition to symptoms at the envenomation site
III	Symptoms of cranial nerve dysfunction such as blurred vision, roving eye movements, hypersalivation, tongue fasciculations, and slurred speech OR Musculoskeletal dysfunction such as jerking of extremities, restlessness, and involuntary shaking
IV	Both cranial nerve and musculoskeletal dysfunction
Other complications	Respiratory failure, aspiration pneumonia, pulmonary edema, rhabdomyolysis

In the review by Curry and colleagues that included 673 patients with scorpion stings, the most frequently seen grade was grade I envenomations, followed by grade II, III, and IV. These amounted to 76.5%, 9.1%, 4.7%, and 3.0% of patients, respectively. In addition, patients with grade III and grade IV envenomations were more likely to belong to the 0 to 5 years and 6 to 10 years age group.[28] Today pediatric cases remain the most common group among those presenting to health care with symptoms related to severe scorpion envenomation.

It should be noted that pancreatitis, commonly held to be an effect of generic scorpion envenomation, does not occur following Bark scorpion envenomation in the United States; rather, this is described following *Tityus* species found in Central and South America.

Assessment

The patient's airway and breathing should be assessed with the understanding that in cases of systemic toxicity, intubation with mechanical ventilation may be necessary. Although this can be seen in adults, most commonly this involves the extremes of age, with younger patients being at highest risk of airway compromise.

In patients who present with grade I or II envenomations, additional workup in the form of laboratory studies or imaging is not necessary unless alternative diagnoses are also being considered. Patients with mild neuromuscular hyperactivity in whom the diagnosis of scorpion sting is secure also do not require laboratory assessment. Those with severe neuromuscular agitation, dehydration, or concern for comorbidities should have electrolytes, renal function, and creatinine phosphokinase assessed.

When patients present with respiratory distress or hypoxia a chest radiograph should be obtained to assess for aspiration or pulmonary edema.[29] In adults with hyperadrenergic effects and comorbid conditions such as coronary artery disease, a cardiac work up including electrocardiogram, serum troponin, and echocardiogram may be warranted.[29]

Management

Grade I and grade II envenomations are managed supportively, with nonopioid analgesics being the mainstay of treatment. Ice packs applied to the sting site may provide some pain relief. Pain can last for approximately 24 hours after sting. Anecdotally, it has been reported that paresthesias associated with scorpion sting can last up to 1 month.

Pain and neuromuscular hyperactivity associated with grade III and IV envenomations are treated with intravenous opioids. Benzodiazepines are also administered to relieve both the hyperadrenergic findings and neurologic symptoms of scorpion sting. Scorpion envenomation can cause respiratory failure without administration of opioids and benzodiazepines, so patients managed with these medications are at increased risk and must be monitored closely. In one study of patients with scorpion envenomation treated without antivenom, 24% of patients required mechanical ventilation.[29]

Patients presenting with grade III or IV symptoms who are provided supportive care typically require admission to the hospital until envenomation resolves. Another option is to administer an equine-derived antivenom called Centruroides immune F(ab')2 or Anascorp.

Indications for Centruroides immune F(ab')2 administration include signs of systemic toxicity such as neuromuscular symptoms, opsoclonus, excessive secretions, and respiratory distress.[30] Although all patients with grade III or grade IV envenomations meet the criteria for treatment with antivenom, the authors prefer to reserve antivenom for those who will require admission to the hospital if they receive only supportive care. The goal of administering Anascorp is complete resolution of envenomation while in the emergency department so that the patient can be discharged home. If the patient already has indications for hospital admission on arrival, such as respiratory failure, we withhold antivenom and provide supportive care.

The FDA-recommended dosage of Anascorp is 3 vials given over approximately 10 minutes. The patient should be monitored for 60 minutes for symptom resolution, and if needed, an additional vial is given until symptoms resolve.

Oftentimes, urgent respiratory symptoms do not allow patients to wait for Anascorp to be mixed and administered. In this case, intubation should be undertaken. Once the patient is intubated, there is no need to give Anascorp.

SUMMARY

Clinicians should be aware of the envenomation syndromes caused by snakes, scorpions, and spiders of North America with special attention paid to both local tissue effects and systemic effects. Envenomation can also mimic other diagnoses, such as exploratory sympathomimetic ingestion in the case of pediatric scorpion toxicity or soft tissue cellulitis in the case of *Loxosceles* envenomation. When the diagnosis is confirmed or highly suspected, physicians should be aware of the indications and potential complications of antivenom treatment in instances where that is available.

CLINICAL PEARLS

- Envenomations from the Crotalinae subfamily can produce local tissue effects, coagulopathy, neurotoxicity, and systemic symptoms; envenomations from snakes of the Elapidae family produce neurotoxicity.
- Two FDA-approved antivenom products are available to treat Crotalinae envenomations; they are both associated with hypersensitivity reactions.
- Envenomation from Loxosceles species can produce cutaneous lesions or a systemic envenomation syndrome involving hemolysis and end-organ damage through the cytotoxic effects of sphingomyelinase D.
- Latrodectus species envenomation produces musculoskeletal pain and autonomic dysfunction through dysregulation of acetylcholine release caused by alpha-latrotoxin.

- *C sculpturatus* is the only North American scorpion species capable of producing a systemic envenomation syndrome; symptoms can range from pain at the site of envenomation to musculoskeletal symptoms and cranial nerve dysfunction.

CLINICS CARE POINTS

- Many envenomations can produce systemic effects. Attention should always be paid first to the patient's airway, breathing, and circulation.
- Pit viper envenomation can be associated with local tissue effects including edema. It can mimic compartment syndrome, and intercompartmental pressures should always be obtained before a fasciotomy is performed.
- Indications for antivenom in the setting of Crotalinae envenomation include progressive swelling, hemotoxicity, systemic envenomation, and neurotoxicity. There are 2 commercially available antivenom products.
- Coral snake envenomation is associated with neurotoxicity; antivenom should be administered if these symptoms are present. Local tissue changes are typically mild, and in these cases antivenom is not indicated if this is the only presenting symptom.
- Bites from Latrodectus and Loxosceles species are rare; infectious cause such as cellulitis and local abscess should be considered whenever this diagnosis is considered.
- The Arizona bark scorpion—Centruroides sculpturatus—is the only scorpion in North America capable of producing an envenomation syndrome. There are grades of envenomation that relate to the distance of pain and paresthesia from the envenomation site and presence or absence of cranial nerve dysfunction and musculoskeletal symptoms.

DISCLOSURE

The authors have nothing to disclose.

REFERENCES

1. Seifert SA, Boyer LV, Benson BE, et al. AAPCC Data database characterization of native U.S. venomous snake exposures, 2001-2005. Clin Toxicol 2009;47(4): 327–35.
2. Tasoulis Theo, Isbister Geoffrey. A Review and Database of Snake Venom Proteomes. Toxins 2017;9(9):290.
3. Ruha Anne-Michelle, Kleinschmidt Kurt C, Greene Spencer, et al. The Epidemiology, Clinical Course, and Management of Snakebites in the North American Snakebite Registry. J Med Toxicol 2017;13(4):309–20.
4. Heise C William, Ruha Anne-Michelle, Padilla-Jones Angela, et al. Clinical Predictors of Tissue Necrosis following Rattlesnake Envenomation. Clin Toxicol (Philadelphia, Pa.) 2018;56(4):281–4.
5. Gerkin Richard, Sergent Kathleen Clem, Curry Steven C, et al. Life-threatening Airway Obstruction from Rattlesnake Bite to the Tongue. Ann Emerg Med 1987; 16(7):813–6.
6. Kerns William, Tomaszewski Christian. Airway Obstruction following Canebrake Rattlesnake Envenomation. J Emerg Med 2001;20(4):377–80.
7. Lewis JV, Portera CA Jr. Rattlesnake bite of the face: case report and review of the literature. The Am Surgeon 1994;60(9):681–2.
8. Lavonas Eric J, Ruha Anne-Michelle, Banner William, Bebarta Vikhyat, Bernstein Jeffrey N, Bush Sean P, Kerns 2nd, William P, Richardson William H, Seifert Steven A, Tanen David A, Curry Steve C, Dart Richard C. Unified

Treatment Algorithm for the Management of Crotaline Snakebite in the United States: Results of an Evidence-informed Consensus Workshop. BMC Emerg Med 2011;11(1):2.
9. Levine Michael, Ruha Anne-Michelle, Padilla-Jones Angela, et al. Bleeding Following Rattlesnake Envenomation in Patients With Preenvenomation Use of Antiplatelet or Anticoagulant Medications. Acad Emerg Med 2014;21(3):301–7.
10. Vohra R, Cantrell FL, Williams SR. Fasciculations after Rattlesnake Envenomations: A Retrospective Statewide Poison Control System Study. Clin Toxicol (Philadelphia, Pa.) 2008;46(2):117–21.
11. Cumpston Kirk L. Is There a Role for Fasciotomy in Crotalinae Envenomations in North America? Clin Toxicol (Philadelphia, Pa.) 2011;49(5):351–65.
12. Gold Barry S, Dart Richard C, Barish Robert A. Bites of Venomous Snakes. New Engl J Med 2002;347(5):347–56.
13. Anavip Package Insert – FDA. Available at: https://www.fda.gov/media/92139/download.
14. Crofab Package insert – FDA Available at: https://www.fda.gov/media/74683/download.
15. Bush Sean P, Ruha Anne-Michelle, Seifert Steven A, et al. Comparison of F(ab')2 versus Fab Antivenom for Pit Viper Envenomation: A Prospective, Blinded, Multicenter, Randomized Clinical Trial. Clin Toxicol (Philadelphia, Pa.) 2015;53(1):37–45.
16. Gummin David D, Mowry James B, Spyker Daniel A, et al. 2018 Annual Report of the American Association of Poison Control Centers' National Poison Data System (NPDS): 36th Annual Report. Clin Toxicol (Philadelphia, Pa.) 2019;57(12):1220–413.
17. Kitchens Craig S, Van Mierop LHS. Envenomation by the Eastern Coral Snake (Micrurus Fulvius Fulvius): A Study of 39 Victims. JAMA 1987;258(12):1615–8.
18. NA Coral Snake Antivenin package insert – FDA. Available at: https://www.fda.gov/files/vaccines%2C%20blood%20%26%20biologics/published/Package-Insert—North-American-Coral-Snake-Antivenin.pdf.
19. German Benjamin T, Hack Jason B, Brewer Kori, et al. Pressure-Immobilization Bandages Delay Toxicity in a Porcine Model of Eastern Coral Snake (Micrurus Fulvius Fulvius) Envenomation. Ann Emerg Med 2005;45(6):603–8.
20. Bucaretchi Fábio, Hyslop Stephen, Ronan José Vieira, Adriana Safioli Toledo, Roberto Madureira Paulo, et al. Bites by Coral Snakes (Micrurus Spp.) in Campinas, State of São Paulo, Southeastern Brazil Acidentes Por Serpentes Corais (Micrurus Spp.) Em Campinas, Estado De São Paulo, Sudeste Do Brasil. Revista Do Instituto De Medicina Trop De São Paulo 2006;48(3):141–5.
21. Hogan Christopher J, Barbaro Katia Cristina, Winkel Ken. Loxoscelism: Old Obstacles, New Directions. Ann Emerg Med 2004;44(6):608–24.
22. Gendron Blake P. Loxosceles Reclusa Envenomation. Am J Emerg Med 1990;51–4.
23. Clark Richard F, Wethern-Kestner Susan, Vance, et al. Clinical Presentation and Treatment of Black Widow Spider Envenomation: A Review of 163 Cases. Ann Emerg Med 1992;782–7.
24. Nordt SP, Clark RF, Lee A, et al. Examination of Adverse Events following Black Widow Antivenom Use in California. Clinical Toxicology (Philadelphia, Pa.) 2012;50(1):70–3.
25. Murphy Christine M, Hong Jeannie J, Beuhler Michael C. Anaphylaxis with Latrodectus Antivenin Resulting in Cardiac Arrest. J Med Toxicol 2011;317–21.

26. Ibister GK, Bawaskar HS. Scorpion envenomation. N Engl J Med 2014;371(5): 457–63.
27. Kang A Min, Brooks Daniel E. Nationwide Scorpion Exposures Reported to US Poison Control Centers from 2005 to 2015. J Med Toxicol 2017;158–65.
28. Curry, Steven, Vance, Michael, Ryan, Patricia, et al. Envenomation by the Scorpion Centruroides Sculpturatus. J Toxicol Clin Toxicol. 1983-1984;21(4-5):417–49.
29. O'Connor Ayrn, Ruha Anne-Michelle. Clinical Course of Bark Scorpion Envenomation Managed Without Antivenom. J Med Toxicol 2012;258–62.
30. Antivenom - FDA. Available at: https://www.fda.gov/media/81093/download.

Toxic Alcohol Poisoning

Jennifer A. Ross, MD, MPH[a], Heather A. Borek, MD[b],
Christopher P. Holstege, MD[c,d,*], Joshua D. King, MD[e]

KEYWORDS

• Toxic alcohol • Methanol • Ethylene glycol • Diethylene glycol • Propylene glycol • Isopropyl alcohol • Acetone • Osmol gap

KEY POINTS

- Toxic alcohols are found in numerous products, and significant exposure can lead to toxicity, which mimics other disease processes.
- The presence of toxic alcohol poisoning may be suggested by an anion gap metabolic acidosis and/or an increased osmol gap, depending on the specific toxic alcohol responsible and the timing of the laboratory analysis in relation to exposure.
- An osmol gap can be useful in determining a toxic alcohol ingestion, but the osmol gap has many limitations, and a normal result does not rule out the presence of a toxic alcohol. Conversely, the test has poor specificity, and most patients with an elevated osmol gap do not have toxic alcohol poisoning.
- With ethylene glycol, methanol, diethylene glycol, and propylene glycol, an increased osmol gap can be present early after toxic exposure, but as metabolism progresses, the osmol gap closes and an anion gap metabolic acidosis develops with eventual loss of the increased osmol gap.

INTRODUCTION

The term “toxic alcohols” refers to several short-chain alcohols with detrimental effects in ingestion related to metabolites that cause metabolic acidosis and/or specific end-organ toxicity. According to the Annual Report of the American Association of

[a] Adolescent Substance Use and Addiction Program (ASAP), Boston Children’s Hospital, Boston, MA 02115, USA; [b] Division of Medical Toxicology, Department of Emergency Medicine, University of Virginia School of Medicine, PO Box 800774, Charlottesville, VA 22908-0774, USA; [c] Division of Medical Toxicology, Department of Emergency Medicine, University of Virginia School of Medicine, Blue Ridge Poison Center, University of Virginia Health System, Charlottesville, VA 22908-0774, USA; [d] Division of Medical Toxicology, Department of Pediatrics, University of Virginia School of Medicine, Blue Ridge Poison Center, University of Virginia Health System, Charlottesville, VA 22908-0774, USA; [e] Medicine and Pharmacy, Maryland Poison Center, Nephrology Fellowship, University of Maryland, Maryland Poison Center, 220 Arch Street, Baltimore, MD 21201, USA

* Corresponding author. Division of Medical Toxicology-Blue Ridge Poison Center, University of Virginia Health System, P.O. Box 800774, Charlottesville, VA 22908-0774.
E-mail address: ch2xf@virginia.edu

Emerg Med Clin N Am 40 (2022) 327–341
https://doi.org/10.1016/j.emc.2022.01.012
emed.theclinics.com
0733-8627/22/

Poison Control Centers' National Poison Data System, there are thousands of toxic alcohol exposures in the United States each year with numerous deaths.[1] This article reviews the topic of toxic alcohols, specifically ethylene glycol, methanol, diethylene glycol, propylene glycol, and isopropyl alcohol. Patients poisoned with toxic alcohols often present without a history of exposure, and it is ancillary testing, specifically the anion gap and osmol gap, that enable clinicians to diagnose these toxins. This article also reviews the significance of an anion gap metabolic acidosis in the poisoned patient, which often is the common laboratory abnormality first noted in patients with specific toxic alcohols, and explores the utility as well as limitations of the osmol gap.

Ethylene Glycol

Ethylene glycol is present in numerous readily available products, including antifreeze, deicers, detergents, paints, and cosmetics. Ethylene glycol toxicity is associated with both accidental and intentional ingestions. It is a colorless, sweet-tasting liquid that can be disguised in other drinks, as has been reported with numerous criminal poisonings.[2] Sodium fluorescein dye is added to some preparations of antifreeze to facilitate identification of radiator leaks; however, this is product dependent, and fluorescence of the patient's oral pharynx or urine is not a reliable indicator of poisoning.[3]

Ethylene glycol is rapidly absorbed through the gastrointestinal (GI) tract, and the volume of distribution is 0.7 L/kg. Ethylene glycol undergoes first-order elimination when concentrations are less than 250 mg/dL, with a half-life of approximately 4 hours. When concentrations are greater than 250 mg/dL, elimination becomes zero-order, thereby prolonging the elimination half-life. When alcohol dehydrogenase (ADH) is competitively inhibited, such as with ethanol ingestion or the use of fomepizole, metabolism of ethylene glycol is delayed and becomes renally dependent, prolonging the elimination half-life to greater than 10 hours.

Metabolism of ethylene glycol occurs primarily in the liver through serial oxidation initially by ADH and aldehyde dehydrogenase (ALDH), with each step reducing NAD+ to NADH (**Fig. 1**). The rate-limiting step in metabolism occurs with the conversion of glycolic acid to glyoxylic acid by lactate dehydrogenase, leading to the development of a marked anion gap metabolic acidosis due to the accumulation of glycolic acid. Glyoxylic acid undergoes conversion to oxalic acid, α-hydroxy-β-ketoadipic acid, or glycine. Thiamine is a cofactor in the production of α-hydroxy-β-ketoadipic

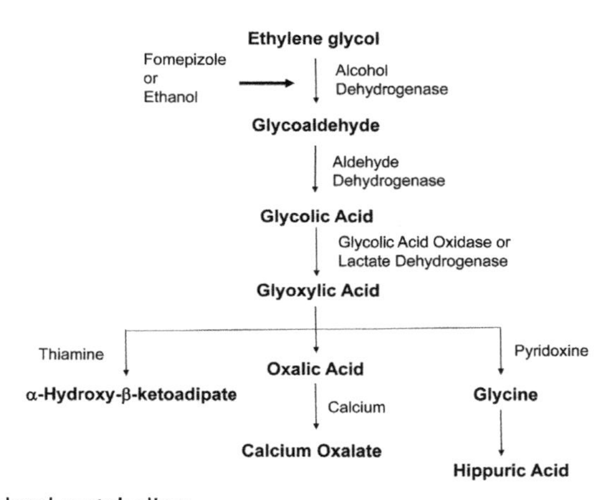

Fig. 1. Ethylene glycol metabolism.

acid, and pyridoxine and magnesium are cofactors in the production of glycine. These cofactors play a role in treating toxicity. Oxalic acid readily precipitates with calcium to form insoluble calcium oxalate crystals. Urine microscopy may reveal the presence of calcium oxalate crystals; although oxalate crystals formation in urine may occur in a variety of conditions, the presence of a large number of calcium oxalate monohydrate crystals may suggest ethylene glycol as a cause of toxicity. Organ injury, especially to the kidneys, is caused by the widespread deposition of calcium oxalate monohydrate crystals. The α-hydroxy-β-ketoadipic acid and glycine pathways are considered nontoxic.

Patients who ingest ethylene glycol may initially seem inebriated, mimicking ethanol intoxication. Immediately following the exposure, the patient will not be acidotic until enough time has passed to allow metabolism; however, an elevated osmol gap may be detected due to ethylene glycol. If ethanol is not coingested (which prevents metabolism of ethylene glycol), an anion gap metabolic acidosis will develop after a delay of hours, leading to potential compensatory hyperventilation. As the acidosis worsens and oxalic acid forms, hypocalcemia, creatinine elevation, seizures, and cardiac dysrhythmias may occur. Acute kidney injury is common in late-presenting or untreated ethylene glycol poisoning. Oxalic acid combined with calcium may lead to hypocalcemia with subsequent tetany, seizures, and QT interval prolongation. Cerebral edema has been reported with deposition of calcium oxalate crystals in the brain.

Patients with ethylene glycol poisoning can have elevations in serum lactate concentration—although they may have a concomitant lactic acidosis, laboratory instruments using lactate oxidase may not be able to differentiate between lactate and glycolic acid due to its structural similarity to lactate, resulting in a (frequently large) falsely elevated lactate.[4,5] This false lactate elevation, sometimes termed the "lactate gap," is common when using blood gas analyzers and point-of-care testing, as these methods typically rely on lactate oxidase.[6] A large difference in the reported lactate concentration between analyzers that use lactate dehydrogenase and lactate oxidase-based testing may help to demonstrate a lactate gap and thus uncover an ethylene glycol poisoning.

Although the serum ethylene glycol concentration itself is not predictive of outcome, the serum concentration of glycolic acid correlates with mortality. Because of the rapid elimination of ethylene glycol, its serum concentration may be low or undetectable at a time when glycolic acid remains elevated. If available, the determination of both ethylene glycol and glycolic acid concentrations provides useful clinical and confirmatory analytical information in ethylene glycol ingestion.[7] However, most hospital laboratories are unable to perform ethylene glycol or glycolic acid levels. According to Porter's study, an initial anion gap greater than 20 mmol/L and pH less than 7.30 are predictors for the development of acute renal failure in ethylene glycol toxicity (sensitivities of 95.6% and 100%, respectively and specificities of 94.4% and 88.5%, respectively).[7]

The mainstay of therapy for ethylene glycol toxicity includes administration of fomepizole (or ethanol if fomepizole is not available), thiamine, pyridoxine, and hemodialysis. Fomepizole has a higher affinity for ADH than ethylene glycol and will compete for metabolism, preventing the breakdown of ethylene glycol into toxic metabolites. Ethanol may also be used to inhibit ADH when fomepizole is unavailable. Fomepizole is the preferred treatment over ethanol, as it is more easily dosed, does not cause further inebriation or sedation, more strongly competitively inhibits ADH, and is associated with less administration errors.[8,9] Fomepizole has been used without dialysis in ethylene glycol poisoning if there is no significant acidosis or renal failure.[10,11] However, because of the significant prolongation of ethylene glycol's elimination half-life with fomepizole, fomepizole treatment without dialysis may prolong the time necessary for monitoring and intensive care unit care.[11] Fomepizole will not prevent the conversion of the acid metabolites to oxalate and the potential development of renal failure.

Fomepizole is administered intravenously with a loading dose of 15 mg/kg, followed by maintenance dosing of 10 mg/kg every 12 hours until the ethylene glycol concentration drops to less than 20 mg/dL.[12] If additional dosing is required beyond 4 maintenance doses, the dose should be increased to 15 mg/kg every 12 hours due to fomepizole's autoinduction of its own metabolism. During dialysis, fomepizole dosing should be increased to every 4 hours. If fomepizole is not available, ethanol can be used to competitively inhibit ADH and is administered via intravenous or oral routes, with blood levels maintained at approximately 100 mg/dL. Ethanol therapy requires more frequent laboratory testing than with fomepizole to assure the ethanol level is maintained at appropriate levels and to ensure that hypoglycemia does not develop. The patient will require closer mental status and respiratory monitoring due to the additional inebriating effects of ethanol. At present, intravenous ethanol is generally not available in the United States.

Pyridoxine and thiamine can theoretically aid in the metabolism of glyoxylic acid away from oxalic acid to nontoxic metabolites (glycine and α-hydroxy-β-ketoadipate). Sodium bicarbonate administration can be considered for patients with significant acidosis. Hemodialysis will remove both ethylene glycol and its acidic toxic metabolites. Ethylene glycol-poisoned patients often present late with marked acidosis and developing renal failure associated with oxalate crystals in the urine. Such cases should not await confirmation of an ethylene glycol level, and instead hemodialysis should be pursued emergently. The indications for hemodialysis depend on the specific case and available local resources.[13] The clinician should discuss the case further with the local poison center (medical toxicologist) and nephrologist and include consideration of the total ethylene glycol level, the degree of metabolic acidosis (eg, anion gap >20 mmol/L or pH < 7.30), and/or the presence of renal failure.[7]

Methanol

Methanol is found in numerous products, including as a solvent in several commercial products and as a constituent in windshield wiper fluid, copy machine fluids, fuel additives (octane boosters), paint remover or thinner, antifreeze, canned heating sources, deicing fluid, shellacs, and varnishes. Toxicity has been reported following consumption, both intentionally (eg, as an ethanol substitute or in suicide attempts) or accidently (eg, present as a contaminant in illegal whiskey.)[14] Although methanol contamination of home-brewed liquor (moonshine) is not currently common in the United States, worldwide outbreaks of methanol poisoning related to illicit liquor occur periodically. Toxicity has also occurred via dermal and inhalational exposure.[15]

Methanol is slowly oxidized by ADH (at about one-tenth the rate of ethanol) to formaldehyde. Formaldehyde in turn is rapidly oxidized by ALDH to formic acid (**Fig. 2**). Formic acid and formaldehyde are mitochondrial toxins, resulting in cellular dysfunction largely occurring in the central nervous system (CNS), especially the optic nerve.

Patients who ingest methanol may initially seem inebriated, similar to ethanol intoxication, although the degree of inebriation is often less due to methanol being a shorter chain alcohol than ethanol. The patient will not immediately develop acidosis due to methanol's slow metabolism; however, an elevated osmol gap may be present. If ethanol is not coingested preventing metabolism of methanol, the patient may develop a progressive anion gap metabolic acidosis after a delay of hours and subsequent optic neuropathy with reported visual disturbances potentially leading to blindness. Methanol toxicity can result in intracranial hemorrhages, as well as infarcts, especially

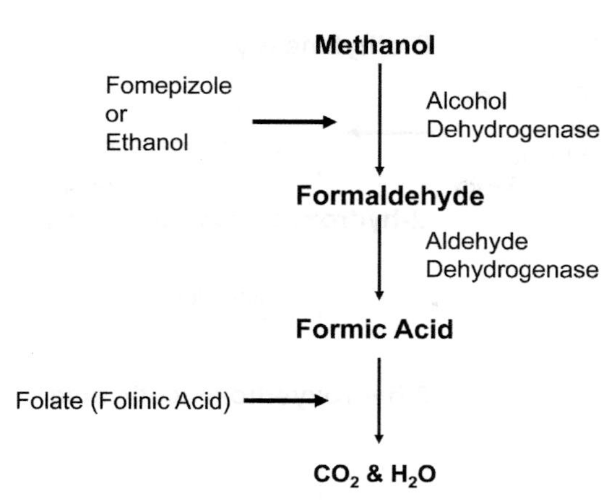

Fig. 2. Methanol metabolism.

of the basal ganglia, with an incidence of abnormal brain computed tomography findings in 67% of methanol poisoned patients in one study.[16]

The mainstay of therapy for methanol toxicity includes administration of fomepizole (or ethanol if fomepizole is not available), folate or folinic acid, and hemodialysis.[17] As a competitive antagonist of ADH, fomepizole will prevent the metabolism of methanol into its toxic metabolite, formic acid.[18] Methanol levels greater than 20 mg/dL are considered toxic. Once ADH is blocked by fomepizole, the half-life of methanol increases to more than 50 hours.[17] Unlike ethylene glycol, there is no significant renal elimination of methanol, and it is thought to be eliminated through exhaled air. Because of its long elimination half-life as well as significant, often irreversible toxicity, treatment with fomepizole in combination with hemodialysis is often recommended. Folate or folinic acid can aid in the conversion of formic acid to nontoxic byproducts and can be considered an adjunct to treatment. Hemodialysis will rapidly remove both methanol and formic acid with indications and associated evidence found at *The Extracorporeal Treatments in Poisoning Working Group* (EXTRIP) Web site (www.extrip-workgroup.org/methanol).

Diethylene Glycol

Diethylene glycol is an industrial solvent used in a variety of products, including antifreeze, brake fluid, wallpaper strippers, and fabric and dye manufacturing. Notoriously, diethylene glycol has been used as an excipient in liquid preparations of medications due to its widespread availability and cheap cost, resulting in multiple historical outbreaks of mass poisoning; the first such incident (the "Massengill disaster") occurred in the United States in 1937. Diethylene glycol is metabolized by ADH and ALDH to 2-hydroxyethoxyacetic acid, after which it is oxidized to diglycolic acid (**Fig. 3**).[19] Diglycolic acid inhibits the citric acid cycle at succinate dehydrogenase, resulting in both nephrotoxicity and neurotoxicity.[20] The development of an anion gap metabolic acidosis may be delayed for longer than 12 hours postingestion.[21,22]

Patients who ingest diethylene glycol may seem inebriated, similar to ethanol intoxication. Toxicity may further progress with metabolism to the development of gastritis, hepatitis, pancreatitis, metabolic acidosis, coma, and delayed neurologic sequelae. Acute kidney injury is consistently reported in human cases.[19]

As with ethylene glycol and methanol, treatment with fomepizole (or ethanol if fomepizole is not available) prevents the breakdown to more toxic acidic metabolites.[23] If

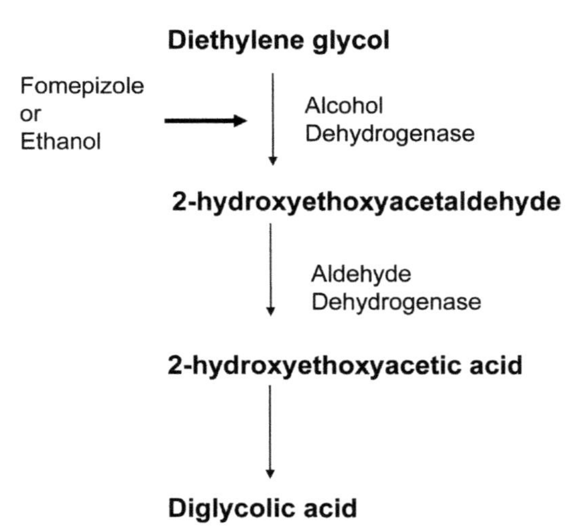

Fig. 3. Diethylene glycol metabolism.

patients develop a significant anion gap metabolic acidosis or renal failure, hemodialysis is indicated.

Propylene Glycol

Propylene glycol is used as a diluent in many pharmaceutical medications, such as lorazepam, diazepam, phenobarbital, and phenytoin.[24] Propylene glycol toxicity is a potentially life-threatening iatrogenic complication that is preventable (see article 9).[25,26] It is also used in other products, such as topical medications, cosmetics, and as a solvent. Propylene glycol is metabolized by ADH to lactaldehyde and then by ALDH to lactate and pyruvate (**Fig. 4**).

Propylene glycol ingestions can also cause inebriation similar to ethanol, and massive exposures have been reported to produce toxic adverse effects, including a marked lactic acidosis (both D- and L-lactate are produced), hypoglycemia, seizures, and coma. Hypotension, dysrhythmias, and cardiovascular decompensation can also occur.[27]

Unlike other toxic alcohols that produce carboxylic acid metabolites, removal from the source of propylene glycol and supportive care alone is often sufficient to treat patients with propylene glycol poisoning, likely due to rapid metabolism of lactate. If the patient develops acidosis, treatment with sodium bicarbonate may be indicated. In massive ingestions where the parent compound is considered to still be present, fomepizole may be of benefit. Hemodialysis is effective but is rarely necessary, as these patients generally do well with supportive care; however, for end-organ toxicity such as seizures and coma, or for patients with significant kidney function impairment, it may be indicated to remove D-lactate and improve acidemia.[24]

Isopropyl Alcohol (Isopropanol)

Isopropanol is readily available as an aqueous solution for use as rubbing alcohol but can also be found in other products such as cleaners, disinfectants, antifreezes, deicers, cosmetics, solvents, inks, and pharmaceuticals. It is used as an ethanol substitute by alcoholics because it is readily available and inexpensive.[28] With the emergence of COVID-19, hand cleansers containing greater than 60% isopropanol are

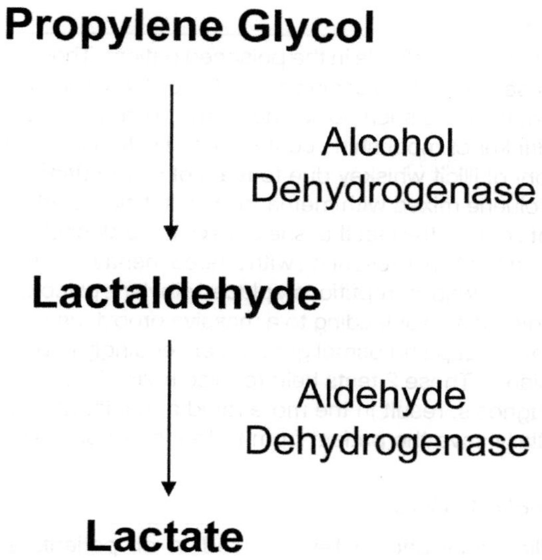

Propylene Glycol

↓ Alcohol Dehydrogenase

Lactaldehyde

↓ Aldehyde Dehydrogenase

Lactate

Fig. 4. Propylene glycol metabolism.

more readily available to the public, and poison centers have documented increasing human exposure calls.[29]

Isopropanol has a short elimination half-life of 3 to 7 hours. It is rapidly metabolized by ADH to acetone, which is eliminated more slowly.[30] The kidneys excrete approximately 80% as acetone; 20% of isopropyl alcohol is eliminated unchanged. Acetone has CNS depressant activity similar to that of ethanol, and because of its longer elimination half-life, it may prolong the apparent CNS effects of isopropanol. Isopropanol is a secondary alcohol (the hydroxyl group is attached to a central, rather than a terminal carbon), and consequently it is metabolized by ADH to a dimethyl ketone (acetone) and not an acid. Ingestions of isopropyl alcohol will not cause significant metabolic acidosis unlike other toxic alcohols.

Patients who ingest isopropyl alcohol may present with inebriation similar to ethanol intoxication.[31] Isopropyl alcohol is a marked GI irritant and can cause hematemesis and hemorrhagic gastritis. Massive ingestions can lead to vasodilation and hypotension. Both isopropyl alcohol and acetone cause CNS depression.

The increased acetone can be detected in the patient's breath and results in a positive test for ketones in the serum and urine, potentially misleading the clinician into making a diagnosis of ethanol intoxication or diabetic ketoacidosis.[28] However, the presence of acetone in the breath (fruity odor) and urine in the absence of glycosuria or hyperglycemia provides a clue to the diagnosis of isopropyl alcohol intoxication. In addition, acetone may falsely elevate serum creatinine by interfering with the most common laboratory method used for creatinine determination (Jaffé reaction), with an elevation in serum creatinine with a normal blood urea nitrogen (eg, a serum creatinine of 2 mg/dL with a blood urea nitrogen level of 5 mg/dL) acting as a prompt to consider isopropanol poisoning.[32]

Supportive care is the mainstay of treatment. Fomepizole or ethanol is not indicated and will likely prolong toxicity. Hemodialysis is effective at removing both isopropyl alcohol and acetone, but is rarely necessary, as these patients generally improve with supportive care.

Laboratory Testing

The history is notoriously unreliable in the poisoned patient. There are numerous reports of patients who presented with poisoning due to toxic alcohols that were only determined by clinicians who maintained such poisoning on their differential diagnosis. Case examples include the drinker of moonshine contaminated with methanol who was not forthcoming on a history of illicit whiskey due to fears of prosecution[14]; the substance user who was huffing toluene mixed with methanol who initially failed to give such history[33]; the suicidal patient who hid the fact that she drank a toxic alcohol along with medications taken in overdose; the patient presenting with altered mental status following the attempted murder by a spouse who surreptitiously placed ethylene glycol in a smoothie[2]; and the unrecognized medication error leading to a massive propylene glycol overdose.[24]

Two tests, the anion gap and osmol gap, are exceedingly important to consider as a critical care clinician.[34] These 2 tests help to raise toxic alcohols as a consideration in the differential diagnosis, result in the more rapid administration of appropriate treatment, and potentially save the patient from further harm or death.

Anion Gap Metabolic Acidosis

A basic metabolic panel should be obtained in all patients suspected of being poisoned. When a low serum bicarbonate is discovered, the clinician should determine if an elevated anion gap exists. The equation most commonly used for the serum anion gap calculation is as follows:[35]

$$\text{Anion gap} = Na^{+} - (Cl^{-} + HCO_3^{-})$$

The primary cation (sodium) and primary anions (chloride and bicarbonate) are represented in the equation.[36] Other serum cations are not commonly included in this calculation because either their concentrations are relatively low (eg, potassium), they may not have been assayed (eg, magnesium), or assigning a number to represent their respective contribution is difficult (eg, cationic serum proteins).[37] Similarly, there are a multitude of other serum anions (eg, sulfate, phosphate, organic anions) that are also difficult to measure or quantify in terms of charge-concentration units (mEq/L).[36,37] The anion gap represents these "unmeasured" ions. The normal range for the anion gap has conventionally been accepted to be 6 to 14 mEq/L.[36,37] Practically speaking, an increase in the anion gap beyond the normal range, accompanied by metabolic acidosis, represents an increase in unmeasured endogenous (eg, lactate) or exogenous (eg, glycolic acid) anions.[35] A list of the more common causes of this phenomenon is organized in the classic *MUDPILES* mnemonic (**Box 1**).

Box 1
Potential toxic causes of increased anion gap metabolic acidosis

*M*ethanol

*U*remia

*D*iabetic, starvation, alcoholic ketoacidosis

*P*ropylene glycol

*I*ron, *I*nhalants (ie, carbon monoxide, cyanide, toluene), *I*soniazid, *I*buprofen

*L*actic acidosis

*E*thylene glycol

*S*alicylates, *S*ympathomimetics

It is imperative that clinicians who care for poisoned patients presenting with an increased anion gap metabolic acidosis investigate the cause in a timely fashion. Many symptomatic poisoned patients may have an initial mild metabolic acidosis due to elevation of serum lactate. This finding can occur for a variety of reasons, including acidosis related to tissue hypoperfusion or a recent seizure. However, with adequate supportive care the anion gap acidosis should improve. If, despite adequate supportive care, an anion gap metabolic acidosis worsens, the clinician should consider either toxins that form acidic metabolites (eg, toxic alcohols) or toxins that worsen lactic acidosis by interfering with aerobic energy production (eg, cyanide, iron).[38] The failure to trend the anion gap in a timely fashion has led to numerous cases of adverse outcomes due to missed toxins, especially toxic alcohols, which would have been diagnosed earlier had the clinician performed serial testing (eg, every 2 hours) of the patient's chemistries.

Osmol gap

The serum osmol gap is a laboratory test that may be useful when evaluating poisoned patients. This test is most often discussed in the context of evaluating the patient suspected of toxic alcohol intoxication. Although this test may have utility in such situations, it has many pitfalls that limit its effectiveness.

Osmotic concentrations may be expressed in terms of either osmolality (milliosmoles per kilogram of solvent [mOsm/kg]) or osmolarity (milliosmoles per liter of solution [mOsm/L]).[39] Osmolality (Osm_M) is measured by an osmometer, a tool that most often uses the technique of freezing point depression.[40] Serum osmolarity (Osm_C) may be estimated clinically by several equations[41] involving the patient's serum glucose, sodium, and urea nitrogen, which normally account for almost all of the measured osmolality.[42] One of the most commonly used calculations is expressed as

$Osm_C = 2(\text{sodium}) + (\text{urea nitrogen})/2.8 + (\text{glucose})/18.$

The numerical factor in the sodium term (expressed in millimoles per liter) accounts for corresponding anions that contribute to osmolarity; the numerical factors in the other 2 terms convert their concentration units from milligrams per deciliter to millimoles per liter.[43] Finding the osmolar contribution of any other osmotically active substance that is reported in milligrams per deciliter (such as urea nitrogen or glucose) is accomplished by dividing by one-tenth of the substance's molecular weight in daltons.[43] For urea nitrogen this conversion factor is 2.8 and for glucose it is 18. Similarly, additional terms, along with corresponding conversion factors, may be added to this equation to account for ethanol and the various toxic alcohols (assuming they have been measured and their results are expressed in milligrams per deciliter):

$Osm_C = 2(\text{sodium}) + (\text{urea nitrogen})/2.8 + (\text{glucose})/18 + (\text{ethanol})/4.6 + (\text{methanol})/3.2 + (\text{ethylene glycol})/6.2 + (\text{isopropanol})/6.0.$

The difference between the measured (Osm_M) and calculated (Osm_C) osmotic concentrations is the osmol gap:[43]

$\text{Osmol gap} = Osm_M - Osm_C$

One problem with this equation is that the units are different, as the measured form is in units of osmolality (milliosmoles per kilogram) and the calculated form is in units of osmolarity (milliosmoles per liter). This unit difference is generally not considered significant for clinical purposes, and the gap may be expressed in either of the units; as a result, the osmol gap is interchangeably referred to as the osmolal or osmolar gap.[41] Another important consideration is the timing of collection of samples. When comparing the measured and calculated osmoles, these samples should be collected at the same time from the same blood draw. Using older samples may not account for changes that have occurred to laboratory values over the course of treatment and could obscure interpretation of the osmol gap.

If a significant elevation of the osmol gap is discovered, the difference in the 2 values may represent presence of foreign substances in the blood.[41] Possible causes of an elevated osmol gap are listed in **Box 2**. Unfortunately, what constitutes a normal osmol gap is widely debated. Conventionally, a normal gap has been defined as less than or equal to 10 mOsm/kg. The original source of this value is an article from Smithline and Gardner, which declared this number as pure convention.[44] Further clinical study has not shown this assumption to be correct. A study of 56 healthy adults reported the normal osmol gap to range from −9 to +5 mOsm/kg.[45] A study examining a pediatric emergency department population (n = 192) found a range from −13.5 to 8.9.[46] Another study looked at the osmol gaps of 177 emergency department patients and reported the range to be from −10 to 20 mOsm/kg.[47] A vital point brought forth by the authors of this study, however, is that the day-to-day coefficient of variation for their laboratory in regard to sodium was 1%. They concluded that this level of imprecision translates to an analytical standard deviation of 9.1 mOsm/kg in regard to the osmol gap. This analytical imprecision alone may account for the variation found in osmol gaps of many patients. This concern that even small errors in sodium, urea nitrogen, glucose, and osmolality assays can result in large variations of the osmol gap has been voiced by other researchers.[48] Overall,

Box 2
Causes of an elevated osmol gap

Toxic alcohols

- Ethanol
- Isopropanol
- Methanol
- Ethylene glycol

Drugs and excipients

- Mannitol
- Propylene glycol
- Glycerol
- Osmotic contrast dyes

Other chemicals

- Ethyl ether
- Acetone
- Trichloroethane

Disease or illness

- Chronic renal failure
- Lactic acidosis
- Diabetic ketoacidosis
- Alcoholic ketoacidosis
- Starvation ketoacidosis
- Circulatory shock
- Hyperlipidemia
- Hyperproteinemia

the clinician should recognize that there is likely a wide range of variability in a patient's baseline osmol gap.

Several concerns exist in regard to using the osmol gap as a screening tool in the evaluation of the potentially toxic alcohol poisoned patient. The lack of a well-established normal range is particularly problematic. For example, a patient may present with an osmol gap of 9 mOsm/kg, which is considered normal by the traditionally accepted upper normal limit of 10 mOsm/kg. If, however, this patient had an osmol gap of −5 mOsm/kg just before ingestion of a toxic alcohol, the patient's osmol gap must have increased by 14 mOsm/kg to reach the new gap of 9 mOsm/kg. If this increase was due to ethylene glycol, it would correspond to a toxic level of 86.8 mg/dL.[49] In addition, if a patient's ingestion of a toxic alcohol occurred at a time distant from the actual blood sampling, the osmotically active parent compound will have been metabolized to the acid metabolites. These metabolites do not influence the osmol gap because they are anions that displace bicarbonate and are accounted for by the doubled sodium term in the equation; hence no osmol gap elevation will be detected.[41,50] Therefore, it is possible that a patient may present at a point after ingestion with only a moderate increase in their osmol gap and anion gap. Steinhart reported a patient with ethylene glycol toxicity who presented with an osmol gap of 7.2 mOsm/L due to a delay in presentation.[51] Darchy and colleagues presented 2 other cases of significant ethylene glycol toxicity with osmol gaps of 4 and 7 mOsm/L.[48] The lack of an abnormal osmol gap in these cases was speculated to be due to either metabolism of the parent alcohol or a low baseline osmol gap that masked the toxin's presence.

In addition to concerns with potential missed toxicity, the osmol gap is a particularly nonspecific test at levels outside the normal range and only approaches high specificity for toxic alcohols greater than 30 to 40 mOsm/L.[52] Case studies have found that patients presenting to emergency care with osmol gaps of 15 mOsm/L or greater were more likely to have a condition other than toxic alcohol poisoning, especially alcoholic ketoacidosis. Moreover, critically ill patients may have elevated osmol gaps due to circulating organic solutes such as amino acids.[52,53]

Given lack of specificity and the risk of late presentations of toxic alcohol poisoning without elevation in the osmol gap, assessing the osmol gap should be used with caution as an adjunct to clinical decision-making and not as a primary determinant to rule out toxic alcohol ingestion. If the osmol gap obtained is particularly large, it suggests an agent from **Box 2** may be present. A "normal" osmol gap should be interpreted with caution, as it may not rule out the presence of such an ingestion. The test result must be interpreted within the context of the clinical presentation. If such a poisoning is suspected, appropriate therapy should be initiated presumptively (ie, fomepizole administration, hemodialysis, and so forth) while confirmation from serum levels of the suspected toxin is pending. If a concomitant anion gap and osmol gap is present in patients without a clear history of toxic alcohol poisoning, however—especially those in whom ethanol is detected (as the presence of ethanol would logically delay metabolism of toxic alcohols and preclude development of anion gap acidosis)—seeking assistance from a medical toxicologist is highly advised, as empirical fomepizole may not be necessary in all cases.

SUMMARY

Toxic alcohol exposures can cause patients to become critically ill, and many products containing toxic alcohols are readily accessible. Ethylene glycol and methanol are found in numerous household products. Diethylene glycol, propylene glycol, and isopropyl alcohol, although less commonly ingested, can lead to unique clinical toxidromes that must be recognized and appropriately treated. It is important for critical care clinicians to know how to calculate, interpret, and identify the differential diagnosis for an anion gap metabolic acidosis. An osmol gap can be useful in identifying toxic alcohol ingestions; however, it has many limitations that must be recognized. It is important for critical care specialists to be familiar with these formulas as well as each toxic alcohol, so that an exposure can be identified promptly and treated appropriately.

CLINICS CARE POINTS

- Although classic teaching informs that toxic alcohol ingestions will present with an elevated osmol gap and anion gap, in reality this may not be the case and depends on the time of ingestion and which toxic alcohol is involved.
- Toxic alcohol levels are not readily available at many hospitals. If there is a high concern, dialysis and fomepizole (or ethanol) should be initiated for suspected poisoned patients with an unresolving anion gap metabolic acidosis who do not have an alternative cause for laboratory abnormalities.
- Laboratory interpretation and management recommendations for toxic alcohol poisonings are complex. Clinicians should consider discussing the case details with a regional poison center or clinical toxicologist.

DISCLOSURE

The authors do not have any commercial or financial conflicts of interest, and there are no funding sources for this article.

REFERENCES

1. Gummin DD, Mowry JB, Beuhler MC, et al. 2019 Annual report of the american association of poison control centers' national poison data system (NPDS): 37th annual report. Clin Toxicol (Phila) 2020;58(12):1360–541.
2. Alsufyani A, Blackshaw A, Holstege C. Surreptitiously administered ethylene glycol resulting in murder. Clin Toxicol 2018;56(10):958–9.
3. Wallace KL, Suchard JR, Curry SC, et al. Diagnostic use of physicians' detection of urine fluorescence in a simulated ingestion of sodium fluorescein-containing antifreeze. Ann Emerg Med 2001;38(1):49–54.
4. Shirey T, Sivilotti M. Reaction of lactate electrodes to glycolate. Crit Care Med 1999;27(10):2305–7.
5. Eder AF, Dowdy YG, Gardiner JA, et al. Serum lactate and lactate dehydrogenase in high concentrations interfere in enzymatic assay of ethylene glycol. Clin Chem 1996;42(9):1489–91.
6. Brindley PG, Butler MS, Cembrowski G, et al. Falsely elevated point-of-care lactate measurement after ingestion of ethylene glycol. CMAJ 2007;176(8):1097–9.
7. Porter WH, Rutter PW, Bush BA, et al. Ethylene glycol toxicity: the role of serum glycolic acid in hemodialysis. J Toxicol-Clin Toxicol 2001;39(6):607–15.
8. Lepik KJ, Levy AR, Sobolev BG, et al. Adverse drug events associated with the antidotes for methanol and ethylene glycol poisoning: a comparison of ethanol and fomepizole. Ann Emerg Med 2009;53(4):439–50.

9. Lepik KJ, Sobolev BG, Levy AR, et al. Medication errors associated with the use of ethanol and fomepizole as antidotes for methanol and ethylene glycol poisoning. Clin Toxicol (Phila) 2011;49(5):391–401.
10. Buller GK, Moskowitz CB. When is it appropriate to treat ethylene glycol intoxication with fomepizole alone without hemodialysis? Semin Dial 2011;24(4): 441–2.
11. Buchanan JA, Alhelail M, Cetaruk EW, et al. Massive ethylene glycol ingestion treated with fomepizole alone-a viable therapeutic option. J Med Toxicol 2010; 6(2):131–4.
12. Brent J, McMartin K, Phillips S, et al. Fomepizole for the treatment of ethylene glycol poisoning. Methylpyrazole for Toxic Alcohols Study Group. N Engl J Med 1999;340(11):832–8.
13. Lavergne V, Nolin TD, Hoffman RS, et al. The EXTRIP (EXtracorporeal TReatments In Poisoning) workgroup: guideline methodology. Clin Toxicol (Phila) 2012;50(5): 403–13.
14. Holstege CP, Ferguson JD, Wolf CE, et al. Analysis of moonshine for contaminants. J Toxicol Clin Toxicol 2004;42(5):597–601.
15. Barceloux DG, Bond GR, Krenzelok EP, et al. American academy of clinical toxicology practice guidelines on the treatment of methanol poisoning. J Toxicol-clin Tox 2002;40(4):415–46.
16. Taheri MS, Moghaddam HH, Moharamzad Y, et al. The value of brain CT findings in acute methanol toxicity. Eur J Radiol 2010;73(2):211–4.
17. Brent J, McMartin K, Phillips S, et al. Methylpyrazole for toxic alcohols study group. Fomepizole for the treatment of methanol poisoning. N Engl J Med 2001;344(6):424–9.
18. Hovda KE, Jacobsen D. Expert opinion: fomepizole may ameliorate the need for hemodialysis in methanol poisoning. Hum Exp Toxicol 2008;27(7): 539–46.
19. Schep LJ, Slaughter RJ, Temple WA, et al. Diethylene glycol poisoning. Clin Toxicol (Phila) 2009;47(6):525–35.
20. Landry GL, Dunning CL, Conrad T, et al. Diglycolic acid inhibits succinate dehydrogenase activity in human proximal tubule cells leading to mitochondrial dysfunction and cell death. Toxicol Lett 2013;221(3):176–84.
21. Conrad T, Landry GM, Aw TY, et al. Diglycolic acid, the toxic metabolite of diethylene glycol, chelates calcium and produces renal mitochondrial dysfunction in vitro. Clin Toxicol (Phila) 2016;54(6):501–11.
22. Landry GM, Martin S, McMartin KE. Diglycolic acid is the nephrotoxic metabolite in diethylene glycol poisoning inducing necrosis in human proximal tubule cells in vitro. Toxicol Sci 2011;124(1):35–44.
23. Brent J. Fomepizole for the treatment of pediatric ethylene and diethylene glycol, butoxyethanol, and methanol poisonings. Clin Toxicol (Phila) 2010;48(5):401–6.
24. Zosel A, Egelhoff E, Heard K. Severe lactic acidosis after an iatrogenic propylene glycol overdose. Pharmacotherapy 2010;30(2):219.
25. Wilson KC, Farber HW. Propylene glycol accumulation during continuous-infusion lorazepam in critically ill patients. J Intensive Care Med 2008; 23(6):413.
26. Wilson KC, Reardon C, Theodore AC, et al. Propylene glycol toxicity: a severe iatrogenic illness in ICU patients receiving IV benzodiazepines: a case series and prospective, observational pilot study. Chest 2005;128(3): 1674–81.

27. Lim TY, Poole RL, Pageler NM. Propylene glycol toxicity in children. J Pediatr Pharmacol Ther 2014;19(4):277–82.
28. Zaman F, Pervez A, Abreo K. Isopropyl alcohol intoxication: a diagnostic challenge. Am J Kidney Dis 2002;40(3):E12.
29. Chang A, Schnall AH, Law R, et al. Cleaning and disinfectant chemical exposures and temporal associations with COVID-19 - National Poison Data System, United States, January 1, 2020-March 31, 2020. MMWR Morb Mortal Wkly Rep 2020; 69(16):496–8.
30. Daniel DR, McAnalley BH, Garriott JC. Isopropyl alcohol metabolism after acute intoxication in humans. J Anal Toxicol 1981;5(3):110–2.
31. Rich J, Scheife RT, Katz N, et al. Isopropyl alcohol intoxication. Arch Neurol 1990; 47(3):322–4.
32. Kroll MH, Roach NA, Poe B, et al. Mechanism of interference with the Jaffé reaction for creatinine. Clin Chem 1987;33(7):1129–32.
33. Frenia ML, Schauben JL. Methanol inhalation toxicity. Ann Emerg Med 1993; 22(12):1919–23.
34. Holstege CP, Borek HA. Toxidromes. Crit Care Clin 2012;28(4):479–98.
35. Chabali R. Diagnostic use of anion and osmolal gaps in pediatric emergency medicine. Pediatr Emerg Care 1997;13(3):204–10.
36. Ishihara K, Szerlip HM. Anion gap acidosis. Semin Nephrol 1998;18(1):83–97.
37. Gabow PA. Disorders associated with an altered anion gap. Kidney Int 1985; 27(2):472–83.
38. Judge BS. Metabolic acidosis: differentiating the causes in the poisoned patient. Med Clin North Am 2005;89(6):1107–24.
39. Kruse JA, Cadnapaphornchai P. The serum osmole gap. J Crit Care 1994;9(3): 185–97.
40. Erstad BL. Osmolality and osmolarity: narrowing the terminology gap. Pharmacotherapy 2003;23(9):1085–6.
41. Glaser DS. Utility of the serum osmol gap in the diagnosis of methanol or ethylene glycol ingestion. Ann Emerg Med 1996;27(3):343–6.
42. Worthley LI, Guerin M, Pain RW. For calculating osmolality, the simplest formula is the best. Anaesth Intensive Care 1987;15(2):199–202.
43. Suchard JR. Osmolal Gap. In: Dart RC, editor. Medical toxicology. 3rd ed. Philadelphia, PA: Lippincott Williams & Wilkins; 2004. p. 106–9.
44. Smithline N, Gardner KD Jr. Gaps–anionic and osmolal. JAMA 1976;236(14): 1594–7.
45. Glasser L, Sternglanz PD, Combie J, et al. Serum osmolality and its applicability to drug overdose. Am J Clin Pathol 1973;60(5):695–9.
46. McQuillen KK, Anderson AC. Osmol gaps in the pediatric population. Acad Emerg Med 1999;6(1):27–30.
47. Aabakken L, Johansen KS, Rydningen EB, et al. Osmolal and anion gaps in patients admitted to an emergency medical department. Hum Exp Toxicol 1994; 13(2):131–4.
48. Darchy B, Abruzzese L, Pitiot O, et al. Delayed admission for ethylene glycol poisoning: lack of elevated serum osmol gap. Intensive Care Med 1999;25(8): 859–61.
49. Hoffman RS, Smilkstein MJ, Howland MA, et al. Osmol gaps revisited: normal values and limitations. J Toxicol Clin Toxicol 1993;31(1):81–93.
50. Eder AF, McGrath CM, Dowdy YG, et al. Ethylene glycol poisoning: toxicokinetic and analytical factors affecting laboratory diagnosis. Clin Chem 1998;44(1): 168–77.

51. Steinhart B. Case report: severe ethylene glycol intoxication with normal osmolal gap–"a chilling thought. J Emerg Med 1990;8(5):583–5.
52. Krasowski MD, Wilcoxon RM, Miron J. A retrospective analysis of glycol and toxic alcohol ingestion: utility of anion and osmolal gaps. BMC Clin Pathol 2012; 12(1):1–10.
53. Inaba H, Hirasawa H, Tadanobu M. Serum osmolality gap in postoperative patients in intensive care. Lancet 1987;329(8546):1331–5.

Updates on the Evaluation and Management of Caustic Exposures

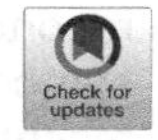

Richard J. Chen, MD[a,*], Rika N. O'Malley, MD[b], Matthew Salzman, MD[c]

KEYWORDS

• Caustic • Alkali • Acid • Exposure • Overdose

KEY POINTS

- Caustics are a class of chemicals capable of causing burns upon contact with tissue and consist of acids and bases.
- Exposure to caustics occur when they are ingested, but ocular, dermal, and pulmonary exposure is possible.
- Gastrointestinal exposure to caustics leads to significant morbidity and mortality, most commonly in the form of stricture formation and malignant transformation of damaged tissues.
- Esophagogastroduodenoscopy remains the gold standard in prognostication and should be considered early after a caustic ingestion, but increasing evidence suggests computed tomographic scan may also have a role.
- Hydrofluoric acid is a weak acid that requires special consideration and management.

INTRODUCTION

A caustic, also referred to as a corrosive, is a chemical capable of causing injury upon tissue contact. Generally, strong acids, with a pH < 3, and strong alkalis, with a pH > 11, are of greatest concern for human exposure. In 2019, the American Association of Poison Control Centers annual report documented more than one hundred eighty thousand exposures.[1] Household cleaners also make up a large portion of pediatric exposures, with more than ninety-seven thousand single substance exposures

[a] Division of Medical Toxicology, Department of Emergency Medicine, Albert Einstein Medical Center, Philadelphia, PA 19141-3098, USA; [b] McLeod Health Seacoast, Little River, SC, USA; [c] Division of Medical Toxicology and Addiction Medicine, Department of Emergency Medicine, Cooper Medical School of Rowan University, Keleman 152, Camden, NJ 08103, USA
* Corresponding author. Division of Medical Toxicology, Department of Emergency Medicine, Albert Einstein Medical Center, 5501 Old York Road, Korman Building B-6, Philadelphia, PA 19141-3098, USA,
E-mail address: chenrich@einstein.edu

Emerg Med Clin N Am 40 (2022) 343–364
https://doi.org/10.1016/j.emc.2022.01.013
emed.theclinics.com

reported in 2019. Reported exposures to caustics occur to the eyes and skin, but poison center calls regarding caustics exposure are most commonly via ingestion.[1] A recent source of exposure comes in the form of detergent capsules or pods, consisting of a mix of anionic and ionic surfactants, propylene glycol contained within a water-soluble polyvinyl alcohol membrane, which are often brightly colored and easily mistaken by children as candy or other edible foods.[2] Clinical consequences of exposure are more severe when compared with typical detergents.[3,4]

Generally speaking, little controversy exists in patient management following dermal or ocular caustic exposure. Immediate water irrigation of the site of exposure, followed by routine burn care, with analgesia, fluid, and electrolyte replacement, is the standard of care. In this article, a thorough review of management of gastrointestinal caustic exposure is explored not only because of the high rates of morbidity and mortality associated with these exposures but also because there remains controversy regarding appropriate management of such exposures. Hydrofluoric acid (HF), a weak acid in its aqueous form, requires special consideration and specific antidotes, and as such, is addressed separately.

CAUSTIC INGESTION

Pathophysiology

The likelihood and severity of esophageal injury after caustic ingestion are related to several factors, including agent pH, titratable acid or alkaline reserve (TAR), physical state (solid, liquid, or gel), and tissue contact time, as well as quantity and concentration of the substance ingested. The pH can be determined in the emergency department by litmus paper testing if there is product available, or by identifying the substance ingested and finding its safety data sheet (formally known as a materials safety data sheet). The TAR, or the amount of acid or base required to titrate a chemical's pH to 8.00, may be a better predictor of esophageal injury than pH, especially after ingestion of near-neutral pH toxicants[2]; however, as this information is often not readily available in the clinical setting, evaluation and risk assessment should be performed using pH, concentration, volume, contact duration, and body surface area of skin involved in the exposure.[2] Tissue contact time may be influenced by the physical state of the toxicant, as ingested solids are more likely to adhere to mucous membranes of the gastrointestinal tract, resulting in prolonged contact. In a rat model, caustic soda (sodium hydroxide, NaOH) has been shown to cause esophageal damage after 10 minutes of contact time, and esophageal perforation after 120 minutes of contact.[5] Furthermore, in this animal study, solution concentration was determined to be the most important predictor of esophageal damage. Caustic soda concentrations of 1.83% were sufficient to cause epithelial necrosis, whereas concentrations of 7.33% induced submucosal damage, and concentrations of 14.33% resulted in muscle and adventitial damage.[5]

Acids and alkalis are known to produce different types of tissue damage. Acids generally cause coagulation necrosis, with eschar formation that may limit substance penetration and injury depth.[6] Alkalis, in contrast, combine with tissue proteins and cause liquefactive necrosis and saponification and are classically taught to penetrate deeper into tissues. In addition, alkali absorption leads to thrombosis in blood vessels, impeding blood flow to already damaged tissue.[7] These mechanisms of injury suggest that alkali ingestion would lead to more serious injury and complications; however, this distinction is probably not clinically relevant in the setting of strong acid or base ingestion, as both are able to penetrate esophageal tissues rapidly, potentially leading to full-thickness damage to the esophageal wall.[8] In 1 study, strong acid ingestion was actually associated with longer hospital stays and increased incidence of systemic complications, such as renal failure, liver dysfunction, disseminated intravascular coagulation (DIC), and hemolysis, when compared with alkali ingestion.[8]

Esophageal injury mechanisms may be more complicated than the chemical burns described above. Reactive oxygen species (ROS) generation with subsequent lipid peroxidation has been implicated as contributing to initial esophageal injury, and subsequent stricture formation seen commonly after caustic ingestion. Investigators have measured concentrations of malondialdehyde (MDA), a known end-product of lipid peroxidation, as well as glutathione (GSH), a known endogenous free-radical scavenger, in esophageal tissue exposed to NaOH. The investigators found significantly higher MDA concentrations, indicating the presence of ROS 24 hours postexposure. These concentrations remained high for 72 hours after exposure compared with noninjured controls. Furthermore, significantly lower GSH concentrations in tissue exposed to NaOH were found in injured esophageal tissue compared with controls, further supporting the presence of ROS and free radical damage.[9]

Esophageal injury may begin within minutes after corrosive ingestion and may persist for hours thereafter.[10] Initially, tissue injury is marked by eosinophilic necrosis with swelling and hemorrhagic congestion.[7] Four to 7 days after ingestion, mucosal sloughing and bacterial invasion occur. This period is further marked by inflammation and the appearance of granulation tissue. During this time, ulcers become covered with a fibrinous layer. Perforation may occur during this time if ulceration exceeds the muscle plane. Fibroblasts appear at injury sites around day 4, and on day 5, roughly, an "esophageal mold" is formed, consisting of dead cells, secretions, and possibly food. On the tenth day after ingestion, esophageal repair begins. Finally, approximately 1 month after exposure, esophageal ulcerations begin to epithelialize.[7]

Clinical Assessment and Studies

Patients who present for medical care following caustic ingestion may have varied signs and symptoms. Patients may be asymptomatic, but may also suffer from nausea, vomiting, dysphagia, odynophagia, drooling, abdominal pain, chest pain, or stridor. Attempts have been made to correlate symptoms and physical findings with esophageal injury, but the literature is inconclusive. One study found that the presence of 2 or more signs or symptoms, including vomiting, drooling, or stridor, predicted serious esophageal injury.[11] A later study suggested that drooling and dysphagia alone correlated with esophageal injury.[12] A following study found that patients with more than 3 signs or symptoms following corrosive ingestion had increased likelihood of esophageal injury.[13] Other studies,[14–17] however, do not support these conclusions and suggest that clinical findings do not correlate with presence or severity of esophageal injury after corrosive ingestion. It has been demonstrated that absence of oropharyngeal injury does not exclude esophageal or gastric lesions,[18] with 1 series finding a 12% incidence of grade II esophageal lesions in asymptomatic patients.[14]

Investigators have attempted to correlate laboratory values with injury severity and outcome following caustic ingestion. One study found a white blood cell count greater than 20,000 cells/mm^3, as well as age, strong acid ingestion, and the presence of deep esophageal ulcers or necrosis, to be predictors of mortality.[19] A subsequent study found no correlation between C-reactive protein or leukocyte counts and esophageal injury and patient outcomes and concluded that these are not useful predictive markers.[13] Despite these findings, hemolysis, DIC, renal failure, and liver failure have all been reported following caustic ingestion,[8] suggesting that laboratory studies may be useful in guiding patient management, but not in predicting morbidity or mortality.

Adult patients with signs of perforated viscous, peritonitis, mediastinitis, or hemodynamic instability may require prompt surgical evaluation and intervention,[20] including exploratory laparotomy or laparoscopy, necrotic tissue resection, or esophagectomy with delayed colonic interposition. Patients presenting with abdominal pain and peritoneal findings should have chest and abdominal radiographs performed to determine the presence of intraperitoneal air or mediastinal air. Criteria for emergent surgery have been proposed, including presence of shock or DIC, need for hemodialysis, acidosis, and degree of esophageal injury seen on endoscopy.[21] One study found that, following a caustic ingestion, an arterial pH < 7.22 or a base excess lower than -12 indicates severe esophageal injury and need for consideration of emergency surgery.[22] Some suggest that the presence of grade 3 lesions, described in later discussion, alone mandate immediate exploratory laparoscopy with removal of necrotic tissue, as this approach has been associated with improved outcomes and decreased mortality.[6,23,24] It is important to note, however, that these criteria are reported in the adult patient literature only. In the pediatric population, these criteria have not been studied, and some investigators recommend exhausting all resources to try to preserve the child's native esophagus.[25] Recent evidence,[26] however, suggests that computed tomography (CT) imaging may be helpful in limiting unnecessary surgical intervention, potentially reducing morbidity and mortality associated with radical procedures, such as esophagectomy, which is discussed later in this article.

At present, esophagogastroduodenoscopy (EGD) remains the gold standard in evaluation of patients with corrosive ingestions.[16,27] Initial endoscopes were rigid, and endoscopy was associated with increased incidence of esophageal perforation. However, flexible EGD has been established as a safe and reliable tool for assessing esophageal damage up to 96 hours after caustic ingestion,[28,29] so long as gentle insufflation is used during the procedure. Only clinical or radiological suspicion for perforated viscous is a contraindication for EGD.[29] Lesions are defined as follows:

Grade	Endoscopic Findings
Grade 0	Normal esophagus
Grade 1	Mucosal edema and hyperemia
Grade 2a	Friability, hemorrhages, erosions, blisters, whitish membranes, exudates, and superficial ulcerations
Grade 2b	Deep or circumferential ulceration, in addition to 2a lesions
Grade 3a	Small and scattered areas of necrosis
Grade 3b	Extensive necrosis

Classifying burn degree is important for patient prognosis and management. Patients with grade 0 and 1 lesions do not develop delayed sequelae, such as stricture or gastric outlet obstruction.[28] These patients should be able to tolerate oral intake and have complete resolution of their symptoms before they are discharged home or, in the setting of self-harm, medically cleared for further psychiatric evaluation. As lesion severity increases, stricture formation incidence increases. Following a grade 2b burn, stricture incidence may be as high as 71%,[29] and after a grade 3 burn, as high as 100%.[30] In addition, the degree of esophageal injury visualized by endoscopy has been shown to be an accurate predictor of systemic complications and death, with each increased injury grade correlating with a nine-fold increase in morbidity and mortality.[8]

Attempts have been made to determine which patients should undergo EGD after corrosive ingestion. Some investigators[18,20,31] recommend all patients who have ingested a corrosive undergo EGD, in light of the fact that studies have shown that patients who are asymptomatic may still have significant esophageal or gastric injury. One retrospective study, however, found that asymptomatic patients who had unintentionally ingested a corrosive were unlikely to have clinically significant esophageal injury.[32] Another retrospective study of adults with accidental caustic ingestions suggests that early endoscopy is not necessary for management.[33] In addition, a retrospective review of children who had ingested hair relaxer, which often contains sodium or lithium hydroxide and may have a pH > 11, found that, despite the presence of lip and oropharyngeal injury, of the patients who underwent EGD, none had greater than grade 1 esophageal or gastric injury, and none had an adverse clinical outcome.[34] In a study performed in Turkey, the investigators proposed a DROOL score[35] to help management of pediatric caustic ingestions without endoscopy. The score evaluates the presence of drooling, reluctance of oral intake, presence of oropharyngeal burns, presence of other signs/symptoms (persistent fever, hematemesis, abdominal tenderness, retrosternal pain, and dyspnea), and leukocytosis. The investigators found that scores less than 4 were 100% sensitive and 96% specific in predicting esophageal strictures.[35] These data suggest that the need for endoscopy should be made on a clinical, case-by-case basis. Typical indications for which EGD should be strongly considered include visible posterior pharyngeal burns, stridor and respiratory distress, vomiting, chest or abdominal pain, or the inability or refusal to drink.[36,37] Perhaps most notably, intentional ingestion of corrosives in a suicide attempt should undergo EGD, as these patients often consume larger volumes of more corrosive agents as compared with unintentional ingestions and are at increased risk for esophageal or gastric injury.[38]

In addition to EGD, other diagnostic modalities have been investigated to determine esophageal injury following caustic ingestion. High-resolution ultrasonography (endoscopic ultrasonography, EUS) can be performed concomitantly with EGD, using a 20-MHz ultrasound mini-probe that is smaller than a traditional transesophageal echocardiogram probe. EUS is better able to define deeper esophageal tissue layers and predict late complications, such as stricture formation. Early investigators[39] have proposed an injury grading system based on ultrasound findings, with grade 0 demonstrating intact muscle layers; grade I demonstrating well-defined, but thickened layers; grade II demonstrating indistinct muscle layers; and grade III showing completely indistinguishable muscle layers. The investigators further subdivide grade II and III lesions into a and b, with grade a showing noncircumferential injury, and grade b showing full-circumference injury. A subsequent study confirmed that EUS was able to identify deeper tissue injury than conventional EGD.[40] However, the investigators also concluded that this procedure does not add prognostic value over EGD alone. EUS remains under investigation in utility for management of caustic injuries. An additional diagnostic tool for determining esophageal injury is the Technetium-99m sucralfate swallowing study. This tool was found to be useful in detecting esophageal injury in humans when performed within 24 hours of ingestion, as well as being useful in documenting healing on repeat studies.[41]

Although flexible EGD is considered the gold standard in prognosis and management of caustic injuries, it possesses several limitations. First, it is an invasive procedure and carries the risk, albeit low, of iatrogenic esophageal perforation. Furthermore, it is unable to assess the depth of necrosis, potentially subjecting patients to unnecessary surgical intervention.[42,43] As a result, finding an alternative noninvasive method of prognostication is desirable. Recently, more research has been done in evaluating CT imaging, which may be used as an alternative prognostic strategy. CT is noninvasive and quicker and can characterize deeper tissues that would not be visualized on an EGD.[44]

The standard protocol is to obtain a CT scan of the neck down to the iliac crests with intravenous (IV) and oral contrast administration.[45] Initial imaging with a noncontrast study should be performed, followed by a study with contrast.[46] Two grading systems have been proposed in current literature. Both systems use a graded scale, similar to the Zargar classification used in EGD. The first system was proposed to be used to help predict risk of stricture formation. Grade I lesions are associated with the lowest risk, and grade IV lesions are associated with highest risk of stricture formation.[44]

Grading Scale Proposed by Ryu and colleagues[44]

Grade	CT Finding
Grade I	No definite swelling of esophagus wall (<3 mm, within normal limit)
Grade II	Edematous wall thickening (>3 mm) without periesophageal soft tissue infiltration
Grade III	Edematous wall thickening with periesophageal soft tissue infiltration plus well-demarcated tissue interface
Grade IV	Edematous wall thickening with periesophageal soft tissue infiltration plus blurring of tissue interface or localized fluid collection around esophagus or descending aorta

In this study, the authors determined that CT imaging had a higher sensitivity and specificity for predicting stricture formation when compared with endoscopic grading.[44] The authors additionally found that grade III and IV were significantly correlated with higher incidence of esophageal stricture formation. A subsequent study used a modified grading system (grade I, IIa, IIb, III). Using this modified scale, the authors found that CT scan grading alone outperformed endoscopy in prediction of stricture formation and performed equally as well as a combined CT-endoscopy classification.[47] Transmural necrosis of the esophagus is defined on CT as having at least 2 of the following criteria: esophageal-wall blurring, periesophageal-fat blurring, or absence of esophageal wall enhancement. Full-thickness necrosis of the stomach is defined as an absence of postcontrast gastric-wall enhancement. There currently are no studies comparing these 2 grading systems, so it is unclear which performs better in prediction of stricture formation.

Grading Scale Proposed by Bruzzi and colleagues,[47] 2019

Grade	CT Finding
Grade I	Clearly delineated esophageal wall; homogenous postcontrast enhancement with absent edema and fat stranding
Grade IIa	Internal enhancement of esophageal mucosa and significant edema of esophageal wall, appearing hypodense; "target" aspect may be seen; mediastinal fat stranding
Grade IIb	Fine rim of esophageal enhancement, but mucosa does not enhance; esophageal lumen is dilated; mediastinal fat stranding
Grade III	Transmural necrosis as shown by absence of postcontrast wall enhancement

CT imaging may provide additional guidance in determining need for surgical intervention in patients with high-grade esophageal injury on EGD. In a study by Chirica and colleagues, patients with confirmed grade 3b injury on endoscopy and compared survival after emergent esophagectomy versus CT-directed management.[48] They found limiting esophagectomy to those with full-thickness necrosis on CT scan improved overall survival, resulted in no deaths in those patients managed conservatively, and improved subsequent self-sufficiency and resuicide rates.

In a follow-up investigation by the same investigators, use of CT to direct management of esophagogastric injury was studied.[26] They demonstrated that limiting emergent esophagectomy or gastrectomy to those with both CT scan findings of full-thickness necrosis and high-grade injury on EGD prevented unnecessary surgical intervention when compared with an endoscopy-alone algorithm. The results validated their previous findings that CT scan is a suitable method in selecting patients requiring emergent surgery after caustic ingestions. This conclusion is supported by a consensus statement by the World Society of Emergency Surgery.[49]

Additional studies suggest that, although useful in further characterization of caustic injury, CT scan cannot replace endoscopy and that all patients with caustic esophagitis should still receive endoscopy.[50,51] In 1 study, CT scan was found to have high specificity, but lower sensitivity in predicting stricture formation and overall underestimated severity of injury. [50] Another study found similar results, with CT scan having high specificity but low sensitivity and low correlation between endoscopy findings and CT scan findings concerning severity of caustic injury.[51]

CT scan is a noninvasive, rapid diagnostic method with evidence suggesting that it may have a more significant role in the evaluation and management of caustic ingestions. There is evidence that it can provide additional information concerning degree of esophageal or gastric injury and can help guide necessity of surgical intervention. Despite this, conflicting evidence prevents CT scan from being the sole diagnostic method for management of these patients and should not replace EGD.

Special consideration for the pediatric population should be given when deciding on pursuing CT scan. Radiation exposure is a known exposure risk for development of cancer in the future, and increased rates of future cancer in pediatric patients has been demonstrated.[52,53] In addition, there is limited evidence in the utility of CT scan in pediatric populations after caustic injury. As a result, EGD remains the primary modality for evaluation of the esophagus and stomach after a caustic injury in the pediatric population.

Treatment

Initial treatment of patients after caustic ingestion includes hemodynamic stabilization and airway assessment, with possible endotracheal or nasotracheal intubation, or surgical airway management if there is evidence of upper-airway compromise. Although activated charcoal administration is common after toxicant ingestion, this practice is absolutely contraindicated after caustic ingestion, as activated charcoal does not adsorb caustics and interferes with endoscopic evaluation.

A potential early intervention might include pH neutralization, with a patient consuming either a weak acid or a weak base. This practice is generally not recommended for fear of compounding injury by inducing an exothermic reaction. This concern, however, is not borne out in animal studies, which demonstrate that intraluminal temperatures do not increase dangerously with neutralization therapy, and that there is no additive damage from an exothermic reaction.[54,55] Furthermore, Homan and colleagues[56] demonstrated that early neutralization therapy decreases esophageal injury on a histopathological level in a rat model, and that delayed neutralization therapy results in increased esophageal damage. There are, however, no data to support this practice in humans and is currently not routinely recommended.

In addition to pH neutralization, dilution has been suggested as a possible technique for mediating esophageal injury after caustic ingestion. One study investigated dilution with milk and water after exposing rat esophagi to 50% NaOH. The investigators concluded that early dilution with milk or water decreased esophageal injury from alkali exposure.[57] No human clinical data exist to support this practice, and, as such, it is currently not recommended routinely due to potential for emesis, obscuring EGD evaluation and increasing luminal pressure and subsequent perforation.

Other treatments that have been suggested immediately following corrosive ingestions include enteral or parenteral proton-pump inhibitors and H-2 blockers. These agents are used to suppress reflux of gastric contents back into the esophagus, thereby minimizing esophageal injury.[20] However, 1 study found increased gastric injury when H-2 blockers were administered immediately following corrosive ingestion.[7] The investigators postulated that this increase in gastric injury was a result of stomach acid suppression and decreased caustic neutralization, leading them to recommend starting this treatment 24 hours after caustic ingestion. In a prospective study by Cakal and colleagues,[58] IV omeprazole therapy correlated with improvement in Zargar classification on EGD after 72 hours. Further clinical studies are needed to confirm efficacy.

Use of nasogastric (NG) tubes in caustic ingestion is controversial. Some investigators recommend the insertion of an NG tube early in the course of a caustic ingestion to maintain the patency of the esophageal lumen and avoid stricture formation.[59–61] There are, however, concerns for local irritation of the esophageal mucosa, perforation, bacterial infection, and exacerbation of gastroesophageal reflux by placement of the tube.[60] A recent international survey indicated that most participating practitioners would perform NG tube insertion only when there is visual oropharyngeal or endoscopic esophageal damage and would do so under endoscopic accompaniment.[62] For a safer and more conservative practice, Shikowitz and colleagues[63] recommend NG tube insertion should not be performed in the emergency department and should only be inserted under direct visualization with endoscopy in the setting of caustic ingestion.

The most concerning chronic complications after caustic ingestions include stricture formation and esophageal malignant transformation. As strictures may develop in 26% to 55% of patients who ingest caustic substances,[23,64] early interventions are aimed at preventing or minimizing this complication. The most common, and perhaps most controversial, treatments used to prevent stricture formation are parenteral corticosteroids and antibiotics. Corticosteroids are thought to attenuate inflammation and granulation and fibrous tissue formation.[65] One prospective study found no benefit from systemic steroid administration in children who had ingested caustic substances, and that the development of strictures was related only to severity of esophageal injury.[66] A subsequent study found that high doses of methylprednisolone were beneficial in patients with grade 2b esophageal lesions, with a decreased incidence of stricture formation and decreased need for bougienage after stricture formation.[67] A subsequent randomized control trial by Usta in 2014 found that administration of a 3-day course of high-dose methylprednisolone (1/1.73 m^2) in grade 2b esophageal burns resulted in significantly lower rates of esophageal stricture formation.[68] However, some animal studies have demonstrated increased morbidity and mortality associated with corticosteroid use.[69] In addition, a meta-analysis of studies published between 1991 and 2004 ultimately found that corticosteroids are of no benefit and do not significantly decrease the incidence of strictures after corrosive ingestion[70] and recommends the abandonment of this practice. This conclusion is further supported by the findings in a Fulton's pooled analysis of studies from 1956 to 2006 that also found limited data to support routine use of steroids in patients with grade 2b caustic esophagitis. Other investigators have supported this conclusion, finding that systemic steroid treatment has no beneficial effect on esophageal wound healing following caustic esophageal burns.[71] Of note, there have been no prospective clinical trials evaluating the utility of antibiotics alone, and their value in the setting of caustic ingestion without signs of concomitant infection, such as peritonitis or mediastinitis, is unknown. Despite the 1000 times greater incidence of esophageal cancer in patients who have ingested caustics over the general population,[72] routine screening is not currently recommended.[20]

There remain potential treatment modalities for stricture formation prevention. Because of the ROS generated after caustic ingestion, investigators have been focusing on antioxidant treatment in order to prevent esophageal strictures. In a rat model, treatment with vitamin E caused decreased collagen synthesis and stricture formation.[73] In addition, ketotifen, an H-1 blocker and mast-cell stabilizer, when given either orally or intraperitoneally to rats, decreased stricture formation and fibrosis after caustic ingestion.[74] Phosphatidylcholine, which stimulates collagenase activity and prevents excessive collagen accumulation, when given to rats after caustic ingestion, prevented stricture formation.[75] Halofuginone, a collagen type 1 synthesis inhibitor, reduced esophageal stricture occurrence in rats exposed to NaOH.[76] Other treatments, such as 5-fluorouracil, octreotide, and interferon-alfa-2b, also show possible benefit in experimental settings.[77,78] Data in humans are lacking with respect to these treatments but may represent interesting options worthy of further investigation.

Other treatment modalities exist for the prevention and treatment of strictures, including bougienage, esophageal stent placement, intralesional corticosteroid injection, and endoscopic dilatation after stricture formation. Instrumentation of the esophagus can lead to perforation, especially during days 7 to 21 after ingestion, at which time the burn area is weakest, as necrotic tissue begins to slough.[16] Despite this, Tiryaki and colleagues[64] found early, prophylactic, dilatation with bougienage to be safe as well as effective at reducing time for stricture resolution. Esophageal stents have also been shown to reduce the incidence of stricture formation.[79–81]

Once strictures have formed, patients often require endoscopic balloon dilatation, or bougienage. Multiple dilatations may be required long term in order for strictures to resolve; however, stable patients may be able to perform this task at home, eliminating the need for frequent hospital admissions.[82] In addition, some investigators advocate intralesional corticosteroid injections as augmentation to stricture dilation and have found that using this technique, although technically difficult, reduces the number or dilatations required for stricture resolution.[83] Surgical intervention may be necessary if these treatments fail, in the presence of malignant transformation, or lengthy or tight strictures.[84] Surgical options include colonic or small bowel interposition and gastric transposition.[80] Although these procedures are often highly invasive, a minimally invasive technique has been described, using thoracoscopic and laparoscopic technique.[84]

CAUSTIC ENEMAS

Although less common than caustic ingestion, caustic enema use and abuse have been reported, at times with devastating consequences. Caustic enemas have been used in suicide and homicide attempts, as abortifacients, as tribal therapeutics, or by accident.[85] Patients with underlying psychiatric disorders reportedly have used alkali enemas in a misguided attempt to purge parasites from their intestines.[86] Caustics that have been rectally administered include car battery acid (sulfuric acid), potash, muriatic acid, acetic acid, HF, ammonia, and hydrogen peroxide (Haroz R, personal communication, 2006).[85,87–89] Corrosive enemas may be more damaging than corrosive ingestion, as the agent has increased tissue contact time in the lower gastrointestinal tract than in the upper gastrointestinal tract.[87] Despite the potentially devastating consequences associated with caustic enemas, less is known about treatment and prognosis.

Patients presenting after rectal caustic administration may have varied symptoms, including anorectal pain, abdominal pain or colic, and tenesmus. In 1 report, a

5-year-old boy who had received an acetic acid enema presented with lethargy and cyanosis.[87] Clinical findings may include hematochezia, hypotension, hypogastric tenderness, flank tenderness, and a hypertonic or hypotonic anal sphincter.[85,87] Frank peritonitis has never been reported immediately following rectal caustic administration.

Patients who present following caustic enemas may require hemodynamic stabilization and should be assessed for potential intestinal bleeding and the need for emergent transfusion. Chest and abdominal radiographs may need to be obtained to determine the presence of free air. In the absence of peritoneal findings, lower endoscopy, such as sigmoidoscopy or colonoscopy, should be considered in order to determine the extent and depth of injury. However, some investigators suggest that this may be of little help and may increase risk of perforation.[85] There is no injury grading system for corrosive enema injuries as described for corrosive esophagitis. Injury may range from none to friable mucosa, to extensive, full-thickness necrosis, extending as far proximally as the terminal ileum. Surgical management with exploration and resection of bowel may be necessary if there is evidence of necrotic tissue, peritonitis, or pneumoperitoneum. It is important to note, however, that postoperative mortalities have been reported as greater than 50%.[85]

Similar to patients with corrosive esophagitis, patients with corrosive colitis are at risk for significant morbidity and mortality, including strictures, fistulas, bowel perforation, peritonitis, renal and hepatic dysfunction, and DIC.[87,89] Early interventions to alleviate pain and minimize sequelae include mesalamine enema, beclomethasone enema,[90] and parenteral steroids and antibiotics. To date, no clinical studies have been done to evaluate the efficacy of these treatments. Supportive care remains the mainstay of treatment, with early surgical and gastroenterology consultation for endoscopic evaluation and possible surgical intervention. Patients may also require prolonged observation or close follow-up, as delayed viscous perforation has been reported, and patients with strictures may require dilatation, as well as possible surgical resection, should dilatation fail.[85]

HYDROFLUORIC ACID

HF is marketed in several formulations for both industrial and commercial use. It is available as an anhydrous acid in concentrations greater than 99%, as well as in aqueous solution in concentrations up to 70%.[91] In its anhydrous form, it is considered a strong acid, but in aqueous solution is considered a weak acid. Even in its aqueous form as a weak acid, HF exposure may have devastating consequences. Industrial uses include the manufacturing of refrigerants, herbicides, pesticides, pharmaceuticals, high-octane gasoline, aluminum, plastics, electrical components, and light bulbs. It can also be found in commercial products for rust removal, brass and crystal cleaning, and enamel etching.[92] Ammonium bifluoride is also available in over-the-counter products, especially in car wheel cleaners, and exposure to it should be treated in a similar manner to as an exposure to HF.

Mechanism of Action

HF, in its aqueous form, is a weak acid that slowly dissociates into hydrogen and fluoride ions, resulting in tissue penetration via a nonionic diffusion gradient potentially causing extensive liquefaction necrosis, behaving more like an alkali than an acid.[93] In addition, fluoride ions penetrate tissues and form insoluble salts with positively charged ions, such as calcium and magnesium, causing tissue injury, hypocalcemia, hypomagnesemia, and pain that is often out of proportion to visible tissue injury.[94]

Clinical Manifestations and Initial Assessment

Dermal contact with HF is the most common route of exposure, especially injuries to the hands with the use of low-concentration rust remover and aluminum-cleaning products.[95] After HF skin contact, symptoms may be immediate or delayed. HF concentrations greater than 50% may cause immediate, severe, and throbbing pain and a whitish discoloration of the skin. Concentrations of 20% to 50% generally produce pain and swelling on the exposed areas that may be delayed up to 8 hours. HF solutions less than 20% may cause no immediate symptoms on skin contact but may cause serious injury that may be delayed 12 to 24 hours.[96]

Aqueous HF solutions are highly volatile and produce vapors that are lighter than ambient air, often resulting in concomitant inhalational and dermal injury, especially with head and neck exposures.[93] Pulmonary effects include upper-airway irritation, narrowing, swelling, and obstruction of the upper airway that may be immediate or delayed up to 36 hours.[96] Physical findings may include stridor, wheezing, or rhonchi, as well as erythema and ulceration of the upper-respiratory tract.[97] High concentration HF inhalation may result in rapid onset of noncardiogenic pulmonary edema and death.[98]

Ocular exposure to HF may be the result of aqueous or HF vapor contact. Eye contact may result in pain, corneal sloughing, revascularization, corneal opacification, and occasionally, keratoconjunctivitis sicca as a long-term complication.[99]

HF ingestion can cause gastritis while sparing the remainder of the gastrointestinal tract. After ingestion, patients may present with nausea, vomiting, or abdominal pain. Systemic absorption is rapid and usually fatal within the first 30 minutes after ingestion, but potentially as long as 7 hours after ingestion.[94]

Death following HF exposure is often a result of cardiac dysrhythmias, most notably ventricular fibrillation.[99] These cardiac dysrhythmias are most likely multifactorial, secondary to electrolyte abnormalities, acidosis, or hypoxia.[95] Hypocalcemia alone is probably insufficient to explain the dysrhythmias, as rats exposed to sodium fluoride still died of cardiovascular failure despite calcium replacement.[100] Some investigators postulate that hyperkalemia precipitates cardiac toxicity, as fluoride ions increase intracellular calcium concentration, subsequently causing potassium efflux and systemic hyperkalemia.[101]

Because of concerns for both upper- and lower-airway edema, close inspection of the patient's airway is paramount. Evidence of oropharyngeal edema may prompt early endotracheal or nasotracheal intubation, or surgical airway management. IV access may need to be obtained to monitor serum electrolyte levels, such as calcium, potassium, magnesium, and sodium, as well as to administer analgesia, IV fluids, and electrolytes. An increase in ionized serum fluoride and decrease in total and ionized serum calcium, hyponatremia, and hyperkalemia can occur following moderate HF exposure[102]; however, as there is little correlation between clinical outcomes and serum fluoride levels, monitoring serum fluoride is of little value.[103]

Cardiac monitoring and serial electrocardiography (ECG) may demonstrate electrolyte abnormalities before serum studies are available, although the sensitivity of ECG is unclear.[94] The ECG may show sinus tachycardia, nonspecific ST segment abnormalities, QTc prolongation, QRS widening, or ventricular fibrillation. Patients manifesting pulmonary symptoms such as cough or dyspnea may require chest radiography evaluation.

Decontamination and Topical Treatments

All patients suffering HF exposure require immediate decontamination, with emergency personnel taking care not to contaminate themselves.[104] All areas that have been in contact with HF should be promptly irrigated with copious amounts of water. Contaminated clothing should be removed and stored in sealed plastic bags so as to avoid secondary exposure to care providers.

Topical treatments are aimed at decreasing pain, skin injury, and systemic absorption of fluoride ions. Quaternary ammonium compounds, such as benzalkonium chloride, have been used to decontaminate and irrigate HF burns. These compounds are purported to inactivate fluoride ions on the skin. Exposed skin can be soaked in a 0.13% benzalkonium chloride water solution or dressed in benzalkonium chloride–soaked compression dressings to be changed every 2 to 4 minutes. These compounds are useful in mild burns, but less useful in deeper burns.[93] Of note, these compounds should not be used in the eye.

Calcium-containing gels can also be applied topically to low concentration (less than 20%) HF burns. A 2.5% calcium gel can be prepared by mixing 3.5 g of calcium gluconate powder with 5 ounces of a water-soluble lubricant or mixing 25 mL of 10% calcium gluconate with 75 mL of water-soluble lubricant.[95,104] The gel should be left in place for 15 minutes, rinsed, and reapplied as often as necessary until pain is relieved.[93] Topical magnesium has also been proposed as a treatment for HF burns, but its efficacy is uncertain. Some studies report effectiveness similar to topical calcium,[105,106] while others report little evidence to support the routine use of magnesium to treat low-concentration dermal HF exposure.[104]

Hexafluorine is a hypertonic agent that has been used for many years in Europe to decontaminate skin and ocular HF burns. It is thought to chelate both hydrogen and fluoride ions, thereby decreasing systemic absorption. Despite case reports describing successful HF burn treatment with Hexafluorine,[107,108] animal studies of HF-induced dermal injury treated with Hexafluorine showed no difference in electrolyte disturbances in the Hexafluorine-treated animals compared with those decontaminated with water. Furthermore, animals decontaminated with Hexafluorine had more severe skin burns compared with those treated with water or calcium gluconate gel.[109] More recent evidence suggests that Hexafluorine may be beneficial in HF exposure and may be preferable to other decontamination methods.[110–112]

Regional and Systemic Treatments

Intradermal calcium injection has been recommended when application of topical calcium gel fails to relieve the pain within the first few minutes following HF exposure or following skin exposure to HF of greater than 20% concentration. Recommendations suggest using a 27- or 30-gauge needle; no more than 0.5 mL/cm^2 of 10% calcium gluconate is injected into the subcutaneous tissue surrounding the exposed areas.[96] Calcium chloride should not be used because it can cause further tissue damage. Despite reported successful treatment of HF exposure with local calcium injection, there are several concerns with this technique, and its routine use is discouraged. First, patients may experience more pain from multiple injections. Second, the volume that can be infiltrated into digits is limited, and vascular compromise can occur if too much fluid volume is infiltrated into a closed finite space, such as fingertips. Furthermore, there is concern that digital calcium injection may extend the burn into the subungual area. Finally, local hyperosmolality and tissue toxicity of calcium may cause more damage than the HF itself.[91,95,113]

Following inhalational exposure to HF, nebulized calcium gluconate may attenuate local and systemic toxicity. Calcium gluconate 2.5% (2.5 g or 25 mL of calcium gluconate in 100 mL of water) can be nebulized via conventional means to treat serious HF inhalation with systemic hypocalcemia.[93,96,104,114,115] In an observational cohort, nebulized calcium gluconate appeared to be effective in treating inhalational exposure to HF.[116] Further study is needed to further assess efficacy.

Parenteral calcium can be administered through standard peripheral IV means as well as in combination with a Bier block. Peripheral IV calcium administration of calcium gluconate, which contains 0.45 mEq/mL of calcium, should be limited to 0.1 to 0.2 mL/kg pushed slowly over 5 minutes. Calcium chloride, which contains 1.36 mEq/mL of calcium, should be administered through central venous access slowly, as it is an irritant and can cause tissue injury and necrosis should it extravasate.

The Bier block was originally intended for regional anesthesia of the distal extremities. Its use in the treatment of HF burns was first reported in 1992.[117] This technique involves achieving IV access in the hand or foot of the affected extremity. A tourniquet, such as a blood pressure cuff, is then applied to the proximal portion of the limb and inflated to 50 mm Hg above the patient's systolic blood pressure. The cuff or tourniquet should not be applied on the forearm or lower leg because adequate arterial compression cannot be obtained. The block is more effective if the extremity is exsanguinated before the tourniquet is inflated. This can be done by tightly wrapping the distal part of the extremity with a soft rubber bandage. It is also acceptable to simply elevate the extremity for 20 to 30 seconds while applying firm digital pressure on the brachial or femoral artery.[118] A volume of 25 mL of 2.5% calcium gluconate is then infused slowly while the cuff remains inflated. After 25 minutes, the cuff pressure is decreased gradually over 5 minutes. Of note, this technique should not be used for patients with poor peripheral vascular circulation. In addition, gradual cuff deflation is important so as not to cause systemic hypercalcemia.

Magnesium sulfate has been proposed as a treatment for HF burns, but its efficacy has not been firmly established. One rat study showed that high-dose IV magnesium sulfate infusion decreased mortality.[119] However, a subsequent study of IV magnesium sulfate failed to demonstrate decreased fluoride bioavailability or risk of death after HF exposure.[120]

Intraarterial calcium infusion is an additional treatment option, if the HF burn involves a large part of an extremity or is a high concentration exposure to the hands. An arterial line should be placed ipsilaterally and proximally to the affected area. A solution of 10 mL of 10% calcium gluconate in 40 mL of normal saline or dextrose 5% in water is run through the line over 4 hours. The infusion can be repeated every 4 to 8 hours, with pain relief considered the indication for therapy cessation.[96,113] More recent case reports further suggest clinical efficacy of intraarterial calcium gluconate treatment for hand and finger-related burns.[121,122] The arterial pressure waveform should be monitored continuously after the infusion is completed for as long as the artery is cannulated. Complications of this therapy include ulnar, radial, and median nerve palsy, hematoma formation, and inflammation of the puncture site.[123] One case series of patients suffering HF extremity injuries described a slight decrease in serum magnesium levels requiring correction and clinically insignificant hypercalcemia with this technique.[124] Furthermore, an increased incidence of microperforation of blood vessels with higher-concentration calcium gluconate solutions was described in a rat model of intraarterial calcium infusion.[125] High-concentration intraarterial calcium chloride infusion has been described, but the potential for vessel injury and tissue necrosis from extravasation mandates extreme caution. When cannulating a major artery, such as the brachial artery, consultation with a surgeon or interventional radiologist may be warranted.

Hemodialysis and burn excision are other modalities available for treating patients with HF burns. One case report describes a patient who suffered a 7% body surface area burn with 71% HF. The patient developed fluoride-induced cardiotoxicity and ventricular fibrillation, which was treated successfully with hemodialysis. Utility of hemodialysis for the management of high-concentration HF exposure is otherwise unproven.[126] In addition, 1 case report describes a favorable outcome for a patient treated with aggressive surgical resection of HF burns.[127] Furthermore, a recent rabbit study showed a decrease in the serum fluoride, and in the degree of hypocalcemia and mortality in a group treated with excision of the exposed area 30 minutes after the injury was induced, compared with groups treated conservatively and with calcium gluconate infusion.[128] In most HF exposures, however, surgical treatment should be limited to debridement of blisters and necrotic tissues to enhance the efficacy of medical treatment.[93]

Ocular exposure

Ocular exposure to HF in the form of a liquid splash or vapor requires vigorous irrigation with water, normal saline, or lactated ringer solution. Copious irrigation with nonmineral-containing solutions is the only widely accepted therapy for HF exposure to the eyes. Generally accepted treatment for HF skin exposure, such as calcium or magnesium application, may not be appropriate for ocular burn.[129] Urgent ophthalmology consultation is appropriate once the patient is stabilized. Commercially available calcium gluconate–containing solutions are available[130]; however, an animal study of 1% calcium gluconate irrigation did not show any significant advantage over saline irrigation.[131] Recent evidence suggests that Hexafluorine is a preferred method of irrigation and decontamination for ocular exposures.[111,112] Another animal study suggests possible benefit with magnesium chloride solution irrigation,[129] and there are case reports of successful treatment of ocular HF exposure with calcium gluconate eye drops[132,133]; however, these therapies should only be instituted after emergent consultation with an ophthalmologist.

SUMMARY

Patients who have ingested caustic substances have potential for significant morbidity and mortality. Close evaluation of the patient's airway, with aggressive supportive care, remains paramount. Currently, there is little evidence to support the use of parenteral corticosteroids or systemic antibiotics without concomitant signs of infection following caustic ingestion. Early consultation with a gastroenterologist, otolaryngologist, or surgeon should be considered, as the patient may warrant EGD or surgical intervention. Patients exposed to HF by any route require decontamination, as well as specialized treatments, including topical, regional, and systemic treatments to reduce burns, pain, and systemic complications. These patients may also require early consultation with a surgeon or interventional radiologist, should there be a need for surgical debridement or intraarterial therapies.

CLINICS CARE POINTS

- Initial treatment of caustic exposures should involve hemodynamic stabilization and airway assessment.
- When treating dermal or ocular exposure to caustics, initial management should involve adequate decontamination.
- When treating caustic ingestions, activated charcoal and pH neutralization should not be used.

- Caustic ingestions can present with various symptoms, but it is important to assess for potential airway compromise by looking for findings such as drooling, oropharyngeal swelling, or stridor.
- Findings of critical illness after caustic ingestion, such as acidosis, shock, or high-grade injury on esophagogastroduodenoscopy, should prompt surgical evaluation.
- General care of caustic ingestions is primarily supportive with no specific antidotes available, with exception to hydrofluoric acid.
- Adjunctive treatments include enteral or parenteral proton-pump inhibitors and H-2 blockers.
- Care should be taken to avoid secondary exposure when treating patients with hydrofluoric acid exposure.
- Hydrofluoric acid exposure by any route can cause hypocalcemia, and patients should undergo serum calcium monitoring as well as electrocardiogram monitoring for prolonged QTc, widened QRS, and dysrhythmias.
- Treatment of severe hydrofluoric acid exposure should involve administration of calcium gluconate or calcium chloride.
- Calcium chloride contains a higher milliequivalent of calcium but should only be infused through central venous access.
- Dermal exposure of hydrofluoric acid can cause significant pain, and calcium-containing topical gels should be applied every 15 minutes until pain relief.
  - Mix 3.5 g of calcium gluconate powder with 5 ounces of water-soluble lubricant.
  - Mix 25 mL of 10% calcium gluconate with 75 mL of water-soluble lubricant.
- If topical calcium does not relieve pain, consider calcium administration through intradermal injection (10% calcium gluconate), intravenous, or intraarterial infusion, or via Bier block.
- When performing intradermal injection, care should be taken as to not cause compartment syndrome in smaller areas, such as fingertips.
- When performing intraarterial calcium infusion, access should be placed proximal and ipsilateral to the area of exposure.
- Ocular exposure should be copiously irrigated, and ophthalmologic consultation should be obtained.
- Pulmonary exposure to hydrofluoric acid can be treated with nebulized calcium gluconate 2.5% (2.5 g calcium gluconate in 100 mL of water).

DISCLOSURE

The authors have nothing to disclose.

REFERENCES

1. Gummin DD, Mowry JB, Beuhler MC, et al. Annual report of the American Association of Poison Control Centers' National Poison Data System (NPDS): 37th annual report. Clin Toxicol (Phila) 2020;58(12):1360–541. PMID: 33305966.
2. Hoffman RS, Howland MA, Kamerow HN, et al. Comparison of titratable acid/alkaline reserve and pH in potentially caustic household products. J Toxicol Clin Toxicol 1989;27(4–5):241–6.
3. Claudet I, Honorat R, Casasoprana A, et al. Expositions des enfants aux lessives capsules, écodoses ou pods: plus toxiques que les lessives traditionnelles ? [Pediatric exposures to laundry pods or capsules: more toxic than traditional

laundry products?]. Arch Pediatr 2014;21(6):601–7. French. Epub 2014 May 10. PMID: 24819668.
4. Settimi L, Giordano F, Lauria L, et al. Surveillance of paediatric exposures to liquid laundry detergent pods in Italy. Inj Prev 2018;24(1):5–11.
5. Mattos GM, Lopes DD, Mamede RC, et al. Effects of time of contact and concentration of caustic agent on generation of injuries. Laryngoscope 2006; 116(3):456–60.
6. Havanond C. Is there a difference between the management of grade 2b and 3 corrosive gastric injuries? J Med Assoc Thai 2002;85(3):340–4.
7. Mamede RC, de Mello Filho FV. Ingestion of caustic substances and its complications. Sao Paulo Med J 2001;119(1):10–5.
8. Poley JW, Steyerberg EW, Kuipers EJ, et al. Ingestion of acid and alkaline agents: outcome and prognostic value of early upper endoscopy. Gastrointest Endosc 2004;60(3):372–7.
9. Gunel E, Caglayan F, Caglayan O, et al. Reactive oxygen radical levels in caustic esophageal burns. J Pediatr Surg 1999;34(3):405–7.
10. Satar S, Topal M, Kozaci N. Ingestion of caustic substances by adults. Am J Ther 2004;11(4):258–61.
11. Crain EF, Gershel JC, Mezey AP. Caustic ingestions. Symptoms as predictors of esophageal injury. Am J Dis Child 1984;138(9):863–5.
12. Nuutinen M, Uhari M, Karvali T, et al. Consequences of caustic ingestions in children. Acta Paediatr 1994;83(11):1200–5.
13. Chen TY, Ko SF, Chuang JH, et al. Predictors of esophageal stricture in children with unintentional ingestion of caustic agents. Chang Gung Med J 2003;26(4): 233–9.
14. Gaudreault P, Parent M, McGuigan MA, et al. Predictability of esophageal injury from signs and symptoms: a study of caustic ingestion in 378 children. Pediatrics 1983;71(5):767–70.
15. Gorman RL, Khin-Maung-Gyi MT, Klein-Schwartz W, et al. Initial symptoms as predictors of esophageal injury in alkaline corrosive ingestions. Am J Emerg Med 1992;10(3):189–94.
16. Havanond C, Havanond P. Initial signs and symptoms as prognostic indicators of severe gastrointestinal tract injury due to corrosive ingestion. J Emerg Med 2007;33(4):349–53. Epub 2007 Jul 5. PMID: 17976790.
17. Boskovic A, Stankovic I. Predictability of gastroesophageal caustic injury from clinical findings: is endoscopy mandatory in children? Eur J Gastroenterol Hepatol 2014;26(5):499–503. PMID: 24642691.
18. Previtera C, Giusti F, Guglielmi M. Predictive value of visible lesions (cheeks, lips, oropharynx) in suspected caustic ingestion: may endoscopy reasonably be omitted in completely negative pediatric patients? Pediatr Emerg Care 1990;6(3):176–8.
19. Rigo GP, Camellini L, Azzolini F, et al. What is the utility of selected clinical and endoscopic parameters in predicting the risk of death after caustic ingestion? Endoscopy 2002;34(4):304–10.
20. Katzka DA. Caustic injury to the esophagus. Curr Treat Options Gastroenterol 2001;4(1):59–66.
21. Brun JG, Celerier M, Koskas F, et al. Blunt thorax oesophageal stripping: an emergency procedure for caustic ingestion. Br J Surg 1984;71(9):698–700.
22. Cheng YJ, Kao EL. Arterial blood gas analysis in acute caustic ingestion injuries. Surg Today 2003;33(7):483–5.

23. Estrera A, Taylor W, Mills LJ, et al. Corrosive burns of the esophagus and stomach: a recommendation for an aggressive surgical approach. Ann Thorac Surg 1986;41(3):276–83.
24. Cattan P, Munoz-Bongrand N, Berney T, et al. Extensive abdominal surgery after caustic ingestion. Ann Surg 2000;231(4):519–23.
25. Erdogan E, Eroglu E, Tekant G, et al. Management of esophagogastric corrosive injuries in children. Eur J Pediatr Surg 2003;13(5):289–93.
26. Chirica M, Resche-Rigon M, Zagdanski AM, et al. Computed tomography evaluation of esophagogastric necrosis after caustic ingestion. Ann Surg 2016; 264(1):107–13. PMID: 27123808.
27. Contini S, Scarpignato C. Caustic injury of the upper gastrointestinal tract: a comprehensive review. World J Gastroenterol 2013;19(25):3918–30. PMID: 23840136; PMCID: PMC3703178.
28. Temiz A, Oguzkurt P, Ezer SS, et al. Predictability of outcome of caustic ingestion by esophagogastroduodenoscopy in children. World J Gastroenterol 2012; 18(10):1098–103. PMID: 22416185; PMCID: PMC3296984.
29. Zargar SA, Kochhar R, Mehta S, et al. The role of fiberoptic endoscopy in the management of corrosive ingestion and modified endoscopic classification of burns. Gastrointest Endosc 1991;37(2):165–9.
30. Baskin D, Urganci N, Abbasoglu L, et al. A standardised protocol for the acute management of corrosive ingestion in children. Pediatr Surg Int 2004;20(11–12): 824–8.
31. Squires RH Jr, Colletti RB. Indications for pediatric gastrointestinal endoscopy: a medical position statement of the North American Society for Pediatric Gastroenterology and Nutrition. J Pediatr Gastroenterol Nutr 1996;23(2):107–10.
32. Gupta SK, Croffie JM, Fitzgerald JF. Is esophagogastroduodenoscopy necessary in all caustic ingestions? J Pediatr Gastroenterol Nutr 2001;32(1):50–3.
33. Celik B, Nadir A, Sahin E, et al. Is esophagoscopy necessary for corrosive ingestion in adults? Dis Esophagus 2009;22(8):638–41. Epub 2009 Jun 9. PMID: 19515187.
34. Aronow SP, Aronow HD, Blanchard T, et al. Hair relaxers: a benign caustic ingestion? J Pediatr Gastroenterol Nutr 2003;36(1):120–5.
35. Uygun I, Aydogdu B, Okur MH, et al. Clinico-epidemiological study of caustic substance ingestion accidents in children in Anatolia: the DROOL score as a new prognostic tool. Acta Chir Belg 2012;112(5):346–54. https://doi.org/10.1080/00015458.2012.11680850.
36. Bosnali O, Moralioglu S, Celayir A, et al. Is rigid endoscopy necessary with childhood corrosive ingestion? A retrospective comparative analysis of 458 cases. Dis Esophagus 2017;30:1–7. https://doi.org/10.1111/dote.12458 [PMID: 26822961.
37. Millar AJ, Cox SG. Caustic injury of the oesophagus. Pediatr Surg Int 2015;31: 111–21. https://doi.org/10.1007/s00383-014-3642-3 [PMID: 25432099.
38. Methasate A, Lohsiriwat V. Role of endoscopy in caustic injury of the esophagus. World J Gastrointest Endosc 2018;10(10):274–82. PMID: 30364838; PMCID: PMC6198306.
39. Kamijo Y, Kondo I, Kokuto M, et al. Miniprobe ultrasonography for determining prognosis in corrosive esophagitis. Am J Gastroenterol 2004;99(5):851–4.
40. Chiu HM, Lin JT, Huang SP, et al. Prediction of bleeding and stricture formation after corrosive ingestion by EUS concurrent with upper endoscopy. Gastrointest Endosc 2004;60(5):827–33.
41. Millar AJ, Numanoglu A, Mann M, et al. Detection of caustic oesophageal injury with technetium 99m-labelled sucralfate. J Pediatr Surg 2001;36(2):262–5.

42. Chirica M, Resche-Rigon M, Bongrand NM, et al. Surgery for caustic injuries of the upper gastrointestinal tract. Ann Surg 2012;256(6):994–1001.
43. Ramasamy K, Gumaste VV. Corrosive ingestion in adults. J Clin Gastroenterol 2003;37:119–24.
44. Ryu HH, Jeung KW, Lee BK, et al. Caustic injury: can CT grading system enable prediction of esophageal stricture? Clin Toxicol (Phila) 2010;48(2):137–42. PMID: 20199130.
45. Agarwal A, Srivastava DN, Madhusudhan KS. Corrosive injury of the upper gastrointestinal tract: the evolving role of a radiologist. Br J Radiol 2020; 93(1114):20200528. https://doi.org/10.1259/bjr.20200528. Epub 2020 Jul 24. PMID: 32706982; PMCID: PMC7548375.
46. Chirica M, Bonavina L, Kelly MD, et al. Caustic ingestion. Lancet 2017; 389(10083):2041–52. Epub 2016 Oct 26. PMID: 28045663.
47. Bruzzi M, Chirica M, Resche-Rigon M, et al. Emergency computed tomography predicts caustic esophageal stricture formation. Ann Surg 2019;270(1):109–14. PMID: 29533267.
48. Chirica M, Resche-Rigon M, Pariente B, et al. Computed tomography evaluation of high-grade esophageal necrosis after corrosive ingestion to avoid unnecessary esophagectomy. Surg Endosc 2015;29(6):1452–61. Epub 2014 Aug 27. PMID: 25159655.
49. Chirica M, Kelly MD, Siboni S, et al. Esophageal emergencies: WSES guidelines. World J Emerg Surg 2019;14:26. PMID: 31164915; PMCID: PMC6544956.
50. Lurie Y, Slotky M, Fischer D, et al. The role of chest and abdominal computed tomography in assessing the severity of acute corrosive ingestion. Clin Toxicol (Phila) 2013;51(9):834–7. Epub 2013 Sep 13. PMID: 24032468.
51. Bahrami-Motlagh H, Hadizadeh-Neisanghalb M, Peyvandi H. Diagnostic accuracy of computed tomography scan in detection of upper gastrointestinal tract injuries following caustic ingestion. Emerg (Tehran) 2017;5(1):e61. Epub 2017 Mar 10. PMID: 28894776; PMCID: PMC5585831.
52. Miglioretti DL, Johnson E, Williams A, et al. The use of computed tomography in pediatrics and the associated radiation exposure and estimated cancer risk. JAMA Pediatr 2013;167(8):700–7.
53. Goodman TR, Mustafa A, Rowe E. Pediatric CT radiation exposure: where we were, and where we are now. Pediatr Radiol 2019;49(4):469–78. Epub 2019 Mar 29. PMID: 30923878.
54. Homan CS, Singer AJ, Henry MC, et al. Thermal effects of neutralization therapy and water dilution for acute alkali exposure in canines. Acad Emerg Med 1997; 4(1):27–32.
55. Homan CS, Singer AJ, Thomajan C, et al. Thermal characteristics of neutralization therapy and water dilution for strong acid ingestion: an in-vivo canine model. Acad Emerg Med 1998;5(4):286–92.
56. Homan CS, Maitra SR, Lane BP, et al. Histopathologic evaluation of the therapeutic efficacy of water and milk dilution for esophageal acid injury. Acad Emerg Med 1995;2(7):587–91.
57. Homan CS, Maitra SR, Lane BP, et al. Therapeutic effects of water and milk for acute alkali injury of the esophagus. Ann Emerg Med 1994;24(1):14–20.
58. Cakal B, Akbal E, Köklü S, et al. Acute therapy with intravenous omeprazole on caustic esophageal injury: a prospective case series. Dis Esophagus 2013; 26(1):22–6. Epub 2012 Feb 14. PMID: 22332893.

59. Hawkins Donald B, Demeter Milan J, Barnett Thomas E. Caustic ingestion: controversies in management. A review of 214 cases. Laryngoscope 1980;90(1): 98–109.
60. Mamede RC, De Mello Filho FV. Treatment of caustic ingestion: an analysis of 239 cases. Dis Esophagus 2002;15(3):210–3. PMID: 12444992.
61. Kochhar R, Poornachandra KS, Puri P, et al. Comparative evaluation of nasoenteral feeding and jejunostomy feeding in acute corrosive injury: a retrospective analysis. Gastrointest Endosc 2009;70(5):874–80.
62. Kluger Y, Ishay OB, Sartelli M, et al. Caustic ingestion management: World Society of Emergency Surgery Preliminary Survey of expert opinion. published correction appears in World J Emerg Surg. 2015;10:56. World J Emerg Surg 2015;10:48. Published 2015 Oct 16.
63. Shikowitz MJ, Levy J, Villano D, et al. Speech and swallowing rehabilitation following devastating caustic ingestion: techniques and indicators for success. Laryngoscope 1996;106(2 Pt 2 Suppl 78):1–12. PMID: 8569409.
64. Tiryaki T, Livanelioglu Z, Atayurt H. Early bougienage for relief of stricture formation following caustic esophageal burns. Pediatr Surg Int 2005;21(2):78–80.
65. Jain AL, Robertson GJ, Rudis MI. Surgical issues in the poisoned patient. Emerg Med Clin North Am 2003;21(4):1117–44.
66. Anderson KD, Rouse TM, Randolph JG. A controlled trial of corticosteroids in children with corrosive injury of the esophagus. N Engl J Med 1990;323(10): 637–40.
67. Boukthir S, Fetni I, Mrad SM, et al. [High doses of steroids in the management of caustic esophageal burns in children]. Arch Pediatr 2004;11(1):13–7.
68. Usta M, Erkan T, Cokugras FC, et al. High doses of methylprednisolone in the management of caustic esophageal burns. Pediatrics 2014;133(6):1518–24.
69. Rosenberg N, Kunderman PJ, Vroman L, et al. Prevention of experimental esophageal stricture by cortisone. II. Control of suppurative complications by penicillin. AMA Arch Surg 1953;66(5):593–8.
70. Pelclova D, Navratil T. Do corticosteroids prevent oesophageal stricture after corrosive ingestion? Toxicol Rev 2005;24(2):125–9.
71. Ulman I, Mutaf O. A critique of systemic steroids in the management of caustic esophageal burns in children. Eur J Pediatr Surg 1998;8(2):71–4.
72. Zwischenberger JB, Savage C, Bidani A. Surgical aspects of esophageal disease: perforation and caustic injury. Am J Respir Crit Care Med 2002;165(8): 1037–40.
73. Gunel E, Caglayan F, Caglayan O, et al. Effect of antioxidant therapy on collagen synthesis in corrosive esophageal burns. Pediatr Surg Int 2002;18(1):24–7.
74. Yukselen V, Karaoglu AO, Ozutemiz O, et al. Ketotifen ameliorates development of fibrosis in alkali burns of the esophagus. Pediatr Surg Int 2004;20(6):429–33.
75. Demirbilek S, Aydin G, Yucesan S, et al. Polyunsaturated phosphatidylcholine lowers collagen deposition in a rat model of corrosive esophageal burn. Eur J Pediatr Surg 2002;12(1):8–12.
76. Ozçelik MF, Pekmezci S, Saribeyoğlu K, et al. The effect of halofuginone, a specific inhibitor of collagen type 1 synthesis, in the prevention of esophageal strictures related to caustic injury. Am J Surg 2004;187(2):257–60. PMID: 14769315.
77. Duman L, Büyükyavuz BI, Altuntas I, et al. The efficacy of single-dose 5-fluorouracil therapy in experimental caustic esophageal burn. J Pediatr Surg 2011;46: 1893–7 [PMID: 22008323.

78. Kaygusuz I, Celik O, Ozkaya OO, et al. Effects of interferon-alpha-2b and octreotide on healing of esophageal corrosive burns. Laryngoscope 2001;111: 1999–2004 [PMID: 11801986.
79. Berkovits RN, Bos CE, Wijburg FA, et al. Caustic injury of the oesophagus. Sixteen years experience, and introduction of a new model oesophageal stent. J Laryngol Otol 1996;110(11):1041–5.
80. Zhou JH, Jiang YG, Wang RW, et al. Management of corrosive esophageal burns in 149 cases. J Thorac Cardiovasc Surg 2005;130(2):449–55.
81. Wang RW, Zhou JH, Jiang YG, et al. Prevention of stricture with intraluminal stenting through laparotomy after corrosive esophageal burns. Eur J Cardiothorac Surg 2006;30(2):207–11.
82. Bapat RD, Bakhshi GD, Kantharia CV, et al. Self-bougienage: long-term relief of corrosive esophageal strictures. Indian J Gastroenterol 2001;20(5):180–2.
83. Kochhar R, Ray JD, Sriram PV, et al. Intralesional steroids augment the effects of endoscopic dilation in corrosive esophageal strictures. Gastrointest Endosc 1999;49(4 Pt 1):509–13.
84. Nwomeh BC, Luketich JD, Kane TD. Minimally invasive esophagectomy for caustic esophageal stricture in children. J Pediatr Surg 2004;39(7):e1–6.
85. Diarra B, Roudie J, Ehua Somian F, et al. Caustic burns of rectum and colon in emergencies. Am J Surg 2004;187(6):785–9.
86. da Fonseca J, Brito MJ, Freitas J, et al. Acute colitis caused by caustic products. Am J Gastroenterol 1998;93(12):2601–2.
87. Kawamata M, Fujita S, Mayumi T, et al. Acetic acid intoxication by rectal administration. J Toxicol Clin Toxicol 1994;32(3):333–6.
88. Cappell MS, Simon T. Fulminant acute colitis following a self-administered hydrofluoric acid enema. Am J Gastroenterol 1993;88(1):122–6.
89. Sheibani S, Gerson LB. Chemical colitis. J Clin Gastroenterol 2008;42(2): 115–21. PMID: 18209577.
90. Michopoulos S, Bouzakis H, Sotiropoulou M, et al. Colitis due to accidental alcohol enema: clinicopathological presentation and outcome. Dig Dis Sci 2000;45(6):1188–91.
91. Burd A. Hydrofluoric acid-revisited. Burns. 2004;30(7):720–2.
92. CDC Chemical Emergencies, Facts About Hydrogen Fluoride - https://emergency.cdc.gov/agent/hydrofluoricacid/basics/facts.asp. Accessed May 2021.
93. Kirkpatrick JJ, Enion DS, Burd DA. Hydrofluoric acid burns: a review. Burns. 1995;21(7):483–93.
94. Kao WF, Dart RC, Kuffner E, et al. Ingestion of low-concentration hydrofluoric acid: an insidious and potentially fatal poisoning. Ann Emerg Med 1999;34(1): 35–41.
95. Caravati EM. Acute hydrofluoric acid exposure. Am J Emerg Med 1988;6(2): 143–50.
96. Agency for Toxic Substances and Diseases Registry: Medical management guideline for hydrogen fluoride - https://wwwn.cdc.gov/TSP/MMG/MMGDetails.aspx?mmgid=1142&toxid=250. Accessed May 2021.
97. Wing JS, Brender JD, Sanderson LM, et al. Acute health effects in a community after a release of hydrofluoric acid. Arch Environ Health 1991;46(3):155–60.
98. Dote T, Kono K, Usuda K, et al. Lethal inhalation exposure during maintenance operation of a hydrogen fluoride liquefying tank. Toxicol Ind Health 2003; 19(2–6):51–4.

99. Su M. Hydrofluoric acid and fluorides. In: LR Goldfrank NF, Lewis NA, et al, editors. Goldfrank's Toxicologic Emergencies. 11th edition. New York: McGraw-Hill; 2019. p. 1397–402.
100. Strubelt O, Iven H, Younes M. The pathophysiological profile of the acute cardiovascular toxicity of sodium fluoride. Toxicology 1982;24(3–4):313–23.
101. Cummings CC, McIvor ME. Fluoride-induced hyperkalemia: the role of Ca2+-dependent K+ channels. Am J Emerg Med 1988;6(1):1–3.
102. Murano M. Studies of the treatment of hydrofluoric acid burn. Bull Osaka Med Coll 1989;5:39–48.
103. Saady JJ, Rose CS. A case of nonfatal sodium fluoride ingestion. J Anal Toxicol 1988;12(5):270–1.
104. Kirkpatrick JJ, Burd DA. An algorithmic approach to the treatment of hydrofluoric acid burns. Burns. 1995;21(7):495–9.
105. Burkhart KK, Brent J, Kirk MA, et al. Comparison of topical magnesium and calcium treatment for dermal hydrofluoric acid burns. Ann Emerg Med 1994; 24(1):9–13.
106. Dunn BJ, MacKinnon MA, Knowlden NF, et al. Topical treatments for hydrofluoric acid dermal burns. Further assessment of efficacy using an experimental piq model. J Occup Environ Med 1996;38(5):507–14.
107. Soderberg K, Kuusinen P, Mathieu L, et al. An improved method for emergent decontamination of ocular and dermal hydrofluoric acid splashes. Vet Hum Toxicol 2004;46(4):216–8.
108. Mathieu L, Nehles J, Blomet J, et al. Efficacy of hexafluorine for emergent decontamination of hydrofluoric acid eye and skin splashes. Vet Hum Toxicol 2001;43(5):263–5.
109. Hulten P, Hojer J, Ludwigs U, et al. Hexafluorine vs. standard decontamination to reduce systemic toxicity after dermal exposure to hydrofluoric acid. J Toxicol Clin Toxicol 2004;42(4):355–61.
110. Yoshimura CA, Mathieu L, Hall AH, et al. Seventy per cent hydrofluoric acid burns: delayed decontamination with Hexafluorine® and treatment with calcium gluconate. J Burn Care Res 2011;32(4):e149–54. PMID: 21747332.
111. Atley K, Ridyard E. Treatment of hydrofluoric acid exposure to the eye. Int J Ophthalmol 2015;8(1):157–61. PMID: 25709926; PMCID: PMC4325260.
112. Burgher F, Mathieu L, Lati E, et al. Part 2. Comparison of emergency washing solutions in 70% hydrofluoric acid-burned human skin in an established ex vivo explants model. Cutan Ocul Toxicol 2011;30(2):108–15. https://doi.org/10.3109/15569527.2010.534748. Erratum in: Cutan Ocul Toxicol. 2012 Jun;31(2):175. PMID: 21083510; PMCID: PMC3116720.
113. Vance MV, Curry SC, Kunkel DB, et al. Digital hydrofluoric acid burns: treatment with intraarterial calcium infusion. Ann Emerg Med 1986;15(8):890–6.
114. Schiettecatte D, Mullie G, Depoorter M. Treatment of hydrofluoric acid burns. Acta Chir Belg 2003;103(4):375–8.
115. Kono K, Watanabe T, Dote T, et al. Successful treatments of lung injury and skin burn due to hydrofluoric acid exposure. Int Arch Occup Environ Health 2000; 73(Suppl):S93–7.
116. Choe MSP, Lee MJ, Seo KS, et al. Application of calcium nebulization for mass exposure to an accidental hydrofluoric acid spill. Burns 2020;46(6):1337–46. Epub 2020 Mar 21. PMID: 32209280.
117. Henry JA, Hla KK. Intravenous regional calcium gluconate perfusion for hydrofluoric acid burns. J Toxicol Clin Toxicol 1992;30(2):203–7.

118. Casey W. Intravenous regional anesthesia (Bier's block). Update in Anesthesia 1992;(1).
119. Williams JM, Hammad A, Cottington EC, et al. Intravenous magnesium in the treatment of hydrofluoric acid burns in rats. Ann Emerg Med 1994;23(3):464–9.
120. Heard K, Hill RE, Cairns CB, et al. Calcium neutralizes fluoride bioavailability in a lethal model of fluoride poisoning. J Toxicol Clin Toxicol 2001;39(4):349–53.
121. Capitani EM, Hirano ES, Zuim Ide S, et al. Finger burns caused by concentrated hydrofluoric acid, treated with intra-arterial calcium gluconate infusion: case report. Sao Paulo Med J 2009;127(6):379–81. PMID: 20512294.
122. Thomas D, Jaeger U, Sagoschen I, et al. Intra-arterial calcium gluconate treatment after hydrofluoric acid burn of the hand. Cardiovasc Intervent Radiol 2009; 32(1):155–8. Epub 2008 May 28. PMID: 18506520.
123. McKee D, Thoma A, Bailey K, et al. A review of hydrofluoric acid burn management. Plast Surg (Oakv) 2014;22(2):95–8.
124. Siegel DC, Heard JM. Intra-arterial calcium infusion for hydrofluoric acid burns. Aviat Space Environ Med 1992;63(3):206–11.
125. Dowbak G, Rose K, Rohrich RJ. A biochemical and histologic rationale for the treatment of hydrofluoric acid burns with calcium gluconate. J Burn Care Rehabil 1994;15(4):323–7.
126. Bjornhagen V, Hojer J, Karlson-Stiber C, et al. Hydrofluoric acid-induced burns and life-threatening systemic poisoning–favorable outcome after hemodialysis. J Toxicol Clin Toxicol 2003;41(6):855–60.
127. Buckingham FM. Surgery: a radical approach to severe hydrofluoric acid burns. A case report. J Occup Med 1988;30(11):873–4.
128. Yang SJ, Zhang YH, Liu LP, et al. [Comparison of various methods of early management of hydrofluoric acid burn in rabbits]. Zhonghua Shao Shang Za Zhi 2005;21(1):40–2.
129. McCully J. Ocular hydrofluoric acid burns: animal model. Trans Am Ophthalmol Soc 1990;88:649–84.
130. Recommended medical treatment for hydrofluoric acid exposure. Honeywell International Inc.; 2006.
131. Beiran I, Miller B, Bentur Y. The efficacy of calcium gluconate in ocular hydrofluoric acid burns. Hum Exp Toxicol 1997;16(4):223–8.
132. Bentur Y, Tannenbaum S, Yaffe Y, et al. The role of calcium gluconate in the treatment of hydrofluoric acid eye burn. Ann Emerg Med 1993;22(9):1488–90.
133. Rubinfeld RS, Silbert DI, Arentsen JJ, et al. Ocular hydrofluoric acid burns. Am J Ophthalmol 1992;114(4):420–3.

Chemical Agents Encountered in Protests

Aaron S. Frey, DO[a,*], Paul M. Maniscalco, PhD(c), MPA, MS, EMT/P[b], Christopher P. Holstege, MD[a,c]

KEYWORDS

- Riot control agent • Incapacitating agent • Pepper spray • Tear gas • CS • OC • CN • CR

KEY POINTS

- The most common chemicals used in riot control agents are chlorobenzylidene malononitrile (CS), chloroacetophenone (CN), dibenz[*b,f*]-[1,4]-oxazepine (CR), and oleoresin capsicum (OC).
- Ocular, respiratory, dermal, and gastrointestinal symptoms are the most common. Clinical effects usually occur immediately to within several minutes of exposure, but latency periods of hours to weeks have been documented.
- Effects usually improve within minutes to hours after removal from source, but some may experience more severe effects that require intensive care and long-term management.
- Soft tissue, ocular, and neurologic injuries have been seen from the kinetic impact of launched or thrown riot control agent canisters, sometimes with lethal results.
- Treatment consists of symptomatic management. There is no antidote for these agents.

INTRODUCTION

Riot control agents (RCAs) are chemicals that are touted as producing rapid, nonlethal, incapacitating effects used to protect an individual or group when facing a potentially violent physical confrontation and to control the actions and movements of crowds.[1–4] These agents have been given several names such as "harassing agents," "lacrimators," "demonstration control agents," "less-than-lethal weapons," "incapacitating agents," "irritating agents," "short-term incapacitants," and "crowd control weapons," but they are commonly referred to as "tear gas" or "pepper spray."[1,3–8] The moniker "tear gas" came into use due to the ocular irritation and lacrimation that these chemicals produce.[9] Currently, RCAs are frequently classified as either tear gas or pepper spray. Tear gas is actually not a gas, but rather an aerosol of solid

[a] Division of Medical Toxicology, Department of Emergency Medicine, University of Virginia School of Medicine, PO Box 800774, Charlottesville, VA 22908-0774, USA; [b] International Association EMS Chiefs, 47072 Stillwood Place, Potomac Falls, VA 22520, USA; [c] Division of Medical Toxicology, Department of Emergency Medicine & Pediatrics, University of Virginia School of Medicine, PO Box 800774, Charlottesville, VA 22908-0774, USA
* Corresponding author.
E-mail address: AF3MV@virginia.edu

Emerg Med Clin N Am 40 (2022) 365–379
https://doi.org/10.1016/j.emc.2022.01.007
0733-8627/22/

chemicals. Pepper spray refers to those chemicals that are in a pressurized liquid suspension.

History of Riot Control Agents

Increasing incidents of worldwide civil unrest have resulted in the increased use of RCAs.[2,6,10] The first modern RCA was ethyl bromoacetate, which was deployed in Paris in 1913.[11–13] During World War I, acrolein (Papite), chloropicrin (PS), bromoacetone, benzyl bromide, and bromobenzyl cyanide were developed as tear gas agents.[1,13,14] Tear gas was released in April 1915 before the launching of the infamous battle at Ypres, making it the first chemical warfare agent used in World War I.[12] Since then, multiple chemicals have been developed as RCAs.[4] When discussed, these chemicals are referred to by either their chemical name or their unique 1- to 3-letter and number military designation. The most common agents are depicted in **Table 1**, and their military designations are dibenz[*b,f*]-[1,4]-oxazepine (CR), chloroacetophenone (CN), chlorobenzylidene malononitrile (CS), and oleoresin capsicum (OC).[7,13,15] In addition to their use in RCAs, OC and CS have been used in personal self-defense sprays as well as defense sprays against animals such as dogs and bears ("bear mace" or "bear spray").[16–18]

RCAs and bear spray have been used by rioters against authorities and other civilians.[19] Bear spray is often used by rioters because it is easily obtained at outdoor recreation stores and is usually more powerful and sprays a longer distance than the standard self-defense sprays formulated for use against humans.[20] Protesters used bear spray against a journalist and three counter-protesters during a demonstration in Portland, Oregon in August 2020.[21] Protesters sprayed an unidentified chemical agent and bear spray on police during a protest in Salem, Oregon in December 2020.[22,23] Rioters used bear spray on the US Capitol Police during the January 6, 2021 riot at the US Capitol.[24,25] Eleven rioters were arrested for illegal possession of pepper spray during demonstrations in Sacramento, California on January 6, 2021, and bear spray was found on protestors by police in Portland, Oregon in March 2021.[26,27]

In addition to rioters using their own RCAs and bear spray, they have devised ways of neutralizing police-deployed RCAs or using them against the authorities. Rioters have recently been reported to combat RCAs by breaking formation and placing traffic cones over the discharged device to contain the released chemical and pouring water in the hole at top of cone in an attempt to prevent further chemical release.[28] Leaf blowers are being used to blow back tear gas at officers.[28] Grenades containing RCAs are being smothered with a wet towel or are being placed into a thermos flask full of mud.[28] Rioters are also throwing back devices at officers by using heat-proof gloves.[28]

Riot Control Agents as Chemical Warfare Agents and Arms Control Treaties

The 1925 Geneva Gas Protocol for the Prohibition of the use in War of Asphyxiating, Poisonous or Other Gases, and of Bacteriological Methods of Warfare prohibited the use of chemical agents in warfare.[29] However, in 1975, President of the United States, Gerald Ford, signed Executive Order Number 11850, which permits the use of RCAs in certain defensive situations in warfare, such as controlling rioting prisoners of war and in areas outside of an immediate combat zone to protect convoys.[30]

The Convention on the Prohibition of Development, Production, Stockpiling and Use of Chemical Weapons and on their Destruction, often known as the Chemical Weapons Convention, is an international arms treaty that was approved by the United Nations General Assembly in 1992, opened for signatures in 1993, ratified

Table 1
Common chemicals in riot control agents

Chemical Name	Military Designation	Most Common Use	Mechanism of Action	Chemical Structure
Chloroacetophenone	CN	Tear gas	TRPA1 agonism	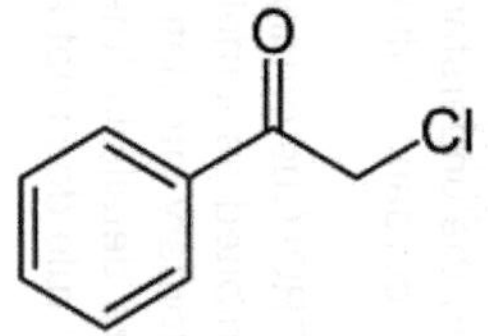
Chlorobenzylidene-malononitrile	CS	Tear gas	TRPA1 agonism	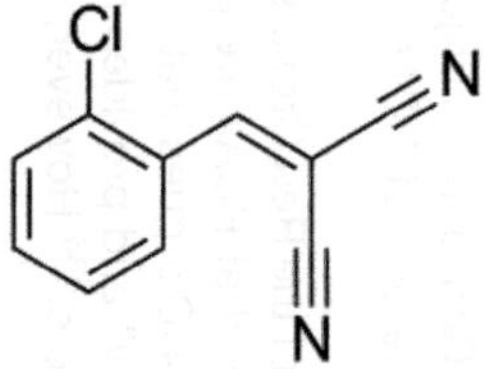
Dibenz[b,f]-[1,4]-oxazepine	CR	Tear gas	TRPA1 agonism	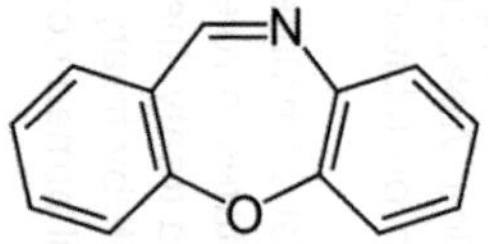
Oleoresin capsicum	OC	Pepper spray	TRPV1 agonism	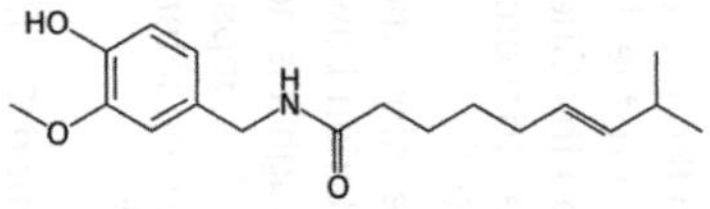 This is capsaicin, the most common ingredient in OC.

by the United States in 1997, and took force in 1997.[31] It states in Article I that RCAs are not to be used in warfare.[32] However, Article II(9) (d) states that the treaty does not apply to "law enforcement including domestic riot control purposes."[32] According to the United States Naval Warfare Publication 1-14M "The Commander's Handbook on the Law of Naval Operations" August 2017 edition: "The United States ratified the Chemical Weapons Convention subject to the understanding that nothing in the Convention prohibited the use of RCAs in accordance with Executive Order 11850."[33]

The International Committee of the Red Cross's (ICRC) Customary International Humanitarian Law states in rule 75 that RCAs are prohibited as a method of warfare.[34] Although it is not a treaty, the ICRC argues that Customary International Humanitarian Law "fills gaps left by treaty law" and provides more details in "the legal framework governing internal armed conflicts."[35] However, this rule does not apply to domestic use.[34]

Common Chemicals in Riot Control Agents

Chloroacetophenone (CN) is a white crystalline solid[1]. It was first investigated as an RCA in the United States in 1917.[12] It was used as a a tear gas agent in the late 1910s and early 1920s, and was adopted by the US Army as the primary active chemical in US Army tear gas munitions in the 1920s.[1,12] By the 1950s, it was the most common RCA in use in the United States.[2] Although it was used by US law enforcement agencies through the 1960s, concerns regarding its toxicity and stability prompted the search for a suitable replacement.[2,14].

Two chemists with the last names of Corson and Stoughton created chlorobenzylidene malononitrile in 1928 and are the namesakes for its military designation CS.[36,37] It is a white solid at room temperature.[38] It was found to be less likely to cause significant adverse health consequences than CN, and it was adopted by the US military as a replacement for CN in tear gas in 1959.[2,14]

Dibenz[*b,f*]-[1,4]-oxazepine (CR) was synthesized in 1962 and is a pale-yellow solid.[1] When used in tear gas, it is mixed in a solution of 80 parts propylene glycol and 20 parts water.[1] CS and CR are both currently deployed worldwide, with CS being the RCA used most in the world.[1,14,39]

Pepper spray is a liquid solution. It was first developed in the 1960s and became popular with US law enforcement agencies in the 1980s.[2] During that time, many pepper spray manufacturers used CN as their active ingredient, including the proprietary brand Mace.[37] Although it is still used in modern pepper sprays, most companies have replaced it with oleoresin capsicum (OC) because it is considered to be a safer chemical.[1,2,7] OC is a mixture of more than 100 compounds derived from chili peppers, with the chemical capsaicin (8-methyl-N-vanillyl-6-nonenamide) being the most common and the most irritating.[1,7] The concentration of OC in pepper spray varies according to the manufacturer and ranges between 1% to 15%.[37]

Although it is often generalized that CN, CS, and CR are tear gas agents and OC is the active ingredient in pepper spray, it is becoming more common for manufacturers to combine OC and CS in RCAs.[4] It is therefore recommended to refer to an agent's safety data sheet to identify the exact active ingredient.

Delivery Methods for Tear Gas and Pepper Spray

Tear gas is not actually a gas, but rather an aerosol of solid particles.[2,40–42] It is usually deployed in canisters that are flung by hand or fired from a launcher.[2] In these devices, CS, CR, or CN is mixed with a pyrotechnic mixture that, on detonation, creates a smoke or fog of the aerosolized solid.[2,7,43] The composition of the pyrotechnic blend varies among manufacturers. They are also delivered as "pepper balls" that resemble and are deployed similarly to paintballs but release the chemical agent on breaking on impact.[4,44,45] They can also be deployed via vehicle-, aircraft-, and drone-mounted delivery systems.[2]

Pepper spray is stored in pressurized containers and released as a stream.[2] Pepper spray is also sometimes deployed in projectiles that are thrown by hand or a launching device.[2]

Effects of Riot Control Agents

The documented clinical effects due to RCAs are highlighted in **Table 2**. CS, CR, CN, and OC primarily cause ocular, respiratory, and dermal irritation.[1,2,10,40] They elicit sensations of pain and burning in the eyes, upper and lower respiratory tract, and skin, which is often described as incapacitating.[1,2] Ocular exposure causes lacrimation, blepharospasm, and conjunctival inflammation.[1,2,46] Unique to OC is its ability to cause a loss of the blink reflex.[1] Corneal abrasions have been reported.[47] More serious ocular injuries such as conjunctival proliferation and corneal erosions have been reported.[48] Rhinal exposure produces mucosal inflammation, rhinorrhea, and sneezing.[46] Respiratory effects include cough, dyspnea, chest tightness, and pulmonary edema.[7,43] If contaminated secretions are swallowed, nausea, vomiting, and gastrointestinal discomfort can occur.[43] Dermal effects include erythema, edema, blistering, chemical burns, and allergic contact dermatitis.[2,49]

Effects usually occur within seconds to minutes of exposure and last several minutes to hours after removal from the source.[2,5,9,37,40,43,49–51] However, reports have described latency periods of days to weeks before symptom onset and symptom

Table 2
Documented potential clinical effects from riot control agents

Organ System	Common Effects	Potential Complications
Neuropsychiatric	Fear Anxiety Headache	Delayed-onset headaches
Ocular	Pain Lacrimation Blepharospasm Conjunctival inflammation	Corneal abrasions Corneal erosions
Rhinic	Inflammation Rhinorrhea Sneezing	
Respiratory	Cough Dyspnea Bronchoconstriction Upper respiratory tract pain and irritation	Pulmonary edema Laryngeal edema Exacerbations of pre-existing pulmonary disease
Gastrointestinal	Nausea Vomiting Discomfort	—
Dermal	Pain Erythema Edema Blistering Chemical burns Allergic contact dermatitis	—

durations of days to weeks after CS exposure.[39,50,52,53] Recently, delayed onset headaches, gastrointestinal effects, and menstrual changes have been reported.[10] The reader is directed to a systematic review of the timing and duration of effects from CS exposure that was published in 2015 for more information.[39]

Although most effects are mild, serious injuries have been reported. A 2017 review of injuries sustained from CS and OC chemical RCAs from January 1, 1990 to March 15, 2015 found 9261 total injuries, with 74.3% being minor (defined as "transient symptoms that may not be present on physical exam or are expected side effects of chemical irritants"), 17% moderate (defined as "those that were unexpected from previous published data on chemical irritants, were evident on physical exam, or lasted longer than expected, but may not require management by a health professional"), and 8.7% being severe (defined as "those that necessitate professional medical management").[4] Out of all injuries from OC, 6% were severe. Of the CS-induced injuries, 27.9% were severe, including 2 deaths and 58 individuals who suffered permanent disabilities including blindness, persistent vegetative state, limb amputations, and functional loss of limbs.[4] One report described an infant who required extracorporeal membrane oxygenation after being accidently sprayed in his face by a pepper spray device that was attached to his mother's keychain.[54] Deaths from laryngeal edema, chemically induced pulmonary edema, and acute necrotizing laryngotracheobronchitis due to CN, CS, and OC exposure have been reported.[3]

Several possible risk factors for the development of more severe adverse clinical affects have been identified (**Box 1**). Longer duration of exposure, higher chemical concentration, and exposure in an enclosed area may result in more severe effects.[2,4,40,41,43,49,54] Those currently with an acute respiratory infection and those with preexisting lung conditions, such as asthma or chronic obstructive pulmonary disease, may have a more severe response following exposure to RCAs.[5,14,55–58] Individuals with a history of cardiac disease or arrhythmias may develop adverse cardiac affects.[2] In addition, a history of rosacea may increase the risk for more serious dermal effects.[53]

One review published in 2017 found that the percentage of people seeking medical care for documented physical injuries after chemical RCA exposure was approximately 9%.[4] However, some posit that this number may underestimate the rate of health care utilization, as a recent survey of people exposed to tear gas during protests in Portland, Oregon found that 54.6% of respondents reported that they received or were planning to seek medical or mental health care following exposure to RCAs.[10] This same survey did not report the number of individuals reporting care at a hospital but did report that 53.4% of those requiring immediate care received it from volunteer medics, 0.6% received immediate care at an onsite medical utility

Box 1
Suspected risk factors for more serious effects from riot control agents

Exposure to high concentrations of riot control agents

Exposure in confined, poorly ventilated areas

Prolonged exposure

Repeated exposure to riot control agents during a single demonstration

Preexisting cardiac and pulmonary disease

Acute respiratory illness

vehicle, and that 6% received professional medical care with "some delay" after the exposure.[10]

Additional Injury Considerations

In addition to the potential for chemical injuries, there are numerous published reports of people being injured from the launched canisters (**Box 2**). Both blunt and penetrating injuries have occurred.[59,60] In 2013, the President of the Turkish Medical Association reported that 10 protesters had lost eyes, one underwent orchiectomy, and others had minor injuries and lacerations after being shot by tear gas canisters.[58] A report detailing injuries occurring at the George Floyd protests in Minneapolis in 2020 describes a person who was struck with a tear gas canister, causing orbital wall fractures, ocular injuries, and legal blindness in one eye.[61] A study detailing injuries from RCAs deployed during protests in Beirut, Lebanon from October 2019 to February 2020 found that although most tear gas exposures did not cause major complications, 8 injuries, including skull fractures, facial fractures, and a subarachnoid hemorrhage, were due to the impact of launched tear gas canisters.[6] One retrospective chart review of patients admitted to the neurosurgery service at the Neurosurgery Teaching Hospital in Baghdad, Iraq in 2019 identified 41 patients with tear gas canister-related head injuries, 10 of which were fatal penetrating head injuries.[60] A systematic review of injuries from chemical RCAs from 1990 to 2015 reported 231 injuries from projectiles, with 63 being severe.[4] Other articles have described various fractures, maxillofacial injuries, soft tissue injuries and lacerations, and ocular injuries resulting from the impact of launched canisters.[5,44,59,62–64]

Both the active ingredient in the RCA as well as the solvents, propellants, and other ingredients, including the "inactive ingredients," may cause toxic effects, especially to the eyes.[4,40] Methyl-isobutyl ketone, which can induce ocular, upper respiratory, and dermal injuries, and tetrachloroethylene, which may cause pulmonary edema, have been used as solvents for OC and CS agents.[37,54,65] Other solvents that have been used include water, alcohols, and nonflammable organic solvents.[37] Various propellants have been used, including nitrogen, butane, propane, carbon dioxide, and halogenated hydrocarbons.[9,37,54] These other substances may induce additional chemical injuries, but a discussion of their toxicities is beyond the scope of this article.[37]

Reports have been published describing burns from those exposed to aerosolized CS.[49] Burn injuries include chemical burns from CS, contact burns from hot tear gas

Box 2
Documented injuries from riot control agent canisters as projectiles

Blunt head trauma

Intracranial hemorrhage

Penetrating head trauma

Blunt and penetrating ocular injuries

Maxillofacial and orbital wall fractures

Soft tissue bruising

Soft tissue lacerations

Bone fractures

Functional loss of limbs from neurovascular injuries

Testicular trauma

canisters and grenades, and thermal burns from the heat released during the of the ignition of the pyrotechnic mixture in the delivery devices.[49]

Mechanism of Action

The effects of CN, CS, CR, and OC are mediated by agonism of transient receptor potential (TRP) ion channels. Several reviews of these channels have been published recently.[15,66] Briefly, TRP ion channels are one of the several types of sensitizing chemosensory receptors found on peripheral sensory neurons.[14,66] Two subfamilies of TRP ion channels are transient receptor potential ankyrin (TRPA) and transient receptor potential vanilloid (TRPV).[14,15] When bound by an agonist, these receptors cause the characteristic pain and effects associated with chemical irritants.[14,15,66] Most research has been focused on the effects mediated by the TRPA1 and TRPV1 receptors.[15] Capsaicin is an agonist of TRPV1.[2,67] CS, CR, and CN are agonists of TRPA1.[13,14]

TRPV1 was discovered in 1997.[67] It is located on the sensory nerves of the trigeminal, vagal, and dorsal root ganglia.[2] Agonists of this receptor include capsaicin, temperatures greater than 43° C, and acids with a pH less than 5.3.[2,15] When stimulated, they elicit pain in the eyes, nose, upper and lower respiratory tract, and skin.[2,15] In addition, TRPV1 stimulation triggers sneezing, cough, and hypersecretion of mucus.[15]

CS, CR, and CN are agonists of TRPA1.[13,14] TRPA1 is found on trigeminal nerve fibers that innervate the skin of the face, mucous membranes, eyes, nose, and respiratory tract. When stimulated, they evoke pain and produce lacrimation, rhinorrhea, blepharospasm, cough, sneezing, bronchospasm, and pulmonary edema.[14,15]

Diagnosis of CS, CN, CR, and OC Exposure

Diagnosis is based on history and clinical examination findings. CN, CR, CS, and OC can be detected by gas-liquid chromatography and mass spectrometry, but its clinical usefulness in the acute setting is limited.[7]

Non-RCA Chemical Agent Use Against Authorities by Rioters

Chemical agents dispersed in a crowd are not always released by the authorities. Some rioters are releasing chemical agents, some with marked human toxicity and intended to cause permanent injury or death. On April 6, 2019, four adult men and a minor threw a chemical weapon at a police officer, causing a spontaneous ignition. The officer lost consciousness, had difficulty breathing, and was taken to the hospital to be treated for chlorine exposure.[68,69] In 2020, a federal case concluded with the defendant sentenced for attempting to purchase dimethylmercury on the darknet for suspected planned use against authorities.[70] On October 17, 2020, violent demonstrators threw an unknown chemical at police officers at a rally in San Francisco, California, which resulted in two officers requiring medical care for ocular, respiratory, and dermal injuries.[68] On April 17, 2021, a Molotov cocktail and liquid bleach was thrown in the face of a New York City Police Department officer.[69] First responders and hospital personnel must be vigilant and not assume that a chemical released during a riot is a traditional RCA.

Decontamination

Steps need to be taken to remove the chemical from the patient and prevent secondary exposure and contamination of unaffected areas. All individuals contaminated with tear gas, pepper spray, or another chemical will require decontamination. Triage should place exposed individuals in a predesignated "dirty" area near the decontamination area.[71] This specialty triage holding area should be augmented by medical personnel to continuously monitor the clinical status of the contaminated individuals. Concurrently, observing patients exposed to these RCAs for exacerbation of underlying medical conditions is highly encouraged. Some patients who have been exposed to these agents may exhibit signs of decompensation while waiting in queue to be processed through the decontamination area. Recognizing this impact and reprioritizing them vis-à-vis moving them to the front of the decontamination line will be critical to expediting patient care intervention. Moreover, the direct threat to medical personnel conducting decontamination includes contact transfer of agents between patient and clinician. All personnel involved with the decontamination and treatment of chemically exposed patients should wear appropriate personal protective equipment to minimize the risk of secondary contamination, which includes a face shield and/or goggles, a chemical-resistant suit, gloves, and respiratory protection such as a respirator with cartridges designed to filter RCAs, a powered air purifying respirator (PAPRs), or a self-contained breathing apparatus (SCBA).[7,71] Reports of prehospital and hospital personnel being secondary contaminated with CS and becoming symptomatic have been published.[9,71]

Various decontamination methods and treatments have been described in the literature. During demonstrations in Turkey in 2013, some applied lemon juice to their eyes in order to protect them from tear gas, but it was not effective.[58] Several studies have shown that Diphoterine, which is a hypertonic, amphoteric, and chelating agent, decreases pain levels and allows for a faster recovery in those prophylactically treated with it before being exposed to CS and decreased pain levels in those treated postexposure to CS.[41,72] However, it is not approved by the Food and Drug Administration in the United States. Topical use of antacid solutions that contain calcium or magnesium have been used to treat dermal pain caused by capsaicin but published studies have produced conflicting results regarding their efficacy.[58,73–75] A randomized control trial published in 2008 compared the efficacy of aluminum-hydroxide-magnesium hydroxide antacid, 2% lidocaine gel, baby shampoo, milk, and water in treating acute pain from topical OC-containing pepper spray and found no statistical difference in pain relief among them.[46] In 2018, a prospective, randomized control trial comparing the efficacy of baby shampoo plus water versus water alone in reducing dermal pain from OC or CS exposure found that irrigation with water plus baby shampoo did not provide better pain relief than water alone.[76] Water is currently the preferred decontamination agent, as no other method has consistently shown superiority.

Treatment

There are no antidotes to chemical RCAs.[46] Standard treatment is removal from the source and decontamination.[2,40] Exposed individuals should be removed from the contaminated area and into a well-ventilated area with free-flowing air.[37,77] Contaminated clothing should be cut off the victim, preferably outside health care facilities.[77] Clothes should not be pulled over the head or face due to the risk of further contaminating those surfaces.[77] Clothing should be sealed in double plastic bags and placed in a safe location away from decontaminated individuals.[40,77] Humidified supplemental oxygen may improve respiratory symptoms.[40] Bronchospasm should be treated with bronchodilators such as beta-2 agonists.[37] Those who have persistent respiratory symptoms may need admission to the hospital.[37] Laryngospasm may occur, and intubation may be necessary for severe respiratory symptoms.[7] Some investigators have suggested that ocular contamination should first be treated by blowing dry air directly onto the eye to vaporize any dissolved CS that may be present, but no randomized control trial has been conducted to determine the efficacy of this practice.[49] Contact lenses should be removed, and the eyes should be irrigated copiously with water or saline.[40,49] If ocular symptoms persist after irrigation, then a thorough eye examination including fluorescein staining, visual acuity, and slit-lamp testing should be considered.[40,49] Ophthalmology consultation should be considered for persistent symptoms or abnormal findings on eye examination.[7,51] The skin should be irrigated with water.[40] Dermal burns and injuries can be managed with standard care.[37] Pain may require analgesics, which may need to be administered intravenously if oral mucous membranes or respiratory symptoms preclude safe oral administration.[46] For those incidents that occur in the United States, emergency medical personnel should notify the US Poison Control Center by calling 1-800-222-1222. They can give clinical management recommendations and will log the incident into the US National Poison Data System for toxin and public health surveillance.

Future Developments

Antagonists of TRPA1 and TRPV1 have been developed.[14,15,78] Animal studies have demonstrated that they can prevent pain and irritation when exposed to CN and CS.[14] Several biopharmaceutical companies are currently researching these substances as possible therapeutics for respiratory disease and chemically induced injuries.[15] However, these agents are not currently available to purchase or prescribe.

The Reactive Skin Decontamination Lotion (RSDL) Kit has been studied as a potential tool for decontamination of CN, CS, and capsaicin. The kit is composed of a sponge impregnated with a lotion containing potassium 2,3-butanedione monoxime (KBDO) dissolved in a polyethylene glycol monomethyl ether (MPEG) solvent.[79,80] The sponge is rubbed on contaminated skin, allowing the toxic substance to mix with the lotion and be neutralized. In addition, the sponge absorbs the toxin, permitting both neutralization and removal of the chemical to occur.[79] A 2020 study evaluating the liquid phase reactivity of the active lotion component found that it effectively and rapidly degrades CN, is moderately effective in degrading CS, and does not breakdown capsaicin.[80] This study did not include the removal effect of the sponge on these chemicals, however. Further studies will need to be conducted to determine the efficacy of the RSDL Kit on CS, CN, and capsaicin exposures.[80]

CRITICAL CARE POINTS

- All patients exposed to chemical RCAs should have contaminated clothes removed. Contact lenses should be removed. Eyes and all affected body surfaces should be copiously irrigated with water.
- All personnel treating patients exposed to chemical RCAs should wear appropriate personal protective equipment such as goggles or a face shield, respiratory protection such as a respirator with cartridges designed to filter RCAs, a PAPRs, or a SCBA, a chemical resistant suit, and gloves.
- There is no antidote to chemical RCAs. Treat all injuries with standard wound care. Specialist care may be needed.

DISCLOSURE

The authors have nothing to disclose.

REFERENCES

1. Olajos EJ, Salem H. Riot control agents: pharmacology, toxicology, biochemistry and chemistry. J Appl Toxicol 2001;21(5):355–91.

2. Rothenberg C, Achanta S, Svendsen ER, et al. Tear gas: an epidemiological and mechanistic reassessment. Ann N Y Acad Sci 2016;1378(1):96–107.
3. Toprak S, Ersoy G, Hart J, et al. The pathology of lethal exposure to the riot control agents: towards a forensics-based methodology for determining misuse. J Forensic Leg Med 2015;29:36–42.
4. Haar RJ, Iacopino V, Ranadive N, et al. Health impacts of chemical irritants used for crowd control: a systematic review of the injuries and deaths caused by tear gas and pepper spray. BMC Public Health 2017;17(1):831.
5. Unuvar U, Ozkalipci O, Irencin S, et al. Demonstration control agents: evaluation of 64 cases after massive use in Istanbul. Am J Forensic Med Pathol 2013;34(2): 150–4.
6. El Zahran T, Mostafa H, Hamade H, et al. Riot-related injuries managed at a hospital in Beirut, Lebanon. Am J Emerg Med 2021;42:55–9.
7. Vaca FE, Myers JH, Langdorf M. Delayed pulmonary edema and bronchospasm after accidental lacrimator exposure. Am J Emerg Med 1996;14(4):402–5.
8. Haar RJ, Iacopino V, Ranadive N, et al. Death, injury and disability from kinetic impact projectiles in crowd-control settings: a systematic review. BMJ Open 2017;7(12):e018154.
9. Hankin SM, Ramsay CN. Investigation of accidental secondary exposure to CS agent. Clin Toxicol (Phila) 2007;45(4):409–11.
10. Torgrimson-Ojerio BN, Mularski KS, Peyton MR, et al. Health issues and health-care utilization among adults who reported exposure to tear gas during 2020 Portland (OR) protests: a cross-sectional survey. BMC Public Health 2021; 21(1):803.
11. West CJ. The history of poison gases. Science 1919;49(1270):412–7.
12. Jones DP. From military to civilian technology: the introduction of tear gas for civil riot control. Technol Cult 1978;19(2):151–68.
13. Brône B, Peeters PJ, Marrannes R, et al. Tear gasses CN, CR, and CS are potent activators of the human TRPA1 receptor. Toxicol Appl Pharmacol 2008;231(2): 150–6.
14. Bessac BF, Sivula M, von Hehn CA, et al. Transient receptor potential ankyrin 1 antagonists block the noxious effects of toxic industrial isocyanates and tear gases. FASEB J 2009;23(4):1102–14.
15. Achanta S, Jordt S-E. Transient receptor potential channels in pulmonary chemical injuries and as countermeasure targets. Ann N Y Acad Sci 2020;1480(1): 73–103.
16. Pepper Spray Frequently Asked Questions. Sabre red. https://www.sabrered.com/pepper-spray-frequently-asked-questions-0. [Accessed 30 August 2021]. Accessed.
17. Bear Spray. Sabre Red. https://www.sabrered.com/bear-spray. [Accessed 30 August 2021]. Accessed.
18. Protector Dog Sprays. Sabre Red. https://www.sabrered.com/protector-dog-sprays. [Accessed 30 August 2021]. Accessed.
19. Unit RSRS is a reporter for the NNI. Unbearable pain: How bear spray became a prized weapon for violent protesters. NBC News. https://www.nbcnews.com/news/us-news/unbearable-pain-how-bear-spray-became-prized-weapon-violent-protesters-n1261615. [Accessed 30 August 2021]. Accessed.
20. Bear spray is showing up at protests and riots. Here's why, and how it affects humans. Wash Post. Available at: https://www.washingtonpost.com/lifestyle/wellness/bear-spray-pepper-riot-dangerous/2021/03/19/053c3870-87fb-11eb-bfdf-4d36dab83a6d_story.html. Accessed August 30, 2021.

21. Oregonian/OregonLive MB| T. Counter-protesters, photojournalist file battery, assault lawsuit against alleged Proud Boys affiliates. Oregonlive 2020. Accessed. https://www.oregonlive.com/crime/2020/09/counter-protesters-photojournalist-file-battery-assault-lawsuit-against-alleged-proud-boy-affiliates.html. [Accessed 30 August 2021]. Available at:.
22. Reporter JT-S. As lawmakers meet, protesters attempt to storm Capitol building. Salem Reporter 2020. Accessed. https://www.salemreporter.com/posts/3322/as-lawmakers-meet-protesters-attempt-to-storm-capitol-building. [Accessed 30 August 2021]. Available at:.
23. Cline S, America AP for. Protestors try to force their way into Oregon Capitol, use bear spray on police. East Ida News 2020. Accessed. https://www.eastidahonews.com/2020/12/protestors-try-to-force-their-way-into-oregon-capitol-use-bear-spray-on-police/. [Accessed 30 August 2021]. Available at:.
24. WJLA KS. Videos show bear spray attack on Capitol officers during Jan. 6 riot. WBMA. Accessed. https://abc3340.com/news/nation-world/videos-show-bear-spray-attack-on-capitol-officers-during-jan-6-riot. [Accessed 30 August 2021]. Available at:.
25. Two charged for pepper-spraying police officer who died after assault on U.S. Capitol. Reuters 2021. Available at: https://www.reuters.com/article/us-usa-capitol-arrests-idUSKBN2B7213. Accessed August 30, 2021.
26. 11 arrested for having pepper spray at Capitol demonstrations | Updates. abc10.com. Accessed. https://www.abc10.com/article/news/local/sacramento/hundreds-gather-at-sacramento-capitol-to-protest-2020-election/103-d2e330bd-1268-404f-8edc-bc97bef71629. [Accessed 30 August 2021]. Available at:.
27. Portland police: detained protesters had bear spray, hammers. AP NEWS. 2021. Available at: https://apnews.com/article/portland-oregon-racial-injustice-5b1374cb4b7eff6d2ab860beaf28d9b7. Accessed August 30, 2021.
28. New Jersey Regional Operarations and Intelligence Center (ROIC) Threat Analysis Unit. Violent Demonstration Tactics and Trends. Reference Guide. Published June 5, 2020.
29. 1925 Geneva Protocol – UNODA. Accessed. https://www.un.org/disarmament/wmd/bio/1925-geneva-protocol/. [Accessed 13 August 2021]. Available at:.
30. Executive orders. National Archives. 2016. Available at: https://www.archives.gov/federal-register/codification/executive-order/11850.html. Accessed August 13, 2021.
31. History. OPCW. Accessed. https://www.opcw.org/about/history. [Accessed 13 August 2021]. Available at:.
32. Chemical weapons convention. OPCW. Available at: https://www.opcw.org/chemical-weapons-convention. Accessed August 13, 2021.
33. http://usnwc.libguides.com USNWCRG. Commander's Handbook on the Law of Naval Operations. In: Homeland security digital library. United States: Office of the Chief of Naval Operations; 2017. Available at: https://www.hsdl.org/?abstract&did=. Accessed August 13, 2021.
34. Customary IHL - rule 75. Riot control agents. Available at: https://ihl-databases.icrc.org/customary-ihl/eng/docs/v1_rul_rule75. Accessed August 13, 2021.
35. Customary international humanitarian law. 2016. Available at: https://www.icrc.org/en/document/customary-international-humanitarian-law-0. Accessed August 13, 2021.
36. Corson BB, Stoughton RW. Reactions OF Alpha, Beta-unsaturated dinitriles. J Am Chem Soc 1928;50(10):2825–37.

37. Smith J, Greaves I. The use of chemical incapacitant sprays: a review. J Trauma 2002;52(3):595–600.
38. Blain PG. Tear gases and irritant incapacitants. 1-chloroacetophenone, 2-chlorobenzylidene malononitrile and dibenz[b,f]-1,4-oxazepine. Toxicol Rev 2003;22(2): 103–10.
39. Dimitroglou Y, Rachiotis G, Hadjichristodoulou C. Exposure to the riot control agent CS and potential health effects: a systematic review of the evidence. Int J Environ Res Public Health 2015;12(2):1397–411.
40. Breakell A, Bodiwala GG. CS gas exposure in a crowded night club: the consequences for an accident and emergency department. J Accid Emerg Med 1998; 15(1):56–7.
41. Viala B, Blomet J, Mathieu L, et al. Prevention of CS "tear gas" eye and skin effects and active decontamination with Diphoterine: preliminary studies in 5 French Gendarmes. J Emerg Med 2005;29(1):5–8.
42. Henry J. CS "gas" is not a gas. J Accid Emerg Med 1998;15(5):365.
43. Hu H, Fine J, Epstein P, et al. Tear gas–harassing agent or toxic chemical weapon? JAMA 1989;262(5):660–3.
44. Ifantides C, Deitz GA, Christopher KL, et al. Less-lethal weapons resulting in ophthalmic injuries: a review and recent example of eye trauma. Ophthalmol Ther 2020;9(3):1–7.
45. Hay A, Giacaman R, Sansur R, et al. Skin injuries caused by new riot control agent used against civilians on the West Bank. Med Confl Surviv 2006;22(4): 283–91. https://doi.org/10.1080/13623690600945180.
46. Barry JD, Hennessy R, McManus JG. A randomized controlled trial comparing treatment regimens for acute pain for topical oleoresin capsaicin (pepper spray) exposure in adult volunteers. Prehosp Emerg Care 2008;12(4):432–7.
47. Watson WA, Stremel KR, Westdorp EJ. Oleoresin capsicum (Cap-Stun) toxicity from aerosol exposure. Ann Pharmacother 1996;30(7–8):733–5.
48. Gerber S, Frueh BE, Tappeiner C. Conjunctival proliferation after a mild pepper spray injury in a young child. Cornea 2011;30(9):1042–4.
49. Agrawal Y, Thornton D, Phipps A. CS gas–completely safe? A burn case report and literature review. Burns 2009;35(6):895–7.
50. Roth VS, Franzblau A. RADS after exposure to a riot-control agent: a case report. J Occup Environ Med 1996;38(9):863–5.
51. Solomon I, Kochba I, Eizenkraft E, et al. Report of accidental CS ingestion among seven patients in central Israel and review of the current literature. Arch Toxicol 2003;77(10):601–4.
52. Hu H, Christiani D. Reactive airways dysfunction after exposure to teargas. Lancet 1992;339(8808):1535.
53. Watson K, Rycroft R. Unintended cutaneous reactions to CS spray. Contact Dermatitis 2005;53(1):9–13.
54. Billmire DF, Vinocur C, Ginda M, et al. Pepper-spray-induced respiratory failure treated with extracorporeal membrane oxygenation. Pediatrics 1996;98(5):961–3.
55. Karagama YG, Newton JR, Newbegin CJR. Short-term and long-term physical effects of exposure to CS spray. J R Soc Med 2003;96(4):172–4.
56. Zholos AV. TRP channels in respiratory pathophysiology: the role of oxidative, chemical irritant and temperature stimuli. Curr Neuropharmacol 2015;13(2): 279–91.
57. Bessac BF, Jordt S-E. Breathtaking TRP channels: TRPA1 and TRPV1 in airway chemosensation and reflex control. Physiology (Bethesda) 2008;23:360–70.

58. Aktan AO. Tear gas is a chemical weapon, and Turkey should not use it to torture civilians. BMJ 2013;346(11 2):f3801.
59. Wani AA, Zargar J, Ramzan AU, et al. Head injury caused by tear gas cartridge in teenage population. Pediatr Neurosurg 2010;46(1):25–8.
60. Hoz SS, Aljuboori ZS, Dolachee AA, et al. Fatal Penetrating Head Injuries Caused by Projectile Tear Gas Canisters. World Neurosurg 2020;138:e119–23.
61. Kaske EA, Cramer SW, Pena Pino I, et al. Injuries from less-lethal weapons during the george floyd protests in Minneapolis. N Engl J Med 2021;384(8): 774–5.
62. Alhillo HT, Arnaout MM, Radhi HS, et al. Direct head injury caused by a tear gas cartridge. Questions on safety: A case report from Iraq and review of the literature. J Clin Neurosci 2018;56:179–82.
63. Clarot F, Vaz E, Papin F, et al. Lethal head injury due to tear-gas cartridge gunshots. Forensic Sci Int 2003;137(1):45–51.
64. Çorbacıoğlu ŞK, Güler S, Er E, et al. Rare and severe maxillofacial injury due to tear gas capsules: report of three cases. J Forensic Sci 2016;61(2):551–4.
65. Wheeler H, MacLehose R, Euripidou E, et al. Surveillance into crowd control agents. Lancet Lond Engl 1998;352(9132):991–2.
66. Dietrich A, Steinritz D, Gudermann T. Transient receptor potential (TRP) channels as molecular targets in lung toxicology and associated diseases. Cell Calcium 2017;67:123–37.
67. Caterina MJ, Schumacher MA, Tominaga M, et al. The capsaicin receptor: a heat-activated ion channel in the pain pathway. Nature 1997;389(6653): 816–24.
68. 4 men sentenced for ambushing Arvada Police officer with chlorine bomb. KUSA.-com. 2020. Available at: https://www.9news.com/article/news/crime/sentencing-arvada-chlorine-bomb/73-4ce54059-fd06-49dd-a986-cd7b1b549a17. Accessed September 1, 2021.
69. Situational Awareness Bulletin. Improvised Chemical Weapons Pose Potential Threat to Law Enforcement Officers. Published online April 11, 2019.
70. First Responder Primer: Dimethylmercury (DMM).
71. Horton DK, Burgess P, Rossiter S, et al. Secondary contamination of emergency department personnel from o-chlorobenzylidene malononitrile exposure, 2002. Ann Emerg Med 2005;45(6):655–8.
72. Brvar M. Chlorobenzylidene malononitrile tear gas exposure: Rinsing with amphoteric, hypertonic, and chelating solution. Hum Exp Toxicol 2016;35(2): 213–8.
73. Kim-Katz SY, Anderson IB, Kearney TE, et al. Topical antacid therapy for capsaicin-induced dermal pain: a poison center telephone-directed study. Am J Emerg Med 2010;28(5):596–602.
74. Herman LM, Kindschu MW, Shallash AJ. Treatment of mace dermatitis with topical antacid suspension. Am J Emerg Med 1998;16(6):613–4.
75. Lee DC, Ryan JR. Magnesium-aluminum hydroxide suspension for the treatment of dermal capsaicin exposures. Acad Emerg Med 2003;10(6):688–90.
76. Stopyra JP, Winslow JE, Johnson JC, et al. Baby Shampoo to relieve the discomfort of tear gas and pepper spray exposure: a randomized controlled trial. West J Emerg Med 2018;19(2):294–300.
77. Carron P-N, Yersin B. Management of the effects of exposure to tear gas. BMJ 2009;338:b2283.

78. Cui M, Gosu V, Basith S, et al. Polymodal transient receptor potential vanilloid type 1 nocisensor: structure, modulators, and therapeutic applications. Adv Protein Chem Struct Biol 2016;104:81–125.
79. Fentabil M, Gebremedhin M, Purdon JG, et al. Degradation of pesticides with RSDL® (reactive skin decontamination lotion kit) lotion: LC-MS investigation. Toxicol Lett 2018;293:241–8. https://doi.org/10.1016/j.toxlet.2017.11.003.
80. Gebremedhin M, Fentabil M, Cochrane L, et al. In vitro decontamination efficacy of the RSDL® (Reactive Skin Decontamination Lotion Kit) lotion component against riot control agents: Capsaicin, Mace™ (CN) and CS. Toxicol Lett 2020;332:36–41.

The Roles of Antidotes in Emergency Situations

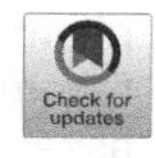

Sasha K. Kaiser, MD, Richard C. Dart, MD, PhD*

KEYWORDS

• Antidote • Methylene blue • Acetylcysteine • Fomepizole • Hydroxocobalamin
• Intralipid • Lipid emulsion • Levocarnitine

KEY POINTS

- Most poisoned patients recover with supportive care; however, when the exposure has been identified, consider specific antidote administration.
- Antidote administration is most effective when given early in the patient course.
- Poison center consultation can provide guidance for selection, dosing, and management of antidote administration. The US national toll-free hotline is 1-800- 222-1222.

ANTIDOTE STOCKING

Antidotes are commonly used to reduce or eliminate the toxic effects of a poison. Often, there is no acceptable substitute. Although recognized over 25 years ago, numerous publications documenting insufficient stocking of antidotes by hospitals in the United States and many other countries continue to be published.[1–4] The medical and financial implications can be enormous. Failing to use the antidote for acetaminophen, for example, can lead to acute liver failure, which may result in liver transplant or death.

In the United States, there is no regulation requiring hospitals to adequately stock antidotes. A joint position statement of the American College of Medical Toxicology and the American Academy of Clinical Toxicology acknowledges the issues and calls for several measures to address the problem. Consensus guidelines for antidote stocking by hospitals that accept emergency patients have been published.[5] These guidelines recommend 44 antidotes for stocking, of which 23 should be available for immediate administration. In most hospitals, this timeframe requires that the antidote be stocked in the emergency department or other location that allows immediate administration. Another 14 antidotes were recommended for availability within 1 hour of the decision to administer, allowing the antidote to be stocked in the hospital

Rocky Mountain Poison and Drug Safety, Denver Health and Hospital Authority, 1391 Speer Boulevard, Suite 600, Denver, CO 80204, USA
* Corresponding author.
E-mail address: Richard.Dart@rmpds.org

Emerg Med Clin N Am 40 (2022) 381–394
https://doi.org/10.1016/j.emc.2022.01.008

pharmacy if the hospital has a mechanism for prompt delivery of antidotes. The panel recommended that each hospital perform a formal antidote hazard vulnerability assessment to determine its specific need for antidote stocking. Antidote administration is an important part of emergency care. These expert recommendations provide a tool for hospitals that offer emergency care to provide appropriate care to poisoned patients.

METHYLENE BLUE

Methylene blue (Provayblue) is commonly used in methemoglobinemia; however, there has been increased interest in utilization for metformin toxicity and cases of refractory vasoplegia.

Mitochondria are the major sites for reactive oxygen species (ROS) production. In metformin toxicity, excessive ROS production overwhelms endogenous clearance capabilities, resulting in impaired bioenergetics and hyperlactatemia.[6,7] In normal oxidative phosphorylation physiology, electrons are fed into complex I or II of the electron transport chain (ETC) from NADH and $FADH_2$. A subsequent series of redox reactions continue the transfer of electrons through different protein complexes. The electron shuttling establishes an electrochemical gradient that is used by complex I to generate adenosine triphosphate (ATP). Supratherapeutic metformin exposure inhibits redox shuttle enzymes, resulting in an altered redox state.[8–11] Methylene blue has been proposed as an alternative electron carrier[7] that bypasses the initial protein complexes with direct delivery of electrons to cytochrome c or ubiquinone. This direct transfer reduces electron leakage and diminishes ROS production.[12] This mechanism has been proposed for the improved hemodynamic response in cases of severe metformin toxicity when used in addition to other resuscitative modalities.[13–16]

Improved hemodynamic stability with the addition of methylene blue in refractory vasoplegia has been reported in cardiopulmonary bypass literature,[17–28] septic shock,[29–32] and radiocontrast anaphylaxis.[33] In addition to acting as an alternative electron carrier, methylene blue inhibits endothelial nitric oxidase synthase (eNOS) and guanylate cyclase (GC) activation, resulting in improved vascular tone.[34,35] Excessive formation of nitric oxide (NO) in distributive shock states leads to profound vasodilation, decreased catecholamine response, and potential myocardial depression through multiple mechanisms. Toxicity from cardioactive xenobiotics with additional vasodilatory mechanisms beyond traditional adrenergic receptor antagonism may benefit from direct GC inhibition. In a systematic review of refractory shock following systemic poisoning, 9 of 17 patients treated with methylene blue demonstrated hemodynamic improvement after failing to adequately respond to intravenous fluid and vasopressor administration.[36]

Caution and Contraindications

Caution should be utilized in patients with known glucose-6-phosphate dehydrogenase deficiency, as these patients are at risk of hemolytic anemia.[37] Additionally, methylene blue is a monoamine oxidase inhibitor and should be used in caution in patients with serotoninergic toxicity.[38]

Dosage and Available Formulations

Intravenous methylene blue is supplied in 5 and 10 mg/mL solutions. Dosing is often based on methemoglobinemia treatment: 1 to 2 mg/kg over 5 to 30 minutes. Local pain and irritation can be minimalized by dilution in 50 mL of 5% dextrose in water. Sodium chloride should be avoided, as this can decrease methylene blue solubility.[39]

Methylene blue can be repeated in 1 hour if there are persistent clinical signs or symptoms.[40] Doses greater than 7 mg/kg have been associated with decreased splanchnic flow and are not recommended.[30]

In a systematic review, patients who received intralipid administration prior to methylene blue were less likely to have hemodynamic improvement,[36] perhaps due to lipophilic sequestration.[41]

Adverse Reactions

Adverse effects associated with methylene blue administration include blue/green urine discoloration,[42] skin discoloration, dysgeusia, hyperhidrosis, nausea, dizziness, and headache.[40]

Skin necrosis and fat necrosis have been reported in tissue extravasation[43] or when used in lymph node biopsy.[44] Methylene blue interferes with oxygen monitoring, resulting in transient factitious low pulse oximetry saturation readings.[37]

HYDROXOCOBALAMIN

Hydroxocobalamin has US Food and Drug Administration (FDA) indications for cyanide toxicity.[45] It has been suggested for treatment of refractory vasoplegic states as an adjunctive, catecholamine-sparing, modality.[46] In cyanide toxicity, hydroxocobalamin resuscitates oxidative phosphorylation by forming cyanocobalamin, resulting in removal of cyanide from the mitochondrial ETC.[47] The mechanism behind hydroxocobalamin is similar to methylene blue: scavenging NO, thus mitigating vasodilatation.[48,49] In a healthy volunteer study, transient increase in blood pressure following hydroxocobalamin administration occurred, with return to baseline 4 hours after infusion.[50]

Clinical experience with hydroxocobalamin in refractory shock is limited but has shown promise in animal models.[51,52] Case reports with improved hemodynamic response following hydroxocobalamin administration are reported in cardiac surgery,[53–55] liver transplantation,[56,57] and vascular surgery.[58] In a case series of patients undergoing cardiopulmonary bypass, administration of hydroxocobalamin was associated with a 24% reduction in vasopressor requirements within 30 minutes.[59]

Caution and Contraindications

Specific contraindications have not been determined.[45,60]

Dosage and Available Formulations

Hydroxocobalamin is available as a vial containing 5 g of lyophilized hydroxocobalamin as a crystalized powder. In adults, the initial dose is 5 g delivered over 15 minutes; this can be repeated for a total of 10 g depending on the patient's response.[60] In a systematic review of patients being treated for refractory vasoplegia, most patients received 5 g of hydroxocobalamin.[46,61]

Adverse Reactions

Administration of high-dose hydroxocobalamin is generally well tolerated. Hydroxocobalamin can result in red-orange skin discoloration that resolves in 24 to 48 hours.[46,62] Chromaturia has been reported to last up to 6 weeks and may interfere with routine urinalysis.[46,61] Hydroxocobalamin has been associated with the development of oxalate nephropathy and acute kidney injury in critically ill burn patients.[63–65]

Allergic reactions have been reported with chronic use but not known to occur in single-dose therapy.[62] Hydroxocobalamin is associated with laboratory interference resulting in inaccurate hemoglobin, aspartate aminotransferase, creatinine, bilirubin, and international normalized ratio (INR), among others.[46,62] Finally, in certain hemodialysis machines, a false blood leak alarm may be triggered.[66]

N-ACETYLCYSTEINE

Acetylcysteine is a highly effective antidote for acetaminophen poisoning. As with most antidotes, efficacy depends on timing of administration with increased benefit when administered 8 hours from acute acetaminophen ingestion.[67]

Caution and Contraindications

The primary contraindication is previous hypersensitivity to acetylcysteine.[68] It should be used with caution in patients with history of severe asthmatic disease.[69]

Dosage and Available Formulations

Acetylcysteine is supplied in an intravenous solution of 200 mg/mL, as well as in oral capsules and powders that range from 500 to 1700 mg.[68] The intravenous solution is diluted with 5% dextrose.[69] Intravenous dosing in the United States is based on a 2- or 3-bag approach. In both of these regimens, the patient receives 300 mg/kg.[70]

3-bag approach[71]

- 150 mg/kg over 1 hour
- 50 mg/kg/h for 4 hours (12.5 mg/kg/h for 4 hours)
- 100 mg/kg/h for 16 hours (6.25 mg/kg/h for 16 hours)

2-bag approach[70]

- 200 mg/kg over 4 hours (50 mg/kg/h for 4 hours)
- 100 mg/kg over 16 hours (6.25 mg/kg/h for 16 hours)

Increased understanding of acetaminophen toxicity has led to a proposal of alternate dosing regimens. Patients with massive acetaminophen ingestions may still go on to develop hepatotoxicity despite treatment with acetylcysteine.[72,73] Acetylcysteine dosing modifications have been proposed to meet glutathione depletion in higher toxic burdens.[71,74] Although dose recommendations vary, adjustments are often advocated when the serum concentration exceeds 300 μg/mL.[74,75] Proposed administration options include increasing the concentration administered or the maintenance infusion rate. In these situations, consultation with a poison center is strongly encouraged.

Additional changes in acetylcysteine administration have centered around duration of therapy. In acute ingestions the patients may still have actionable acetaminophen concentrations following completion of the 20-hour or 21-hour protocol. Patients with persistent detectable acetaminophen concentrations or abnormal aminotransferase may benefit from ongoing acetylcysteine. Again, consultation with a poison center is highly recommended.[71,72] In the United States, the national toll-free hotline number is 1-800-222-1222.

Adverse Reactions

Intravenous acetylcysteine is well tolerated, but has several adverse effects including maculopapular rash, nausea, vomiting, diarrhea, and cutaneous anaphylactoid reactions. Anaphylactoid reactions are more common in the first hour of therapy, during which time the patient is exposed to the most concentrated acetylcysteine. Symptoms can be mitigated with antihistamines, beta agonists in asthmatics, and temporary discontinuation of the infusion with resumption at a lower rate.[76] The rate of adverse drug reactions is decreased in patients treated with the 2-bag protocol compared with the 3-bag protocol without increase in hepatotoxicity.[77]

FOMEPIZOLE

Fomepizole is an effective first-line antidote for the treatment of ethylene glycol and methanol poisoning. Mechanistically, it competitively inhibits hepatic alcohol dehydrogenase, curtailing the formation of toxic metabolites.[78,79] Fomepizole has recently gained interest as a potential therapeutic adjunct in the treatment of acetaminophen toxicity.

Fomepizole inhibits CYP2E1, a key enzyme mediator in acetaminophen toxicity. After a therapeutic dose, greater than 90% of acetaminophen undergoes glucuronidation and sulfation to form inactive metabolites. Approximately 5% of acetaminophen is oxidized via CYP2E1 to form the toxic metabolite N-acetyl-p-benzoquinoneimine (NAPQI).[80] Anecdotal evidence for fomepizole was first described in 2013 in a patient presenting with severe metabolic derangements and alteration in mental status. The patient recovered with a benign clinical course following early treatment with acetylcysteine and a single dose of fomepizole.[81] Fomepizole reduces oxidative metabolism of acetaminophen to NAPQI [82] and likely decreases amplification of NAPQI-induced injury by reducing the activation of c-Jun N-terminal kinase (JNK).[83] Although multiple case reports support its use, use with acetylcysteine, clinical trials have not yet been performed.[84–91]

Caution and Contraindications

Hypersensitivity to pyrazoles is a relative contraindication.[92]

Dosage and Available Formulations

Fomepizole is available in 1.5 mL vials containing 1 g/mL that is diluted with a 100 mL of normal saline or 5% dextrose in water. Case reports have used single doses of 15 mg/kg or repeated doses that mirror treatment for ethylene glycol or methanol:[84–89]

Initial dose: 15 mg/kg intravenously over 30 minutes

Maintenance doses (no hemodialysis): 12 hours after the initial dose, administer 10 mg/kg intravenously over 30 minutes every 12 hours for 4 doses

Subsequent doses: 15 mg/kg intravenously over 30 minutes every 12 hours[92,93]

Adjustment of dose during hemodialysis to similar dosing administration as per ethylene glycol or methanol toxicity should be considered.[92]

Adverse Reactions

Fomepizole is generally well tolerated. Reported side effects include phlebitis, transient eosinophilia, transient rash, headache, nausea, dizziness, and agitation.[78,94–96]

LEVOCARNITINE

Levocarnitine is an essential cofactor in mitochondrial energy production and metabolism of fatty acids. Carnitine has a critical role in β-oxidation of long-chain fatty acids in the mitochondria; it also regulates coenzyme A concentration and removal of toxic acyl-CoA compounds.[97,98] Primary carnitine deficiency is unusual and is often caused by dysfunctional plasma membrane carnitine transporters resulting in deficiency of carnitine transport.[98] More common is secondary carnitine depletion from increased losses (chronic renal failure on dialysis), or iatrogenic pharmacologic exposure. Additionally, malabsorptive states, cirrhosis, diabetes mellitus, and heart failure may result in carnitine depleted states.[97–99]

Carnitine depletion impairs transport of long chain fatty acids resulting in impaired β-oxidation with subsequent decreased production of acetyl-CoA and ATP. Additional effects include excessive production and accumulation of ω-oxidation products, impaired urea cycle, and intracellular accumulation of toxic acyl -CoA.[99]

Valproic acid (VPA) is an antiepileptic agent with a chemical structure similar to short chain fatty acids. Complications of use include hepatotoxicity and encephalopathy. Valproate is extensively metabolized in the liver through glucuronidation, β-oxidation, and ω-oxidation.[99] One of the most important mediators in the metabolism of valproic acid is carnitine. During the process of mitochondrial β-oxidation, VPA depletes carnitine stores. Carnitine supplementation is well tolerated and may be beneficial in acute and chronic valproate exposure.[100–104] Additionally, the supplementation of levocarnitine may be beneficial in high-risk patients.[99]

Caution and Contraindications

Specific contraindications have not been determined.[105]

Dosage and Available Formulations

Levocarnitine is supplied as an oral preparation of 100 mg/mL solution, as well as tablets that range from 250 to 500 mg. Intravenous solutions of 250 and 500 mg/mL vials can be diluted with normal saline or lactated ringers.[105]

In patients presenting with severe metabolic crisis, valproic acid–induced symptomatic hepatotoxicity, symptomatic hyperammonemia, metabolic acidosis, or encephalopathy should receive a loading dose of 100 mg/kg intravenously (up to 6 g) over 30 minutes. Subsequent doses are 15 mg/kg every 6 hours over 10 to 30 minutes.[106] Daily dosing should be 50mg/kg/d divided into doses every 3 to 4 hours.[105]

Oral dosing is reserved for noncritically ill patients with 50 to 100 mg/kg/d up to 3 g/d.[106,107]

Adverse Reactions

Levocarnitine has few adverse effects, with the majority being transient gastrointestinal distress, and a fishy body odor. Additionally, seizures have been reported.[105]

LIPID EMULSION

Various terminologies exist to describe lipid emulsion (Intralipid, Liposyn) administration including intravenous lipid emulsion, lipid resuscitation therapy, lipid rescue, intravenous fat emulsion, and intralipid. Toxicologic (off-label) use includes local anesthetic systemic toxicity (LAST) and lipophilic drug overdose.[108,109] The 2015 American Heart Association Guidelines Update opines "It may be reasonable to administer ILE, concomitant with standard resuscitative care, to patients with local anesthetic systemic toxicity and particularly to patients who have premonitory neurotoxicity or cardiac arrest caused by bupivacaine toxicity. It may be reasonable to administer ILE to patients with other forms of drug toxicity who are failing standard resuscitative measures."[110]

The exact mechanism of action for lipid emulsion efficacy in poisoning is unclear. The main touted mechanism for intralipid is the lipid sink theory; lipid emulsion reduces the volume of distribution of lipophilic xenobiotics by sequestration.[108,111] A concentration gradient develops between the tissue and vascular compartments, drawing the agent away from areas of higher concentration (myocardium or brain).[112] A component of cardiovascular toxicity in LAST may be dysfunctional myocyte oxidative phosphorylation due to decreased fatty acid transport and oxidation. Lipid emulsion may provide sufficient intracellular fatty acid content to overcome the decreased cardiac ATP, improving cardiac contractility and facilitating mitochondrial fatty acid uptake.[111] Other hypothetical mechanisms include the use of intralipid to inhibit eNOS and decrease the NO-mediated vasodilation.[113] Finally, some studies support direct cardiotonic effects of lipid emulsion.[114]

In LAST, patients can develop fulminant refractory cardiovascular collapse that is resistant to other therapeutic modalities. A rat model in 1998 demonstrated potential efficacy in a bupivacaine-induced cardiac arrest.[115] Since then, improved survivability in LAST has been attributed to lipid emulsion administration.[111,115–119]

There are few high-quality studies demonstrating the efficacy of lipid emulsion therapy beyond utility in LAST. The timing of lipid emulsion toward the end of resuscitative efforts with multiple concomitant therapies limits extrapolation of the singular efficacy of ILE. Mechanistically, xenobiotics more likely to respond to lipid rescue therapy are ones with high lipid solubility; this is often defined as an octanol: water partition coefficient (log P) of greater than 2.[111]

Caution and Contraindications

Intralipid is a synthetic fat emulsion composed of soybean oil, glycerin, egg phospholipids, glycerol, and water. Potential relative contraindications include history of hypersensitivity to lipid emulsion or ingredients (ie, eggs, soy, or peanut protein).[109]

Dosage and Available Formulations

Intralipid is available as a 10%, 20%, or 30% emulsion:[109]

Initial dose: 20% lipid emulsion as a 1.5 mL/kg intravenous bolus over 2 to 3 minutes followed by an infusion of 0.25 mL/kg/min[116]

Repeat bolus dosing if there is persistent cardiovascular collapse. The infusion rate may also be doubled in cases of severe hemodynamic compromise.[109,116] Recommended upper limits are 10 to 12 mL/kg of 20% lipid emulsion over the first 30 minutes.[112]

Adverse Reactions

Adverse reactions associated with lipid emulsion are minimal. A systematic review reported pancreatitis, hypertriglyceridemia, and lipemia that may result in laboratory interference and macroscopic hematuria.[108,116] This analytical interference can be managed with brief ultracentrifugation of the samples.[108] Patients receiving intralipid are critically ill, and thus, other adverse events have a temporal relationship with administration but may not be causal.[119,120]

CLINICS CARE POINTS

- Methylene blue and hydroxocobalamin can be considered in poisoned patients with refractory vasoplegic shock.
- Methylene blue administration may result in factitiously low pulse oximetry reading immediately after administration.
- Consider increased acetylcysteine dosing if the patient is presenting with acetaminophen concentration greater than over the 300 μg/mL line.
- Fomepizole has been shown in case reports and animal models to be a potential adjunctive treatment of acetaminophen toxicity in addition to acetylcysteine.

- Consider intravenous levocarnitine administration in patients presenting with valproic acid-induced hepatotoxicity or neurotoxicity.
- Administer intravenous lipid emulsion in addition to standard resuscitative care to patients with local anesthetic systemic toxicity.
- If considered, intravenous lipid emulsion is more likely to be efficacious in overdoses of lipophilic drugs (log *P*>2).

DISCLOSURE

Rocky Mountain & Drug Safety, part of Denver Health and Hospital Authority, has received an Investigator Initiated Study grant regarding the use of fomepizole in the treatment of acetaminophen overdose from Johnson & Johnson Consumer Inc., McNeil Healthcare Division.

REFERENCES

1. Dart RC, Duncan C, McNally J. Effect of inadequate antivenin stores on the medical treatment of crotalid envenomation. Vet Hum Toxicol 1991;33(3):267–9.
2. Dart RC, Stark Y, Fulton B, et al. Insufficient stocking of poisoning antidotes in hospital pharmacies. JAMA 1996;276(18):1508–10.
3. Bailey GP, Rehman B, Wind K, et al. Taking stock: UK national antidote availability increasing, but further improvements are required. Eur J Hosp Pharm 2016; 23(3):145–50.
4. AlTamimi A, Malhis NK, Khojah NM, et al. Antidote availability in Saudi Arabia hospitals in the Riyadh province. Basic Clin Pharmacol Toxicol 2018;122(2): 288–92.
5. Dart RC, Goldfrank LR, Erstad BL, et al. Expert consensus guidelines for stocking of antidotes in hospitals that provide emergency care. Ann Emerg Med 2018;71(3):314–25.e311.
6. Lin AL, Poteet E, Du F, et al. Methylene blue as a cerebral metabolic and hemodynamic enhancer. PLoS One 2012;7(10):e46585.
7. Wen Y, Li W, Poteet EC, et al. Alternative mitochondrial electron transfer as a novel strategy for neuroprotection. J Biol Chem 2011;286(18):16504–15.
8. Madiraju AK, Erion DM, Rahimi Y, et al. Metformin suppresses gluconeogenesis by inhibiting mitochondrial glycerophosphate dehydrogenase. Nature 2014; 510(7506):542–6.
9. Bridges HR, Jones AJ, Pollak MN, et al. Effects of metformin and other biguanides on oxidative phosphorylation in mitochondria. Biochem J 2014;462(3): 475–87.
10. El-Mir MY, Nogueira V, Fontaine E, et al. Dimethylbiguanide inhibits cell respiration via an indirect effect targeted on the respiratory chain complex I. J Biol Chem 2000;275(1):223–8.
11. Owen MR, Doran E, Halestrap AP. Evidence that metformin exerts its anti-diabetic effects through inhibition of complex 1 of the mitochondrial respiratory chain. Biochem J 2000;348(Pt 3):607–14.
12. Wang GS, Hoyte C. Review of Biguanide (Metformin) Toxicity. J Intensive Care Med 2019;34(11–12):863–76.
13. Heredia D, Mancl E, Sayegh B, et al. Successful use of methylene blue for hemodynamically unstable metformin toxicity. Chest 2014;253a.

14. Livshits Z, Nelson LS, Hernandez SH, et al. Severe metformin toxicity: role of methylene blue and CVVHD as therapeutic adjuncts. Clin Toxicol 2010;611–2.
15. Graham RE, Cartner M, Winearls J. A severe case of vasoplegic shock following metformin overdose successfully treated with methylene blue as a last line therapy. BMJ Case Rep. 2015. https://doi.org/10.1136/bcr-2015-210229.
16. Plumb B, Parker A, Wong P. Feeling blue with metformin-associated lactic acidosis. BMJ Case Rep. 2013. https://doi.org/10.1136/bcr-2013-008855.
17. Yiu P, Robin J, Pattison CW. Reversal of refractory hypotension with single-dose methylene blue after coronary artery bypass surgery. J Thorac Cardiovasc Surg 1999;118(1):195–6.
18. Pagni S, Austin EH. Use of intravenous methylene blue for the treatment of refractory hypotension after cardiopulmonary bypass. J Thorac Cardiovasc Surg 2000;119(6):1297–8.
19. Kofidis T, Strüber M, Wilhelmi M, et al. Reversal of severe vasoplegia with single-dose methylene blue after heart transplantation. J Thorac Cardiovasc Surg 2001;122(4):823–4.
20. Leyh RG, Kofidis T, Strüber M, et al. Methylene blue: the drug of choice for catecholamine-refractory vasoplegia after cardiopulmonary bypass? J Thorac Cardiovasc Surg 2003;125(6):1426–31.
21. Dagenais F, Mathieu P. Rescue therapy with methylene blue in systemic inflammatory response syndrome after cardiac surgery. Can J Cardiol 2003;19(2):167–9.
22. Del Duca D, Sheth SS, Clarke AE, et al. Use of methylene blue for catecholamine-refractory vasoplegia from protamine and aprotinin. Ann Thorac Surg 2009;87(2):640–2.
23. Maslow AD, Stearns G, Butala P, et al. The hemodynamic effects of methylene blue when administered at the onset of cardiopulmonary bypass. Anesth Analg 2006;103(1):2–8.
24. McRobb CM, Holt DW. Methylene blue-induced methemoglobinemia during cardiopulmonary bypass? A case report and literature review. J Extra Corpor Technol 2008;40(3):206–14.
25. Mora-Ordóñez JM, Sánchez-Llorente F, Galeas-López JL, et al. [Use of methylene blue in the treatment of vasoplegic syndrome of post-operative heart surgery]. Med Intensiva 2006;30(6):293–6.
26. Ozal E, Kuralay E, Yildirim V, et al. Preoperative methylene blue administration in patients at high risk for vasoplegic syndrome during cardiac surgery. Ann Thorac Surg 2005;79(5):1615–9.
27. Taylor K, Holtby H. Methylene blue revisited: management of hypotension in a pediatric patient with bacterial endocarditis. J Thorac Cardiovasc Surg 2005;130(2):566.
28. Weissgerber AJ. Methylene blue for refractory hypotension: a case report. AANA J 2008;76(4):271–4.
29. Dumbarton TC, Minor S, Yeung CK, et al. Prolonged methylene blue infusion in refractory septic shock: a case report. Can J Anaesth 2011;58(4):401–5.
30. Juffermans NP, Vervloet MG, Daemen-Gubbels CR, et al. A dose-finding study of methylene blue to inhibit nitric oxide actions in the hemodynamics of human septic shock. Nitric Oxide 2010;22(4):275–80.
31. Kirov MY, Evgenov OV, Evgenov NV, et al. Infusion of methylene blue in human septic shock: a pilot, randomized, controlled study. Crit Care Med 2001;29(10):1860–7.

32. Preiser JC, Lejeune P, Roman A, et al. Methylene blue administration in septic shock: a clinical trial. Crit Care Med 1995;23(2):259–64.
33. Oliveira Neto AM, Duarte NM, Vicente WV, et al. Methylene blue: an effective treatment for contrast medium-induced anaphylaxis. Med Sci Monit 2003; 9(11):CS102–6.
34. Lenglet S, Mach F, Montecucco F. Methylene blue: potential use of an antique molecule in vasoplegic syndrome during cardiac surgery. Expert Rev Cardiovasc Ther 2011;9(12):1519–25.
35. Ginimuge PR, Jyothi SD. Methylene blue: revisited. J Anaesthesiol Clin Pharmacol 2010;26(4):517–20.
36. Warrick BJ, Tataru AP, Smolinske S. A systematic analysis of methylene blue for drug-induced shock. Clin Toxicol (Phila) 2016;54(7):547–55.
37. Clifton J, Leikin JB. Methylene blue. Am J Ther 2003;10(4):289–91.
38. Ng BK, Cameron AJ. The role of methylene blue in serotonin syndrome: a systematic review. Psychosomatics 2010;51(3):194–200.
39. Howland M. Methylene Blue. In: Nelson LS, Howland M, Lewin NA, Smith SW, Goldfrank LR, Hoffman RS. eds. Goldfrank's Toxicologic Emergencies, 11e. McGraw Hill; 2019. 1713–1716.
40. Methylene Blue. Micromedex Solutions. Greenwood Village, CO: Truven Health Analytics. http://micromedex.com/. Accessed February 18, 2022.
41. French D, Smollin C, Ruan W, et al. Partition constant and volume of distribution as predictors of clinical efficacy of lipid rescue for toxicological emergencies. Clin Toxicol (Phila) 2011;49(9):801–9.
42. Prischl FC, Hofinger I, Kramar R. Fever, shivering...and blue urine. Nephrol Dial Transplant 1999;14(9):2245–6.
43. Dumbarton TC, Gorman SK, Minor S, et al. Local cutaneous necrosis secondary to a prolonged peripheral infusion of methylene blue in vasodilatory shock. Ann Pharmacother 2012;46(3):e6.
44. Salhab M, Al Sarakbi W, Mokbel K. Skin and fat necrosis of the breast following methylene blue dye injection for sentinel node biopsy in a patient with breast cancer. Int Semin Surg Oncol 2005;2:26.
45. Hydroxocobalamin. Micromedex Solutions. Greenwood Village, CO: Truven Health Analytics. http://micromedex.com/. Accessed February 18, 2022.
46. Shapeton AD, Mahmood F, Ortoleva JP. Hydroxocobalamin for the treatment of vasoplegia: a review of current literature and considerations for use. J Cardiothorac Vasc Anesth 2019;33(4):894–901.
47. Fortin JL, Giocanti JP, Ruttimann M, et al. Prehospital administration of hydroxocobalamin for smoke inhalation-associated cyanide poisoning: 8 years of experience in the Paris Fire Brigade. Clin Toxicol (Phila) 2006;44(Suppl 1): 37–44.
48. Howland M. Hydroxocobalamin. In: Nelson LS, Howland M, Lewin NA, Smith SW, Goldfrank LR, Hoffman RS. eds. Goldfrank's Toxicologic Emergencies, 11e. McGraw Hill; 2019. 1694–1697.
49. Sacco AJ, Cunningham CA, Kosiorek HE, et al. Hydroxocobalamin in refractory septic shock: a retrospective case series. Crit Care Explor 2021;3(4):e0408.
50. Uhl W, Nolting A, Gallemann D, et al. Changes in blood pressure after administration of hydroxocobalamin: relationship to changes in plasma cobalamins-(III) concentrations in healthy volunteers. Clin Toxicol (Phila) 2008;46(6):551–9 [discussion: 576-557].

51. Greenberg SS, Xie J, Zatarain JM, et al. Hydroxocobalamin (vitamin B12a) prevents and reverses endotoxin-induced hypotension and mortality in rodents: role of nitric oxide. J Pharmacol Exp Ther 1995;273(1):257–65.
52. Sampaio AL, Dalli J, Brancaleone V, et al. Biphasic modulation of NOS expression, protein and nitrite products by hydroxocobalamin underlies its protective effect in endotoxemic shock: downstream regulation of COX-2, IL-1β, TNF-α, IL-6, and HMGB1 expression. Mediators Inflamm 2013;2013:741804.
53. Roderique JD, VanDyck K, Holman B, et al. The use of high-dose hydroxocobalamin for vasoplegic syndrome. Ann Thorac Surg 2014;97(5):1785–6.
54. Cai Y, Mack A, Ladlie BL, et al. The use of intravenous hydroxocobalamin as a rescue in methylene blue-resistant vasoplegic syndrome in cardiac surgery. Ann Card Anaesth 2017;20(4):462–4.
55. Burnes ML, Boettcher BT, Woehlck HJ, et al. Hydroxocobalamin as a rescue treatment for refractory vasoplegic syndrome after prolonged cardiopulmonary bypass. J Cardiothorac Vasc Anesth 2017;31(3):1012–4.
56. Woehlck HJ, Boettcher BT, Lauer KK, et al. Hydroxocobalamin for vasoplegic syndrome in liver transplantation: restoration of blood pressure without vasospasm. A A Case Rep 2016;7(12):247–50.
57. An SS, Henson CP, Freundlich RE, et al. Case report of high-dose hydroxocobalamin in the treatment of vasoplegic syndrome during liver transplantation. Am J Transplant 2018;18(6):1552–5.
58. Warner MA, Mauermann WJ, Armour S, et al. Red urinary discolouration following hydroxocobalamin treatment for vasoplegic syndrome. Can J Anaesth 2017;64(6):673–4.
59. Shah PR, Reynolds PS, Pal N, et al. Hydroxocobalamin for the treatment of cardiac surgery-associated vasoplegia: a case series. Can J Anaesth 2018;65(5): 560–8.
60. Cyanokit Package Insert. In: Meridian Medical Technologies. Available at: https://www.accessdata.fda.gov/drugsatfda_docs/label/2006/022041lbl.pdf. Accessed February 18, 2022.
61. Boettcher BT, Woehlck HJ, Reck SE, et al. Treatment of vasoplegic syndrome with intravenous hydroxocobalamin during liver transplantation. J Cardiothorac Vasc Anesth 2017;31(4):1381–4.
62. DesLauriers CA, Burda AM, Wahl M. Hydroxocobalamin as a cyanide antidote. Am J Ther 2006;13(2):161–5.
63. Legrand M. Hydroxocobalamin as a cause of oxalate nephropathy. Kidney Int Rep 2019;4(1):185.
64. Dépret F, Hoffmann C, Daoud L, et al. Association between hydroxocobalamin administration and acute kidney injury after smoke inhalation: a multicenter retrospective study. Crit Care 2019;23(1):421.
65. Legrand M, Michel T, Daudon M, et al. Risk of oxalate nephropathy with the use of cyanide antidote hydroxocobalamin in critically ill burn patients. Intensive Care Med 2016;42(6):1080–1.
66. Cheungpasitporn W, Hui J, Kashani KB, et al. High-dose hydroxocobalamin for vasoplegic syndrome causing false blood leak alarm. Clin Kidney J 2017;10(3): 357–62.
67. Smilkstein MJ, Knapp GL, Kulig KW, et al. Efficacy of oral N-acetylcysteine in the treatment of acetaminophen overdose. Analysis of the national multicenter study (1976 to 1985). N Engl J Med 1988;319(24):1557–62.
68. Acetylcysteine. Micromedex Solutions. Greenwood Village, CO: Truven Health Analytics. http://micromedex.com/. Accessed February 18, 2022.

69. Acetadote (acetylcysteine) Injection Package Insert. In: Cumberland Pharmaceuticals. Available at: https://www.accessdata.fda.gov/drugsatfda_docs/label/2006/021539s004lbl.pdf. Accessed February 18, 2022.
70. Hoyte C, Dart RC. Transition to two-bag intravenous acetylcysteine for acetaminophen overdose: a poison center's experience. Clin Toxicol (Phila) 2019;57(3):217–8.
71. Rumack BH, Bateman DN. Acetaminophen and acetylcysteine dose and duration: past, present and future. Clin Toxicol (Phila) 2012;50(2):91–8.
72. Doyon S, Klein-Schwartz W. Hepatotoxicity despite early administration of intravenous N-acetylcysteine for acute acetaminophen overdose. Acad Emerg Med 2009;16(1):34–9.
73. Marks DJB, Dargan PI, Archer JRH, et al. Outcomes from massive paracetamol overdose: a retrospective observational study. Br J Clin Pharmacol 2017;83(6):1263–72.
74. Chiew AL, Isbister GK, Kirby KA, et al. Massive paracetamol overdose: an observational study of the effect of activated charcoal and increased acetylcysteine dose (ATOM-2). Clin Toxicol (Phila) 2017;55(10):1055–65.
75. Cairney DG, Beckwith HK, Al-Hourani K, et al. Plasma paracetamol concentration at hospital presentation has a dose-dependent relationship with liver injury despite prompt treatment with intravenous acetylcysteine. Clin Toxicol (Phila) 2016;54(5):405–10.
76. Sandilands EA, Bateman DN. Adverse reactions associated with acetylcysteine. Clin Toxicol (Phila) 2009;47(2):81–8.
77. Schmidt LE, Rasmussen DN, Petersen TS, et al. Fewer adverse effects associated with a modified two-bag intravenous acetylcysteine protocol compared to traditional three-bag regimen in paracetamol overdose. Clin Toxicol (Phila) 2018;56(11):1128–34.
78. Brent J, McMartin K, Phillips S, et al. Fomepizole for the treatment of ethylene glycol poisoning. Methylpyrazole for Toxic Alcohols Study Group. N Engl J Med 1999;340(11):832–8.
79. Brent J. Fomepizole for ethylene glycol and methanol poisoning. N Engl J Med 2009;360(21):2216–23.
80. Jaeschke H. Toxic responses of the liver. In: Casarret & Doull's toxicology: the basic science of poisons. McGraw-Hill Education; 2019. p. 557–82.
81. Zell-Kanter M, Coleman P, Whiteley PM, et al. A gargantuan acetaminophen level in an acidemic patient treated solely with intravenous N-acetylcysteine. Am J Ther 2013;20(1):104–6.
82. Kang AM, Padilla-Jones A, Fisher ES, et al. The effect of 4-methylpyrazole on oxidative metabolism of acetaminophen in human volunteers. J Med Toxicol 2020;16(2):169–76.
83. Akakpo JY, Ramachandran A, Duan L, et al. Delayed treatment with 4-methylpyrazole protects against acetaminophen hepatotoxicity in mice by inhibition of c-Jun n-terminal kinase. Toxicol Sci 2019;170(1):57–68.
84. Rampon G, Wartman H, Osmon S, et al. Use of fomepizole as an adjunct in the treatment of acetaminophen overdose: a case series. In: Toxicology communications 2020. p. 1-4.
85. Colon Hidalgo D, Shah S, Rech M. Use of fomepizole and hemodialysis for massive acetaminophen toxicity. Crit Care Med 2020;454.
86. Shah KR, Beuhler MC. Fomepizole as an adjunctive treatment in severe acetaminophen toxicity. Am J Emerg Med 2020;38(2):410–e415.

87. Shah KR, Fox C, Geib AJ, et al. Fomepizole as an adjunctive treatment in severe acetaminophen ingestions: a case series. Clin Toxicol (Phila) 2021;59(1):71–2.
88. Woolum JA, Hays WB, Patel KH. Use of fomepizole, n-acetylcysteine, and hemodialysis for massive acetaminophen overdose. Am J Emerg Med 2020; 38(3):692–e695.
89. Kiernan EA, Fritzges JA, Henry KA, et al. A case report of massive acetaminophen poisoning treated with a novel "triple therapy": n-acetylcysteine, 4-methylpyrazole, and hemodialysis. Case Rep Emerg Med 2019;2019:9301432.
90. Villano JH, O'Connell CW, Ly BT, et al. Case files from the University of California San Diego health system fellowship coma and severe acidosis: remember to consider acetaminophen. J Med Toxicol 2015;11(3):368–76.
91. Althwanay A, Alharthi MM, Aljumaan M, et al. Methanol, paracetamol toxicities and acute blindness. Cureus 2020;12(5):e8179.
92. Antizol (fomepizole) Injection [package insert]. In. Paladin Labs Inc. St-Laurent, Quebec. https://www.accessdata.fda.gov/drugsatfda_docs/label/2020/020696s006lbl.pdf. Accessed February 18, 2022.
93. Bestic M, Blackford M, Reed M. Fomepizole: a critical assessment of current dosing recommendations. J Clin Pharmacol 2009;49(2):130–7.
94. Mégarbane B, Borron SW, Trout H, et al. Treatment of acute methanol poisoning with fomepizole. Intensive Care Med 2001;27(8):1370–8.
95. Brent J, McMartin K, Phillips S, et al, Group MfTAS. Fomepizole for the treatment of methanol poisoning. N Engl J Med 2001;344(6):424–9.
96. Jacobsen D, Sebastian CS, Blomstrand R, et al. 4-Methylpyrazole: a controlled study of safety in healthy human subjects after single, ascending doses. Alcohol Clin Exp Res 1988;12(4):516–22.
97. Evangeliou A, Vlassopoulos D. Carnitine metabolism and deficit–when supplementation is necessary? Curr Pharm Biotechnol 2003;4(3):211–9.
98. Flanagan JL, Simmons PA, Vehige J, et al. Role of carnitine in disease. Nutr Metab (Lond) 2010;7:30.
99. Lheureux PE, Penaloza A, Zahir S, et al. Science review: carnitine in the treatment of valproic acid-induced toxicity - what is the evidence? Crit Care 2005; 9(5):431–40.
100. Bohan TP, Helton E, McDonald I, et al. Effect of L-carnitine treatment for valproate-induced hepatotoxicity. Neurology 2001;56(10):1405–9.
101. Ohtani Y, Endo F, Matsuda I. Carnitine deficiency and hyperammonemia associated with valproic acid therapy. J Pediatr 1982;101(5):782–5.
102. Böhles H, Sewell AC, Wenzel D. The effect of carnitine supplementation in valproate-induced hyperammonaemia. Acta Paediatr 1996;85(4):446–9.
103. Ishikura H, Matsuo N, Matsubara M, et al. Valproic acid overdose and L-carnitine therapy. J Anal Toxicol 1996;20(1):55–8.
104. Murakami K, Sugimoto T, Woo M, et al. Effect of L-carnitine supplementation on acute valproate intoxication. Epilepsia 1996;37(7):687–9.
105. Carnitor (levocarnitine) Injection [package insert]. In: Bedford Laboratories. Available at: https://www.accessdata.fda.gov/drugsatfda_docs/label/2006/021539s004lbl.pdf. Accessed February 18, 2022.
106. Howland M, Carnitine L. In: Nelson LS, Howland M, Lewin NA, et al. editors. Goldfrank's toxicologic emergencies, 11th edition . McGraw-Hill. https://accesspharmacy-mhmedical-com.proxy.hsl.ucdenver.edu/content.aspx?bookid=2569§ionid=210262359.
107. Levocarnitine (Carnitine). In. Greenwood Village, CO: Truven Health Analytics. http://micromedex.com/. Accessed February 18, 2022.

108. Kostic MA, Gorelick M. Review of the use of lipid emulsion in nonlocal anesthetic poisoning. Pediatr Emerg Care 2014;30(6):427–33.
109. Intralipid. Micromedex Solutions. Greenwood Village, CO: Truven Health Analytics. http://micromedex.com/. Accessed February 18, 2022.
110. Lavonas EJ, Drennan IR, Gabrielli A, et al. Part 10: special circumstances of resuscitation: 2015 American heart association guidelines update for cardiopulmonary resuscitation and emergency cardiovascular care. Circulation 2015; 132(18 Suppl 2):S501–18.
111. Weinberg GL. Lipid emulsion infusion: resuscitation for local anesthetic and other drug overdose. Anesthesiology 2012;117(1):180–7.
112. American College of Medical Toxicology. ACMT Position Statement: Guidance for the Use of Intravenous Lipid Emulsion [published correction appears in J Med Toxicol. 2016 Dec;12 (4):416]. J Med Toxicol 2017;13(1):124–5.
113. Ok SH, Sohn JT, Baik JS, et al. Lipid emulsion reverses Levobupivacaine-induced responses in isolated rat aortic vessels. Anesthesiology 2011;114(2): 293–301.
114. Levine M, Hoffman RS, Lavergne V, et al. Systematic review of the effect of intravenous lipid emulsion therapy for non-local anesthetics toxicity. Clin Toxicol (Phila) 2016;54(3):194–221.
115. Weinberg GL, VadeBoncouer T, Ramaraju GA, et al. Pretreatment or resuscitation with a lipid infusion shifts the dose-response to bupivacaine-induced asystole in rats. Anesthesiology 1998;88(4):1071–5.
116. Jamaty C, Bailey B, Larocque A, et al. Lipid emulsions in the treatment of acute poisoning: a systematic review of human and animal studies. Clin Toxicol (Phila) 2010;48(1):1–27.
117. Hoegberg LC, Bania TC, Lavergne V, et al. Systematic review of the effect of intravenous lipid emulsion therapy for local anesthetic toxicity. Clin Toxicol (Phila) 2016;54(3):167–93.
118. Stellpflug SJ, Harris CR, Engebretsen KM, et al. Intentional overdose with cardiac arrest treated with intravenous fat emulsion and high-dose insulin. Clin Toxicol (Phila) 2010;48(3):227–9.
119. Geib AJ, Liebelt E, Manini AF, ToxIC) TIC. Clinical experience with intravenous lipid emulsion for drug-induced cardiovascular collapse. J Med Toxicol 2012; 8(1):10–4.
120. Levine M, Skolnik AB, Ruha AM, et al. Complications following antidotal use of intravenous lipid emulsion therapy. J Med Toxicol 2014;10(1):10–4.

Cardiotoxic Medication Poisoning

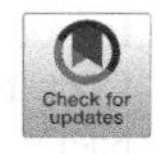

Jon B. Cole, MD[a,b,*], Ann M. Arens, MD[a,b]

KEYWORDS

- Beta-blocker • Calcium channel blocker • Digoxin • Flecainide • High-dose insulin • ECMO • Poisoning

KEY POINTS

- Cardiovascular medications represent a disproportionate share of morbidity and mortality from poisonings in the United States.
- High-dose insulin should be used in most cases of severe beta-blocker and calcium channel blocker poisoning and is likely synergistic when combined with vasopressors.
- Flecainide is the prototypical sodium-channel blocker likely to be encountered by emergency clinicians and is best managed with hypertonic sodium bicarbonate, vasopressors, and inotropes.
- Digoxin is the prototypical cardioactive steroid, and digoxin poisoning rarely requires a complete reversal with fab fragments. Cardioactive steroids from botanic sources are being used as weight loss agents; poisoning in such cases requires high doses of fab fragments.
- Extracorporeal membrane oxygenation use for cardiovascular medication poisoning is increasing, and appears to be an effective nonspecific salvage therapy for refractory poison-induced cardiogenic shock.

Video content accompanies this article at http://www.emed.theclinics.com

INTRODUCTION

Cardiovascular toxins are one of the most commonly reported drug overdoses in the United States. In 2019, 118,287 cardiovascular toxin exposures were reported to the National Poison Data System (NPDS), including 20,341 pediatric exposures.[1] Calcium channel blockers and beta-blockers were the number 6 and 7 causes of drug poisoning and overdose deaths reported in 2019, respectively.[1] That same year, cardiovascular toxins were one of the top 10 categories of poisons evaluated by medical

[a] Department of Emergency Medicine, Hennepin Healthcare, 701 Park Ave, Mail Code: RL.240, Minneapolis, MN 55415, USA; [b] Department of Emergency Medicine, University of Minnesota, Minneapolis, MN, USA
* Corresponding Author.
E-mail addresses: Jon.cole@hcmed.org; jonbcole@gmail.com

Emerg Med Clin N Am 40 (2022) 395–416
https://doi.org/10.1016/j.emc.2022.01.014

toxicologists.[2] Calcium channel blockers and beta-blockers in particular can cause toxicity with a single extra dose[3] and accounted for 12% of patients reported to NPDS who were treated with extracorporeal membrane oxygenation (ECMO) from 2000 to 2018.[4] Given the potential for severe cardiovascular compromise and mortality associated with cardiovascular toxins, understanding the pharmacology, pathophysiology, and treatment strategies for these exposures is paramount.

PHARMACOLOGY AND PATHOPHYSIOLOGY OF POISONING

Normal Cardiac Myocyte Physiology and Cycle

Cardiotoxic xenobiotics exhibit their effects by exploiting the intricate mechanisms regulating cardiac output including heart rate, contractility, peripheral vascular resistance, and cardiac conduction.[5] Complex systems regulate each of these aspects, including the autonomic nervous system and the physiology of cardiac contractility and conduction.

Autonomic nervous system regulation relies primarily on adrenergic receptor activity. Adrenergic xenobiotics take advantage of the normal secondary signaling pathways that alter autonomic tone, including the interactions between adrenergic receptors, including alpha and beta receptors, G-protein complexes, and cyclic AMP synthesized by the enzyme adenylate cyclase.[5] Alpha and beta adrenergic receptors are found on various smooth muscle and adipose tissues throughout the body. Beta adrenergic receptors are a group of G-protein coupled transmembrane receptors with 3 separate subtypes, beta-1, beta-2, and beta-3, each with different affinities for various xenobiotics.[6,7] For example, beta-1 receptor agonists result primarily in increased heart rate and inotropy, whereas beta-2 receptor activation increases heart rate and inotropy to a lesser extent, but primarily results in smooth muscle relaxation. Beta-3 receptor agonism primarily results in lipolysis and thermogenesis and is outside the scope of this review. Alpha receptors interact with their own unique G-protein subtypes, causing different physiologic effects compared with beta receptors. In the periphery, alpha-1 receptor activation results in vasoconstriction. Alpha-2 receptors can be found in both presynaptic and postsynaptic locations. Presynaptic alpha-2 agonism results in negative feedback, decreasing norepinephrine release, and thus may cause hypotension and bradycardia, whereas postsynaptic alpha-2 agonism, similar to alpha-1, results in vasoconstriction.

Cardiac Contractility

Cardiac myocyte function and vascular smooth muscle tone depends on calcium influx across voltage-dependent L-type calcium channels.[5,8] (**Fig. 1**). Several subtypes of L-type calcium channels exist. Medications vary on their affinity for different L-type calcium channels, and thus clinical effects.[8,9]

Depolarization of the myocardial membrane is initiated by voltage-sensitive sodium channels, composed of a single large alpha subunit with multiple receptor sites, as well as several regulatory beta subunits. The receptor sites on the alpha subunit are targeted by different xenobiotics and toxins to alter activity at the sodium channel.[10,11] Voltage-gated fast sodium channels open in response to depolarization of pacemaker cells and are responsible for membrane depolarization. Sodium channels alternate between 1 of 3 states: activated (open), inactivated, or closed.[11]

Voltage-sensitive potassium channels in the myocardium are a group of rectifying channels, meaning the channels change conductance of current based on the transmembrane voltage potential.[12] In the myocardium, the main categories include the delayed rectifier, the iKr (rapidly activating), and the iKs (slowly activating) channels.

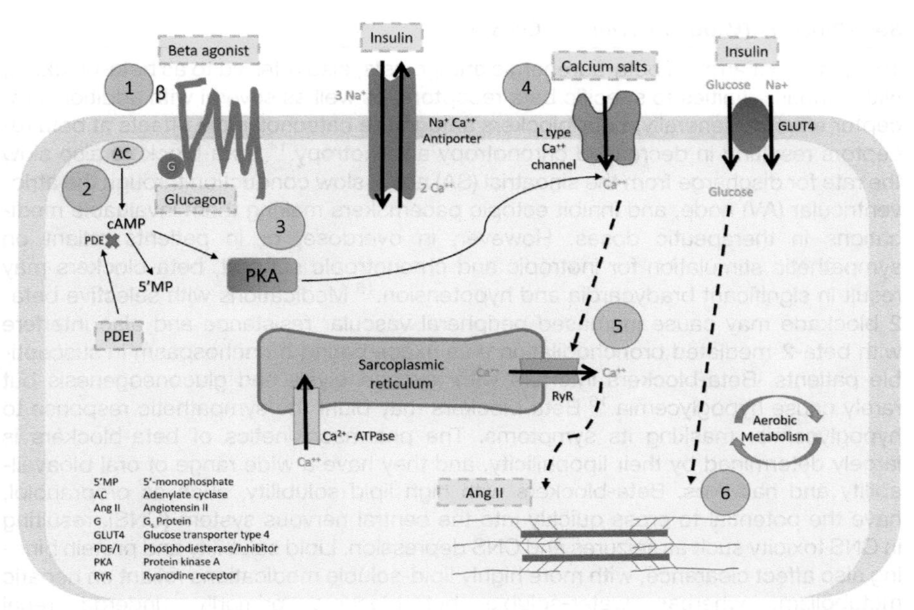

Fig. 1. Beta receptor activation (1): binding of an agonist to a beta receptor results in increased cyclic AMP (cAMP) production (2) via Gs protein-mediated activation of adenylate cyclase (AC). cAMP then interacts with protein kinase A (PKA) (3), which phosphorylates the L-type voltage-sensitive Ca^{2+} channel. Calcium channel activation (4): activation of the L-type Ca^{2+} channel leads to calcium influx, calcium binding to calcium channels located on the sarcoplasmic reticulum. Calcium binding at the sarcoplasmic reticulum results in further calcium release via the ryanodine receptors (RyR) (5). Troponin C, when bound to calcium displaces troponin and tropomyosin from actin allowing actin-myosin binding and myocyte contraction (6). The sensitivity of the contractile elements to calcium is enhanced by angiotensin II. Potential therapies for poison-induced shock are displayed in yellow boxes. (*Figure created by* Samantha Lee, PharmD, DABAT.)

Similar to sodium channels, the potassium channels consist of an alpha subunit, which includes the channel pore, as well as beta subunit proteins. An important subset of the iKr channel includes those with an alpha subunit encoded by the Human Ether-a-go-go Related Gene (hERG). Several xenobiotics exploit the hERG-encoded subunit to reduce current through the channel and thus prolong action potential duration because of specific properties of this particular subunit. The hERG-encoded alpha subunits are able to bind aromatic xenobiotics, and the subunit has a larger pore than other voltage-gated potassium channels allowing larger xenobiotics to enter, and subsequently close the pore.[12] Potassium channel blocking (Vaughan-Williams class III) antidysrhythmics, including amiodarone, ibutilide, dofetilide, and dronedarone, prolong the action potential duration and effective refractory periods by affecting the delayed rectifier potassium current responsible for repolarization of the myocyte; this may result in QT prolongation on an electrocardiography (ECG). Numerous additional medications have QT prolonging properties and may increase the risk of subsequent torsades de pointes. The discussion of this vast array of medications is beyond the scope of this review.[13]

As previously discussed, calcium channels are important for the maintenance of the duration of membrane depolarization and cellular contraction.

Beta-Blockers (Vaughan-Williams Class II)

There is a vast array of beta-adrenergic antagonists, also referred to as beta-blockers, with various affinities to specific beta receptors, as well as several with additional receptor effects. Generally, beta-blockers antagonize catecholamine effects at beta receptors resulting in decreased chronotropy and inotropy.[14] Beta-blockers also slow the rate for discharge from the sinoatrial (SA) node, slow conduction through the atrioventricular (AV) node, and inhibit ectopic pacemakers making them invaluable medications in therapeutic doses. However, in overdose, or in patients reliant on sympathetic stimulation for inotropic and chronotropic support, beta-blockers may result in significant bradycardia and hypotension.[15] Medications with selective beta-2 blockade may cause increased peripheral vascular resistance and also interfere with beta-2-mediated bronchodilation thus exacerbating bronchospasm in susceptible patients. Beta-blockers interfere with glycogenolysis and gluconeogenesis but rarely cause hypoglycemia.[16] Beta-blockers may blunt the sympathetic response to hypoglycemia, masking its symptoms. The pharmacokinetics of beta-blockers is largely determined by their lipophilicity, and they have a wide range of oral bioavailability and half-lives. Beta-blockers with high lipid solubility, such as propranolol, have the potential to cross quickly into the central nervous system (CNS), resulting in CNS toxicity such as seizures and CNS depression. Lipid solubility and protein binding also affect clearance, with more highly lipid-soluble medications reliant on hepatic metabolism, whereas water-soluble beta-blockers primarily undergo renal clearance.[15]

Beta-blockers also differ in their selectivity for beta-1 and beta-2 receptors, and some have additional receptor effects including concomitant alpha receptor blockade, membrane-stabilizing activity ([MSA] also known as sodium channel blockade, or quinidinelike effects), potassium channel blockade, and intrinsic sympathomimetic activity (**Table 1**). Medications with beta-1 selectivity, such as esmolol and metoprolol, primarily result in decreased chronotropy; however, selectivity may be lost in overdose. Beta-blockers with MSA (eg, propranolol) may result in seizure, synergistic

Table 1
Select beta-blockers and receptor selectivity

Beta-1	Beta-1 and Beta-2	Beta-1, Beta-2, Alpha=1
Acebutolol[a,d]	Carteolol	Carvedilol[a]
Atenolol	Nadolol	Labetalol
Betaxolol[a]	Oxprenolol[a]	
Bisoprolol	Penbutolol	
Nebivolol[b]	Pindolol	
	Propranolol[a]	
	Sotalol[a,c]	
	Timolol	
	Ophthalmic only: levobunolol, metipranolol	

[a] Membrane-stabilizing effect.
[b] Also vasodilation secondary to nitric oxide release.[112]
[c] Also class III antidysrhythmic effect.
[d] Also sympathomimetic activity.

bradycardia, QRS prolongation, and ventricular dysrhythmias contributing to morbidity and mortality in overdose. Propranolol has been identified as one of the most fatal beta-blockers in overdose, likely owing to its MSA.[1,17,18] Sotalol and acebutolol also have potassium channel blockade and thus may prolong action potential duration and QT prolongation. Sotalol in particular may result in significant QT prolongation and torsades de pointes. Medications including carvedilol and labetalol are not only nonselective beta receptor antagonists but also alpha-1 antagonists and thus may result in vasodilation in overdose.

Peripheral Alpha-1 Antagonists and Central Alpha-2 Agonists

Peripheral alpha-1 antagonists include prazosin and doxazosin and may result in hypotension secondary to peripheral vasodilation in overdose. As previously discussed, there are some nonselective beta-blockers with additional alpha blockade that may result in vasodilation and thus hypotension in overdose. Many first- and second-generation antipsychotics also cause alpha-1 receptor blockade.

Central alpha-2 agonists, including clonidine, guanfacine, dexmedetomidine, and tizanidine, may cause hypotension and bradycardia as the result of decreased catecholamine release.[19–21] These medications are also unique in that they may result in profound CNS depression as the result of imidazoline receptor agonism. Clonidine also induces beta-endorphin release, which directly stimulates opioid receptors and thus may have opioidlike effects including miosis in overdose and reports of reversal with large doses of naloxone.[19,22,23]

Calcium Channel Blockers (Vaughan-Williams Class IV)

Calcium channel blockers (Vaughan-Williams class IV) are most commonly categorized as dihydropyridines and nondihydropyridines; the unique clinical aspects of each group are due to subtle binding differences of dihydropyridines at the α1c subunit of L-type calcium channels (**Table 2**). At therapeutic doses, dihydropyridines have little direct effect on the myocardium and primarily exert their effect on blood pressure via peripheral vasodilation. These medications include amlodipine, nicardipine, nifedipine, and clevidipine. Amlodipine accounts for a disproportionate number of deaths related to overdose of cardiovascular drugs.[1] Human and animal data suggest that amlodipine may also stimulate nitric oxide release, contributing additionally to vasodilation and potentially increased morbidity.[24–27] Nondihydropyridines include verapamil and diltiazem. These medications are more selective for the heart and have inhibitory effects on the SA and AV nodes.[24] Thus, in addition to their utility in the treatment of hypertension, these medications are also effective rate control agents for

Table 2
Select calcium channel blockers

Dihydropyridines	Nondihydropyridines
Amlodipine[a]	Verapamil
Clevidipine	Diltiazem
Felodipine	
Nicardipine	
Nifedipine	
Nimodipine	

[a] Also vasodilation from nitric oxide release.

tachydysrhythmias such as atrial fibrillation.[24] Diltiazem is second only to amlodipine for cardiovascular drugs resulting in fatality from drug overdoses.[1]

Calcium channel blockers are metabolized extensively in the liver, primarily by CYP3A4, which is responsible for the metabolism of most calcium channel blockers; this makes calcium channel blockers highly susceptible to drug-drug interactions.[24] Calcium channel blockers are also highly protein bound, with a wide range of volume of distribution (from 0.75 L/kg for nifedipine to 21 L/kg for amlodipine). Both these properties make calcium channel blockers poor candidates for extracorporeal removal such as hemodialysis.[24,28]

The clinical effects of overdose are those that would be expected based on the mechanism of action of calcium channel blockers. Toxicity is hallmarked by decreased inotropy, decreased chronotropy including conduction blocks and delays, as well as decreased systemic vascular resistance.[8] Bradycardia and conduction blocks or delays are often seen with nondihydropyridines. Given nondihydropyridine's effects on pacemaker cells and electrical signal propagation in the SA and AV nodes, AV nodal blockade or conduction abnormalities, idioventricular rhythms, complete heart block, or junctional escape rhythms have been described.[24,29–31] In contrast, dihydropyridine overdose often results in hypotension as a result of peripheral vasodilation, thus in overdose, an initial baroreceptor mediated reflex tachycardia may be seen[8]; however, heart rate and contractility both decrease as poisoning becomes more severe.[9] As previously mentioned, amlodipine poisoning in particular may result in a profound vasoplegic shock, resistant to pressor support.[27,32–34] In large overdoses the selectivity of any calcium channel blocker is lost, and bradycardia may also be seen with large dihydropyridine overdoses.[24] Calcium channel blockers can decrease insulin release by inhibiting calcium channels located on the beta-islet cells in the pancreas, thereby decreasing calcium influx into the cell and reducing calcium-mediated insulin release resulting in hyperglycemia. Calcium channel blockers in high dose have also been shown to cause peripheral insulin resistance. Thus, hyperglycemia can be a marker of calcium channel blocker overdose.[35] This hyperglycemic effect is more reliably seen with nondihydropyridines[36] than with dihydropyridines.[27]

FLECAINIDE (AND OTHER CLASS IA AND IC ANTIDYSRHYTHMICS)

Sodium channel blockers (Vaughan-Williams class I antidysrhythmics) all bind to sodium channels and change sodium conductance through fast inward voltage-gated sodium channels by slowing recovery from the open or inactivated state to the resting state. This results in reduction in depolarization rate of the cells and prolonged QRS duration on the ECG. Because a higher proportion of sodium channels are unable to reach a resting state and thus unable to depolarize, the excitability of the myocardium is reduced, and dysrhythmias can be terminated.[13] Sodium channel blockers can further be divided into 3 pharmacologic classes: IA, IB, and IC (**Table 3**). These classes further distinguish the xenobiotic's interaction with sodium channels. Class IC medications, which include flecainide and propafenone, affect activated sodium

Table 3
Sodium channel blockers, by class

Class IA	Class IB	Class IC
Disopyramide	Lidocaine	Flecainide
Procainamide	Mexiletine	Moricizine
Quinidine	Phenytoin	Propafenone

channels or have very slow release from sodium channels resulting in both prolonged channel blockade and decreased channel reactivation. This results in significant increase in toxicity, including QRS prolongation at slow heart rates. Flecainide toxicity in particular has been associated with bradycardia, PR prolongation, QRS and QTc prolongation, AV nodal blockade, and dysrhythmias including ventricular tachycardia and fibrillation.[37,38] Numerous medications, including antidysrhythmics,[37] analgesics,[39] antimalarials,[40] and antihistamines[41] exhibit sodium-channel-blocking effects; however, because of its disproportionate toxicity[4] we focus here on flecainide. Flecainide overdose may also cause a Brugada-like pattern on ECG.[42] In a review of patients treated with ECMO for poisonings over an 18-year period, flecainide was the most common sodium channel blocker in both pediatric and adult patients requiring ECMO with a 12% fatality rate.[4] Fatality rates as high as 22.5% have been reported in patients with any class IC overdose.[43] Dysrhythmia is the most concerning complication following a flecainide, or any class IC overdose, and the mainstay of therapy is close cardiac monitoring, gastrointestinal decontamination, and supportive care. Intravenous (IV) sodium bicarbonate administration is effective to overcome sodium channel blockade and thus prevent or treat dysrhythmias following flecainide overdose.[37,38,44] Flecainide is unique in that urinary alkalinization decreases flecainide clearance.[13] As mentioned earlier, class IC medications may also result in QT prolongation, which may be worsened by hypokalemia caused by sodium bicarbonate administration and intracellular potassium shifts. If sodium bicarbonate cannot be administered for any of these reasons, hypertonic saline boluses may be a reasonable alternative. Magnesium can be considered for patients with QT prolongation or concern for polymorphic ventricular tachycardia. Additional class IA or IC medications should be avoided because of the additional sodium channel blockade. IV lipid emulsion was successful in treating one patient with flecainide overdose.[37] In patients who develop life-threatening or refractory dysrhythmias, venoarterial ECMO (VA-ECMO) or cardiopulmonary bypass should be considered, if available.[38,45,46]

Class IA sodium channel blockers including disopyramide, procainamide, and quinidine are notable for their effects on potassium channels. These medications slow potassium efflux and thus prolong the action potential duration resulting in QT prolongation in addition to QRS prolongation on ECG. Similar to class IC sodium channel blockers, IV sodium bicarbonate to treat QRS prolongation, or magnesium as needed in the setting of QT prolongation are the cornerstones of therapy. Lidocaine is a reasonable alternative to treating dysrhythmias following class IA overdose. Owing to its rapid receptor kinetics, lidocaine may displace class IA antidysrhythmics from receptor sites, reducing sodium channel blockade.

Digoxin

Digoxin is a cardioactive steroid used to increase cardiac contractility in cases of congestive heart failure and to slow conduction in patients with rapid atrial fibrillation. Digoxin's main mechanism of action is inhibition of the membrane Na^+-K^+ ATPase pump on cardiac myocytes. Inhibition of the pump increases intracellular sodium and calcium, enhancing calcium release from the sarcoplasmic reticulum and producing muscle contraction. Secondarily, digoxin potentiates vagal activity depressing sinus node function and decreasing conduction through the AV node.[47] In addition, changes in ventricular repolarization as a result of intracellular calcium accumulation cause classic ECG changes including QT interval shortening and a "scooped" appearance to the ST segment. Delayed afterdepolarizations also occur with increased cytosolic calcium concentrations, resulting in a "U-wave" on the ECG, or premature ventricular contractions.[48] Digoxin has a narrow therapeutic window, with therapeutic concentrations ranging from 0.5 to 1.0 ng/mL.[49] An important consideration in evaluating digoxin concentrations is that digoxin has a very large volume of distribution, and a time period of 6 to 8 hours after digoxin dosing is required for digoxin to completely distribute to tissues, making concentrations drawn before distribution ("predistribution") difficult to interpret.

Digoxin toxicity is often categorized as acute or chronic. Regardless of chronicity, toxicity may result in sedation or altered mental status, nausea and vomiting, electrolyte disturbances, and a multitude of cardiac dysrhythmias. Although there is no specific ECG abnormality that confirms digoxin toxicity, a combination of increased automaticity and impaired conduction (an accelerated junctional rhythm with AV blockade for example) is suggestive.[50] Acute overdose is often marked by pronounced hyperkalemia, which is predictive of mortality.[51] Chronic toxicity often occurs in the face of worsening renal insufficiency given digoxin primarily undergoes renal excretion. While hypokalemia or hyperkalemia may be seen with chronic digoxin toxicity, one study showed that hyperkalemia (>5.0 mEq/L) was also associated with fatality in patients with chronic digoxin toxicity.[52]

In addition to cardiac monitoring and supportive care, there are additional treatment modalities that aid in the treatment of patients with digoxin overdose, including digoxin-specific antibody fragments. Hyperkalemia, particularly in the setting of chronic digoxin toxicity and renal failure can be multifactorial and should be managed similar to any other cause of life-threatening hyperkalemia.[50] Therapies including calcium salts, insulin/glucose, sodium bicarbonate, beta-2 agonists, potassium binders, and hemodialysis if needed are all appropriate therapies to treat hyperkalemia. Older literature suggested that the administration of IV calcium salts to patients with digoxin toxicity could be dangerous and precipitate cardiac tetany or "stone heart."[53–55] However, more recent literature suggests that IV calcium administration is safe in the treatment of digoxin toxicity.[56,57] In the setting of severe bradycardia, atropine may be attempted, but the response is unpredictable and bradycardia may be resistant to atropine. Temporary pacing, including external or transvenous pacing, has been suggested to precipitate fatal dysrhythmias in patients with digoxin toxicity.[58] One study showed that treatment with digoxin-specific antibodies was more effective in preventing life-threatening dysrhythmias in patients with digoxin toxicity compared with patients treated with pacemakers (92% vs 77%), and complications occurred with pacing in 36% of patients.[58] However, it is reasonable to attempt temporary pacing in patients with life-threatening bradydysrhythmias as a temporizing measure, or if digoxin-specific antibody therapy is delayed or unavailable. If digoxin-specific antibodies are unavailable, and a patient has persistent tachydysrhythmias, lidocaine is the most reasonable choice. Lidocaine has not been specifically studied for digoxin poisoning, whereas phenytoin has been described to be effective in treating digoxin-related tachydysrhythmias.[59] Given lidocaine and phenytoin are included in the same medication class (IB), and most clinicians are more familiar with lidocaine as an antidysrhythmic, we recommend lidocaine over phenytoin. In the setting of pulseless ventricular dysrhythmias, electrical cardioversion is reasonable; however, it is unlikely to abort dysrhythmias in otherwise stable patients.

Digoxin-specific antibodies are available for the reversal of digoxin toxicity. There is currently one option available in the United States, ovine digoxin immune fab, or DigiFab. Considerations for digoxin-specific antibodies are listed in **Box 1**. Each vial of digoxin immune fab contains 40 mg, which is able to bind approximately 0.5 mg of digoxin.[49] There are a variety of dosing methods available to treat both acute and chronic digoxin toxicity, if the amount of digoxin is known following an acute ingestion, or if a digoxin concentration is available (**Box 2**). Recent data suggest that a simpler

Box 1
Indications for digoxin immune fab administration

1. Ventricular dysrhythmias more severe than premature ventricular contractions
2. Progressive and hemodynamically significant bradydysrhythmias unresponsive to atropine
3. Serum potassium level greater than 5.0 mEq/L
4. Rapidly progressive rhythm disturbances or increasing potassium levels
5. Coingestion of cardiotoxic drugs, including those discussed in this review
6. Ingestion of plant known to contain cardioactive steroids plus severe dysrhythmia and/or potassium level greater than 5.0 mEq/L
7. Acute ingestion of greater than 10 mg or 0.1 mg/kg in a child *plus* any one of factors 1 to 6
8. Steady-state digoxin concentration greater than 6 ng/mL *plus* any one of the first 6 factors

treatment regimen is reasonable for acute and chronic digoxin toxicity. Pharmacokinetic modeling suggests that 1 to 2 vials (40–80 mg) of digoxin immune fab are sufficient to neutralize digoxin following acute overdoses. A reasonable approach is to treat empirically with 1 vial (40 mg), and repeat doses as needed if symptoms recur.[47] A review of 32 patients with chronic digoxin toxicity showed almost complete free digoxin binding after 1 vial (40 mg) of digoxin immune fab, and 15 of 16 patients treated with 2 vials of digoxin immune fab with free digoxin concentrations of 0 ng/mL after 2 vials of digoxin immune fab, suggesting an empirical treatment with 2 vials (80 mg) of digoxin immune fab for patients with chronic digoxin toxicity is likely sufficient.[49] The investigators comment, however, that although smaller doses of digoxin immune fab were effective in neutralizing digoxin, this did not necessarily correlate to resolution of bradydysrhythmias or hyperkalemia, likely secondary to other underlying complicated comorbidities. The time to onset of reversal of digoxin toxicity is variable. In one study, mean onset to initial response after infusion was 19 minutes (0–60 min), with complete response within a mean of 88 minutes (30–360 min).[60] The investigators noted that 10% of these patients had no response to digoxin immune fab, including patients who were moribund or ultimately determined not to have evidence of significant digoxin toxicity and only 1 patient who truly had no response to digoxin-specific antibody fragments. For patients who are in cardiac arrest, an empirical dose of 10 vials of digoxin immune fab is recommended. It is rare that a single institution would have this amount of antibody available, in which case providers should give the maximum available. There are numerous plants that contain cardiac glycosides similar to digoxin such as yellow oleander (*Cascabela thevetia,* also known as *Thevetia peruviana*) and lily of the valley (*Convallaria majalis*). In the past several years, there have been reports of the use of yellow oleander as a weight loss product, or substituted for benign plant material such as candlenuts.[61–63] For patients with evidence of severe cardiac glycoside poisoning from a weight loss product, an empirical dose of 20 to 30 vials of digoxin immune fab is recommended, if available.

Box 2
Digoxin immune fab dosing

- If dose of digoxin ingested is known but digoxin level is not known:
  - Dose in vials = (amount ingested in mg × 0.8) ÷ 0.5
- If digoxin level *is* known:
  - Dose in vials = (serum digoxin concentration [ng/mL] × patient's weight [kg])/100
    - Round to the nearest vial dosing

Response to digoxin immune fab or need for repeat dosing is predicated on clinical improvement, rather than digoxin concentrations. After digoxin immune fab is administered digoxin concentrations become unreliable and thus cannot be used to follow serum levels unless a laboratory is capable of measuring specifically free digoxin concentrations. When administering digoxin immune fab, exacerbation of the patient's underlying cardiac condition such as atrial fibrillation or congestive heart failure may occur given digoxin is no longer therapeutically active.

GENERAL APPROACH TO THE PATIENT WITH CARDIOTOXIC MEDICATION POISONING

Although cardiotoxic medications each have unique features in poisoning, some universal principles can be applied regardless of the specific medication. All patients with suspected cardiotoxic medication poisoning should receive a prompt evaluation and should be immediately placed on cardiac and pulse oximetry monitoring. IV access should be obtained immediately, and close monitoring of the patient's airway is recommended. If the patient appears drowsy, we recommend the use of end-tidal carbon dioxide monitoring to recognize apnea early. Although gastrointestinal decontamination is controversial for many poisoned patients,[64,65] the risk-benefit ratio in cardiotoxic poisoning favors the use of activated charcoal if there is reasonable suspicion that drug remains in the stomach, or if the drug may be amenable to treatment with multidose activated charcoal.[66] Hypotension should be treated with judicious use of isotonic crystalloid fluids; a 10- to 20-mL/kg bolus is a reasonable starting dose; however, we recommend close monitoring of volume status because volume overload is a common complication in cardiotoxic medication poisoning, particularly with calcium channel blockers.[27] For patients with bradycardia (**Box 3**), atropine (0.02 mg/kg in children with a minimum of 0.1 mg; 1 mg IV in adults) is a reasonable temporizing measure. Because atropine exerts its effects by antagonizing cholinergic input to the myocardium, it may improve the heart rate without appreciable effect on cardiac contractility, rendering it frequently ineffective in severe cardiotoxic medication poisoning.

General Approach to Treatment of Beta-Blocker and Calcium Channel Blocker Poisoning

Stage 1: initial stabilization

Fluid resuscitation, with careful monitoring for volume overload, is the initial treatment of choice for beta-blocker and calcium channel blocker poisoning. Atropine is also recommended for bradycardia at usual doses; a reasonable pulse rate to consider

Box 3
Xenobiotics that cause a combination of bradycardia and hypotension

α_2-adrenergic agonists (eg, clonidine, tizanidine, brimonidine)

Beta-blockers

Calcium channel blockers (particularly diltiazem and verapamil)

Cardioactive steroids (eg, digoxin, oleander, lily of the valley, "nuez de la India")

Cholinergic agents (eg, organophosphates, carbamates, cholinergic mushrooms including. *Clitocybe* and *Inocybe* spp)

Imidazolines (oxymetazoline, tetrahydrozoline, etc.)
Opioids
Withdrawal from sympathomimetic use

the administration of atropine in adults is 50 beats/min; however, atropine should only be administered if bradycardia is likely to be contributing to a lack of perfusion. As the final common pathway for both beta-blocker and calcium channel blocker poisoning is a lack of intracellular calcium (see **Fig. 1**), calcium salts are recommended if hypotension is refractory to fluid resuscitation. We recommend as an initial calcium dose 13 to 25 mEq (3–6 g calcium gluconate, 1–2 g calcium chloride) infused over 10 minutes; moribund patients may receive calcium more rapidly. If a response occurs, repeated doses may be given in 20 minutes, and a constant infusion may be started at 60 mg/kg/h of calcium gluconate (20 mg/kg/h of calcium chloride). If ionized calcium is measured instead of total calcium, we recommend not to exceed 1.5 times the upper limit of normal to minimize the risk of calciphylaxis.[67] The serum calcium concentration can be as high as 18 mg/dL within 15 minutes after a bolus of 5 mL of 10% calcium chloride, therefore calcium concentrations should be measured at least 30 minutes after dosing has concluded.

Although glucagon has been touted as the traditional "antidote" to beta-blocker poisoning, evidence supporting its use is limited.[68] Multiple studies show that glucagon is not superior to other traditional therapies, such as vasopressors and inotropes, for beta-blocker poisoning,[69–75] and glucagon is inferior to high-dose insulin (HDI).[76] Glucagon's hemodynamic effects are often transient, and glucagon frequently causes vomiting. Owing to glucagon's price, hospitals also rarely stock an adequate supply to treat a beta-blocker overdose, further limiting its utility. From clinical experience, we find glucagon most useful in treating small accidental overdoses of beta-blockers, or as a transient therapy to bridge patients to more definitive therapies in beta-blocker poisoning. If glucagon is used, we recommend 5 to 10 mg IV bolus (0.05–0.1 mg/kg for children). Glucagon has no role in calcium channel blocker poisoning. There is no mechanistic reason to believe it would be superior to beta-agonists (see **Fig. 1**), and it has several drawbacks as noted earlier. Patients not responding to these therapies should move to stage 2 (**Table 4**)

Stage 2: vasoactive infusions

Controversy exists on the optimal next therapy for patients refractory to IV fluids, calcium salts, atropine, and (in select cases of beta-blocker poisoning) glucagon. Some experts recommend vasopressors,[77] whereas others recommend HDI.[78] Vasopressors work typically via agonism of adrenergic, vasopressin, or angiotensin II receptors. In contrast, HDI is not a vasopressor, acting rather as both an inotrope and vasodilator. HDI treats shock via 3 mechanisms: increased inotropy via augmentation of calcium processing leading to improved myocardial contractility, maximization of

Table 4
Stages of treatment for beta-blocker and calcium channel blocker poisoning

Stage 1: Initial Stabilization	Stage 2: Vasoactive Infusions	Stage 3: Shock Refractory to HDI & 3 or More Vasopressors/Inotropes
• GI decontamination (if appropriate) • Judicious IV fluid resuscitation • IV calcium • Atropine • Glucagon (in select beta-blocker cases only)	• High-dose insulin • Other inotropes • Vasopressors	• Methylene blue • Intravenous lipid emulsion • Pacemaker • ECMO or other mechanical devices

Abbreviation: GI, gastrointestinal.

myocardial energy availability via optimization of intracellular myocardial glucose transport, and vasodilation via augmentation of endothelial nitric oxide to address microvascular dysfunction secondary to cardiogenic shock.[79] Recall cardiac output is defined by the following equation:

$$\text{Cardiac Output (CO)} = \text{heart rate (HR)} \times \text{stroke volume (SV)}$$

HDI results in a dose-dependent (from 1 U/kg/h to 10 U/kg/h) increase in CO; over a 6-h resuscitation CO may increase 50% comparing 1 U/kg/h versus 10 U/kg/h[80] As heart rate only increases modestly with HDI,[80–82] the vast majority of the increase in CO from HDI comes from an increase in stroke volume, best followed clinically via point-of-care ultrasound (POCUS), although serial echocardiograms is also a reasonable approach (Video 1).

A conundrum exists regarding vasopressors, in that the available evidence supporting their use is extremely limited, yet they are commonly used.[83] Animal data generally show vasopressors to be inferior to HDI,[76,84–86] and in some cases that vasopressors are inferior even to placebo,[81] whereas human case experience with vasopressors is generally positive.[77,83] Recently published large animal data suggest that whereas HDI is superior to vasopressors, in deep shock norepinephrine improves both brain perfusion and mortality.[86] As HDI and vasopressors seem to be synergistic, and vasopressors have a more immediate effect, our recommended strategy for patients with shock refractory to IV fluids, calcium salts, and atropine is to simultaneously start infusions of both low-dose norepinephrine (0.04 μg/kg/min) and HDI (1 U/kg IV bolus, followed by infusion of 1 U/kg/h). Norepinephrine is our recommended vasopressor of choice given its association with improved outcomes in cardiogenic shock,[87] and because of its synergism with HDI.[86] We then recommend close monitoring of pulse, cardiac contractility via POCUS, and mean arterial pressure (MAP) to determine the next optimal step in therapy (**Fig. 2**).

Once HDI and norepinephrine have been initiated, cardiac contractility, heart rate, and MAP should be reevaluated. If, after 30 minutes of HDI infusion at 1 U/kg/h cardiac contractility is still poor, we recommend titrating HDI up to 10 U/kg/h, based on reassessment of cardiac contractility and overall shock state (see HDI titration protocol, **Box 4**). Increasing infusion rates of HDI are associated with increased cardiac output; however, a dose-response phenomenon also occurs with HDI-induced vasodilation.[80] Particularly in dihydropyridine poisoning, HDI-induced vasodilation could, at some point, actually contribute to worsening shock.[82] It is therefore critical, from a hemodynamic standpoint, to establish the optimal HDI dose for each individual patient by carefully monitoring both cardiac output and systemic vascular resistance to optimize HDI dosing. HDI is also associated with other adverse effects that require careful monitoring in a critical care environment, including hypoglycemia, hypokalemia, and volume overload.[78,88,89] Unlike vasodilation, hypoglycemia and hypokalemia associated with HDI do not seem to be dose dependent.[80,88] Nevertheless, they both regularly occur during HDI infusions. Prolonged infusions of HDI can result in hypoglycemia even after HDI infusions cease on recovery.[90] The use of concentrated dextrose solutions via a central line (up to stock 70% dextrose) is associated with fewer hypoglycemic events,[78] and hypokalemia can be managed with typical intensive care unit replacement protocols. Because mild hypokalemia is expected to occur throughout the duration of HDI infusion, caution should be exercised when using HDI for drugs that are also known to prolong the QT interval, such as sotalol. Last, we also recommend concentrating infusions early in resuscitation, including the insulin solution itself (we recommend 10 U/mL) to avoid volume overload. Although HDI provides life-saving

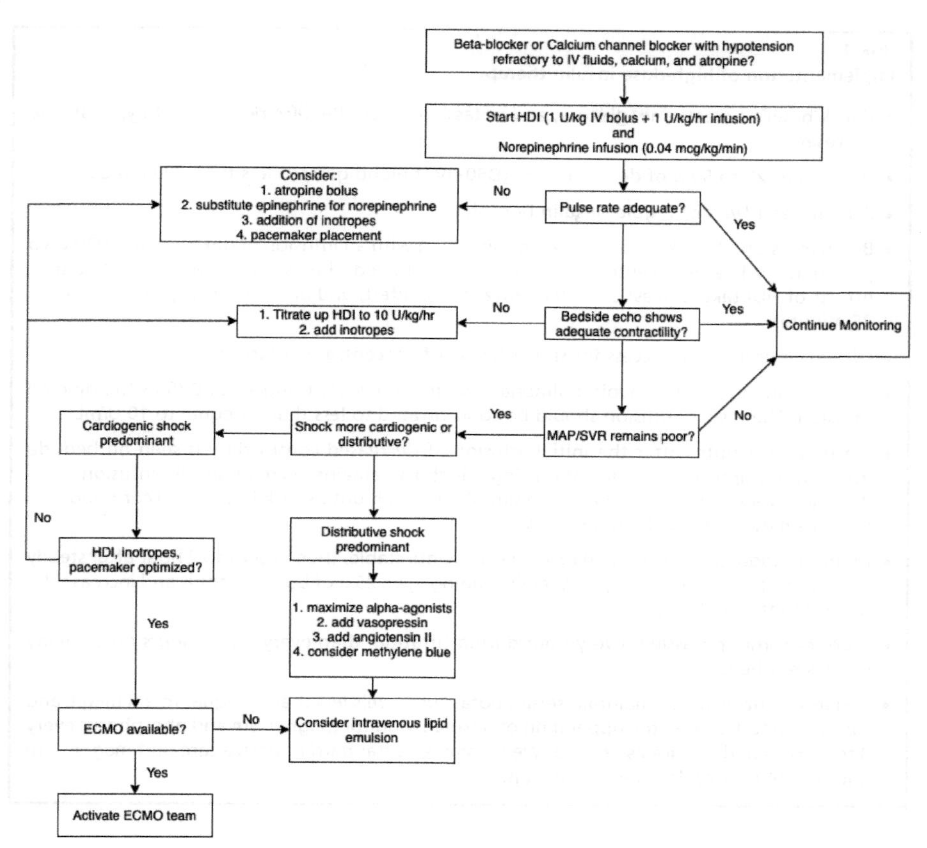

Fig. 2. A comprehensive algorithm for treating beta-blocker or calcium-channel blocker poisoning refractory to IV fluids, calcium, and atropine.

inotropic support in cardiotoxic poisoning, judicious use of the lowest effective dose and close monitoring for adverse events are both critical to optimize patient outcomes.

If bradycardia continues to contribute significantly to shock, therapies focused on increasing heart rate should be pursued, such as additional atropine doses or swapping epinephrine for norepinephrine to take advantage of epinephrine's additional beta-1 agonist effects. Pure inotropes and chronotropes, such as phosphodiesterase inhibitors, dobutamine, and isoproterenol, may also be considered for persistent bradycardia, although most of these medications also cause vasodilation, which could worsen shock. Cardiac pacemakers may be considered for refractory bradycardia, although evidence for pacemakers in poisoning-induced shock is mixed at best. We recommend a pacemaker only in cases in which all other therapies to increase both ejection fraction and heart rate have failed. If MAP continues to be poor after maximizing heart rate and cardiac contractility, it is important to reassess if shock at that point is primarily cardiogenic or distributive. If shock is predominantly cardiogenic, reassessment of therapies to maximize heart rate and contractility should be pursued. If shock is predominantly distributive, we recommend maximizing alpha-adrenergic agonists (typically norepinephrine). No true maximum dose of norepinephrine exists; however, at 0.5 μg/kg/min it is reasonable to add a second vasopressor. Our

Box 4
Implementation of high-dose insulin therapy

- Check baseline creatinine, glucose, and potassium levels. Replace potassium if hypokalemia is present.
- Administer 25 to 50 g of dextrose 50% (D50) IV if blood glucose less than 200 mg/dL.
- Administer 1 U/kg of regular insulin IV push.
- Begin infusion of 1 U/kg/h of regular insulin along with an infusion of dextrose; use D20 via a peripheral IV line until central access has been obtained, then start D50 at 25 g/h. Initial effects of HDI take at least 5 to 10 minutes to manifest, and are not reliably seen for 20 to 25 minutes.
- Obtain central venous access for safe infusion of concentrated glucose.
- Concentrate all fluids to avoid pulmonary edema. Consider using stock D70 as the glucose infusion. The insulin infusion should be concentrated to less than or equal to 10 U/mL.
- Starting 30 minutes after the initial infusion, if decreased contractility is seen on bedside echocardiography or evidence of cardiogenic shock remains, increase insulin infusion 1 to 2 U/kg/h every 15 minutes to a maximum of 10 U/kg/h until shock improves. Moribund patients may be titrated more rapidly.
- Monitor blood glucose every 10 to 15 minutes until stable, then every 1 to 2 hour after steady state is reached. For every hypoglycemic reading, give 25 g of D50 as a bolus and increase the dextrose infusion by 25 g/h.
- Monitor serum potassium every hour during titration, then every 4 to 6 hours once steady state is reached.
- Regarding electrolytes, maintain serum potassium levels less than or equal to 2.8 mEq/L and calcium up to 1.5 times the upper limit of normal. Monitor magnesium and phosphorus every 4 to 6 hours and replace as needed. We recommend standard intensive care unit magnesium and phosphorus replacement protocols.

recommended medication at that time would be vasopressin, dosed at 0.04 U/min in adults. For vasoplegia refractory to high-dose norepinephrine and vasopressin, angiotensin II would be a logical choice because it works via a unique mechanism of action compared with norepinephrine and vasopressin; however, its use in poisoning is poorly described at this time and is limited primarily to case reports.[91]

Stage 3: salvage therapies for shock refractory to high-dose insulin and 3 or more vasopressors

The treatment of beta-blocker or calcium channel blocker poisoning refractory to fluid resuscitation, calcium, atropine, HDI, and 3 or more vasopressors is a unique and profoundly critically ill patient population. As noted in stage 2, treatment depends on the predominant form of shock. For profound vasoplegia refractory to multiple vasopressors, recently methylene blue has gained favor. Methylene blue inhibits the enzyme guanylyl cyclase, resulting in decreased production of cyclic guanosine monophosphate (cGMP) and inhibition of endothelial smooth muscle relaxation, causing an increase in systemic vascular resistance.[92,93] Methylene blue is particularly intriguing for the treatment of amlodipine poisoning, because amlodipine uniquely causes an increase in nitric oxide production, leading to increased cGMP and vasodilation, although in animal models it has not proven superior to standard therapies.[94] Because methylene blue is an oxidant stressor and can lead to hemolysis and paradoxic methemoglobinemia, infusions are time limited. Dosing involves a 1- to 2-mg/kg bolus of a 1% methylene blue solution followed by an infusion of 1 mg/kg for up to 6 hours.

Intravenous fat emulsion (IFE) is an adjunctive therapy for cardiotoxic shock. IFE was first described for use in local anesthetic toxicity; however, its use soon spread to oral cardiotoxic overdoses,[37,95,96] including beta-blockers and calcium channel blockers.[97,98] IFE therapy has multiple proposed mechanisms, including lipid shuttling of offending poisons, providing free fatty acids as fuel for cardiac myocytes, and direct opening of cardiac calcium channels.[99] Although initial case reports and animal studies involving the use of IFE for cardiotoxic overdose were promising, support for IFE in treating oral cardiotoxic overdoses has waned recently.[100,101] A systematic review and expert panel found the evidence for nonlocal anesthetic poisoning to be of very low quality, and did not recommend for or against the use of IFE, even as a salvage therapy.[102] IFE is also associated with numerous adverse effects, including acute lung injury, pancreatitis, and cardiac arrest.[103,104] As such, we recommend IFE in patients with persistent shock not responding to IV fluids, calcium, HDI, and at least 3 vasopressors or inotropes at maximum recommended infusion rates if ECMO is unavailable. IFE dosing is not uniformly agreed upon.[105] We recommend an initial bolus of 1.5 mL/kg of 20% lipid solution administered over 2 to 3 minutes, followed immediately by an infusion of 0.25 mL/kg/min. If a response occurs at this infusion rate, the infusion dose may be decreased to 0.025 mL/kg/min (one-tenth the initial rate) to sustain lipemic serum for a longer period.[101,105]

Last, for patients with profound shock refractory to all other therapies, mechanical cardiovascular support, if available, is indicated. Although various methods, including intra-aortic balloon pumps,[78] left ventricular assist devices,[40,106] and cardiac bypass have been tried, owing to the proliferation of extracorporeal cardiopulmonary resuscitation programs[107] the availability of VA-ECMO for overdose has increased substantially in the past decade[4,108–111] and is therefore our recommended modality. VA-ECMO works nonspecifically to augment cardiac output to preserve organ function and allow for time to metabolize. As such we recommend VA-ECMO in moribund patients with evidence of persistent cardiogenic shock or refractory life-threatening dysrhythmias. The use of VA-ECMO for patients with distributive shock or shock from metabolic dysfunction is controversial and should be made on a case-by-case basis.

SUMMARY

Beta-blockers and calcium channel blockers result in a disproportionate number of fatalities from cardiac medication overdoses, and share similar characteristics. HDI is a superior therapy for both overdoses, but is likely synergistic with vasopressors; therefore we recommend starting vasopressors and HDI simultaneously. Digoxin remains an important cardiac poison and can likely be safely treated with smaller doses of fab fragments than in the past, except for patients in extremis. In patients with features of cardioactive steroid poisoning after ingestion of weight loss products, occult yellow oleander poisoning should be suspected. Flecainide is also a major cause of drug-induced cardiogenic shock and should be treated with hypertonic sodium bicarbonate in addition to usual therapies for cardiotoxic overdoses. ECMO is an invasive but promising nonspecific therapy for refractory shock from cardiotoxic overdose and should be considered primarily in cases of refractory cardiogenic shock.

CLINICS CARE POINTS

- HDI is an inotrope that improves cardiac output primarily via increased cardiac contractility, best monitored with bedside echocardiography.
- In most cases of digoxin poisoning, 2 vials of fab fragments are adequate to treat acute poisoning, and 1 vial is typically adequate in chronic poisoning.

- A pitfall patients and clinicians can make regarding weight loss supplements is confusing benign candlenuts (*Aleurites moluccana*) for yellow oleander (*Cascabela thevetia*), which contains potent cardioactive steroids. Yellow oleander poisoning, in contrast to digoxin poisoning, requires large doses of fab fragments (20–30 vials for acute poisoning).
- Flecainide poisoning should be treated with hypertonic sodium bicarbonate or hypertonic saline; close monitoring for iatrogenic alkalemia and hypernatremia is critical.
- For patients with any cardiotoxic poisoning not responding to HDI and 3 other vasopressors or inotropes, consider methylene blue for refractory vasoplegia and IFE or VA-ECMO for refractory cardiogenic shock.

DISCLOSURE

The authors have nothing to disclose.

SUPPLEMENTARY DATA

Supplementary data related to this article can be found online at https://doi.org/10.1016/j.emc.2022.01.014.

REFERENCES

1. Gummin DD, Mowry JB, Beuhler MC, et al. 2019 Annual Report of the American Association of Poison Control Centers' National Poison Data System (NPDS): 37th Annual Report. Clin Toxicol 2020;58(12):1360–541.
2. Spyres MB, Farrugia LA, Kang AM, et al. The Toxicology Investigators Consortium Case Registry-the 2019 Annual Report. J Med Toxicol 2020;16(4):361–87.
3. Correia MS, Whitehead E, Cantrell FL, et al. A 10-year review of single medication double-dose ingestions in the nation's largest poison control system. Clin Toxicol 2019;57(1):31–5.
4. Cole JB, Olives TD, Ulici A, et al. Extracorporeal Membrane Oxygenation for Poisonings Reported to U.S. Poison Centers from 2000 to 2018: an analysis of the national poison data system. Crit Care Med 2020;48(8):1111–9.
5. Wightman RSHRA. Cardiologic Principles II: Hemodynamics. In: Nelson LS, Howland MA, Lewin NA, et al, editors. Goldfrank's toxicologic emergencies. 11th Edition. New York City, NY: McGraw Hill; 2019. p. 260–7.
6. Levine M, Brent. Beta-Receptor Antagonists. In: Brent J, Burkhart K, Daragan P, et al, editors. Critical care toxicology. New York City, NY: Mosby; 2017. p. 771–86.
7. Wallukat G. The beta-adrenergic receptors. Herz 2002;27(7):683–90.
8. Ranniger C, Roche C. Are one or two dangerous? Calcium channel blocker exposure in toddlers. J Emerg Med 2007;33(2):145–54.
9. Schoffstall JM, Spivey WH, Gambone LM, et al. Effects of calcium channel blocker overdose-induced toxicity in the conscious dog. Ann Emerg Med 1991;20(10):1104–8.
10. Grant AO. Cardiac ion channels. Circ Arrhythm Electrophysiol 2009;2(2):185–94.
11. Bruccoleri RE, Burns MM. A Literature Review of the Use of Sodium Bicarbonate for the Treatment of QRS Widening. J Med Toxicol 2016;12(1):121–9.
12. Clancy C. Cardiologic Principles I: Electrophysiologic and Electrocardiographic Potentials. In: Nelson LS, Howland MA, Lewin NA, et al, editors. Goldfrank's

toxicologic emergencies. 11th Edition. New York City, NY: McGraw Hill; 2019. p. 244–59.
13. Mazer-Amirshahi M, Nelson LS. Antidysrhythmics. In: Nelson LS, Howland MA, Lewin NA, et al, editors. Goldfrank's toxicologic emergencies. 11th Edition. New York City, NY: McGraw Hill; 2019. p. 865–75.
14. Wax PM, Erdman AR, Chyka PA, et al. beta-blocker ingestion: an evidence-based consensus guideline for out-of-hospital management. Clin Toxicol 2005; 43(3):131–46.
15. Brubacher JR. Beta-adrenergic Antagonists. In: Nelson LS, Howland MA, Lewin NA, et al, editors. Goldfrank's toxicologic emergencies. 11th Edition. New York City, NY: McGraw Hill; 2019. p. 926–40.
16. Love JN, Howell JM, Klein-Schwartz W, et al. Lack of toxicity from pediatric beta-blocker exposures. Hum Exp Toxicol 2006;25(6):341–6.
17. Reith DM, Dawson AH, Epid D, et al. Relative toxicity of beta blockers in overdose. J Toxicol Clin Toxicol 1996;34(3):273–8.
18. Love JN, Litovitz TL, Howell JM, et al. Characterization of fatal beta blocker ingestion: a review of the American Association of Poison Control Centers data from 1985 to 1995. J Toxicol Clin Toxicol 1997;35(4):353–9.
19. Isbister GK, Heppell SP, Page CB, et al. Adult clonidine overdose: prolonged bradycardia and central nervous system depression, but not severe toxicity. Clin Toxicol 2017;55(3):187–92.
20. Weerink MAS, Struys MMRF, Hannivoort LN, et al. Clinical Pharmacokinetics and Pharmacodynamics of Dexmedetomidine. Clin Pharmacokinet 2017;56(8): 893–913.
21. Spiller HA, Bosse GM, Adamson LA. Retrospective review of Tizanidine (Zanaflex) overdose. J Toxicol Clin Toxicol 2004;42(5):593–6.
22. Gugelmann HMDFJ. Miscellaneous Antihpertensives and Pharmacologically Related Agents. In: Nelson LS, Howland MA, Lewin NA, et al, editors. Goldfrank's toxicologic emergencies. 11th Edition. New York City, NY: McGraw Hill; 2019. p. 959–68.
23. Seger DL, Loden JK. Naloxone reversal of clonidine toxicity: dose, dose, dose. Clin Toxicol 2018;56(10):873–9.
24. Jang DH. Calcium channel blockers. In: Nelson LS, Howland MA, Lewin NA, et al, editors. Goldfrank's toxicologic emergencies. 11th Edition. New York City, NY: McGraw Hill; 2019. p. 945–52.
25. Zhang X, Kichuk MR, Mital S, et al. Amlodipine promotes kinin-mediated nitric oxide production in coronary microvessels of failing human hearts. Am J Cardiol 1999;84(4A):27L–33L.
26. Zhang X, Hintze TH. Amlodipine releases nitric oxide from canine coronary microvessels: an unexpected mechanism of action of a calcium channel-blocking agent. Circulation 1998;97(6):576–80.
27. Lindeman E, Ålebring J, Johansson A, et al. The unknown known: non-cardiogenic pulmonary edema in amlodipine poisoning, a cohort study. Clin Toxicol 2020;1–8.
28. Wong A, Hoffman RS, Walsh SJ, et al. Extracorporeal treatment for calcium channel blocker poisoning: systematic review and recommendations from the EXTRIP workgroup. Clin Toxicol 2021;59(5):361–75.
29. Watling SM, Crain JL, Edwards TD, et al. Verapamil overdose: case report and review of the literature. Ann Pharmacother 1992;26(11):1373–8.

30. Mégarbane B, Karyo S, Abidi K, et al. Predictors of mortality in verapamil overdose: usefulness of serum verapamil concentrations. Basic Clin Pharmacol Toxicol 2011;108(6):385–9.
31. Beno JM, Nemeth DR. Diltiazem and metoclopramide overdose. J Anal Toxicol 1991;15(5):285–7.
32. Kumar S, Thakur D, Gupta RK, et al. Unresponsive shock due to amlodipine overdose: An unexpected cause. J Cardiovasc Thorac Res 2018;10(4):246–7.
33. Chudow M, Ferguson K. A case of severe, refractory hypotension after amlodipine overdose. Cardiovasc Toxicol 2018;18(2):192–7.
34. Nordmark Grass J, Ahlner J, Kugelberg FC, et al. A case of massive metoprolol and amlodipine overdose with blood concentrations and survival following extracorporeal corporeal membrane oxygenation (ECMO). Clin Toxicol 2019;57(1):66–8.
35. Ashraf M, Chaudhary K, Nelson J, et al. Massive overdose of sustained-release verapamil: a case report and review of literature. Am J Med Sci 1995;310(6):258–63.
36. Levine M, Boyer EW, Pozner CN, et al. Assessment of hyperglycemia after calcium channel blocker overdoses involving diltiazem or verapamil. Crit Care Med 2007;35(9):2071–5.
37. Ellsworth H, Stellpflug SJ, Cole JB, et al. A life-threatening flecainide overdose treated with intravenous fat emulsion. Pacing Clin Electrophysiol 2013;36(3):e87–9.
38. Brumfield E, Bernard KRL, Kabrhel C. Life-threatening flecainide overdose treated with intralipid and extracorporeal membrane oxygenation. Am J Emerg Med 2015;33(12):1840, e3-e5.
39. Cole JB, Sattiraju S, Bilden EF, et al. Isolated tramadol overdose associated with Brugada ECG pattern. Pacing Clin Electrophysiol 2012;35(8):e219–21.
40. Laes JR, Hendriksen S, Cole JB. Use of hyperbaric oxygen therapy in quinine-associated visual disturbances. Undersea Hyperb Med 2018;45(4):457–61.
41. Cole JB, Stellpflug SJ, Gross EA, et al. Wide complex tachycardia in a pediatric diphenhydramine overdose treated with sodium bicarbonate. Pediatr Emerg Care 2011;27(12):1175–7.
42. Soni S, Gandhi S. Flecainide overdose causing a Brugada-type pattern on electrocardiogram in a previously well patient. Am J Emerg Med 2009;27(3):375.e1–3.
43. Köppel C, Oberdisse U, Heinemeyer G. Clinical course and outcome in class IC antiarrhythmic overdose. J Toxicol Clin Toxicol 1990;28(4):433–44.
44. Wilgenhof A, Michiels V, Cosyns B. An irregular, extremely broad QRS complex rhythm. Am J Emerg Med 2019;37(10):1989.e1–3.
45. Reynolds JC, Judge BS. Successful treatment of flecainide-induced cardiac arrest with extracorporeal membrane oxygenation in the ED. Am J Emerg Med 2015;33(10):1542.e1–2.
46. Auzinger GM, Scheinkestel CD. Successful extracorporeal life support in a case of severe flecainide intoxication. Crit Care Med 2001;29(4):887–90.
47. Chan BSH, Buckley NA. Digoxin-specific antibody fragments in the treatment of digoxin toxicity. Clin Toxicol 2014;52(8):824–36.
48. Hack JB. Cardioactive Steroids. In: Nelson LS, Howland MA, Lewin NA, et al, editors. Goldfrank's toxicologic emergencies. 11th Edition. New York City, NY: McGraw Hill; 2019. p. 969–76.

49. Chan BS, Isbister GK, O'Leary M, et al. Efficacy and effectiveness of anti-digoxin antibodies in chronic digoxin poisonings from the DORA study (ATOM-1). Clin Toxicol 2016;54(6):488–94.
50. Hauptman PJ, Kelly RA. Digitalis. Circulation 1999;99(9):1265–70.
51. Smith TW, Butler VP Jr, Haber E, et al. Treatment of life-threatening digitalis intoxication with digoxin-specific Fab antibody fragments: experience in 26 cases. N Engl J Med 1982;307(22):1357–62.
52. Manini AF, Nelson LS, Hoffman RS. Prognostic utility of serum potassium in chronic digoxin toxicity: a case-control study. Am J Cardiovasc Drugs 2011; 11(3):173–8.
53. Gold H, Edwards DJ. The effects of ouabain on the heart in the presence of hypercalcemia. Am Heart J 1927;3(1):45–50.
54. Nola GT, Pope S, Harrison DC. Assessment of the synergistic relationship between serum calcium and digitalis. Am Heart J 1970;79(4):499–507.
55. Bower JO, Mengle HAK. The additive effect of calcium and digitalis: a warning, with a report of two deaths. JAMA 1936;106(14):1151–3.
56. Hack JB, Woody JH, Lewis DE, et al. The effect of calcium chloride in treating hyperkalemia due to acute digoxin toxicity in a porcine model. J Toxicol Clin Toxicol 2004;42(4):337–42.
57. Levine M, Nikkanen H, Pallin DJ. The effects of intravenous calcium in patients with digoxin toxicity. J Emerg Med 2011;40(1):41–6.
58. Taboulet P, Baud FJ, Bismuth C, et al. Acute digitalis intoxication–is pacing still appropriate? J Toxicol Clin Toxicol 1993;31(2):261–73.
59. Rumack BH, Wolfe RR, Gilfrich H. Phenytoin (diphenylhydantoin) treatment of massive digoxin overdose. Br Heart J 1974;36(4):405–8.
60. Antman EM, Wenger TL, Butler VP Jr, et al. Treatment of 150 cases of life-threatening digitalis intoxication with digoxin-specific Fab antibody fragments. Final report of a multicenter study. Circulation 1990;81(6):1744–52.
61. Cole JB, Corcoran JN. Yellow Oleander (Thevetia peruviana), a source of toxic cardiac glycosides, may be substituted for candlenuts (Aleurities moluccana) when taken as a weight-loss supplement. Cardiol Young 2020;30(11):1755–6.
62. Corcoran J, Gray T, Bangh SA, et al. Fatal yellow oleander poisoning masquerading as benign candlenut ingestion taken for weight loss. J Emerg Med 2020;59(6):e209–12.
63. González-Stuart A, Rivera JO. Yellow Oleander Seed, or "Codo de Fraile" (Thevetia spp.): A Review of Its Potential Toxicity as a Purported Weight-Loss Supplement. J Diet Suppl 2018;15(3):352–64.
64. Olson KR. Activated charcoal for acute poisoning: one toxicologist's journey. J Med Toxicol 2010;6(2):190–8.
65. American Academy of Clinical Toxicology. European Association of Poisons Centres and Clinical Toxicologists. Position paper: single-dose activated charcoal. Clin Toxicol 2005;43(2):61–87.
66. de Silva HA, Fonseka M, Pathmeswaran A, et al. Multiple-dose activated charcoal for treatment of yellow oleander poisoning: a single-blind, randomised, placebo-controlled trial. Lancet 2003;361(9373):1935–8.
67. Sim MT, Stevenson FT. A fatal case of iatrogenic hypercalcemia after calcium channel blocker overdose. J Med Toxicol 2008;4(1):25–9.
68. Bailey B. Glucagon in beta-blocker and calcium channel blocker overdoses: a systematic review. J Toxicol Clin Toxicol 2003;41(5):595–602.

69. Love JN, Leasure JA, Mundt DJ. A comparison of combined amrinone and glucagon therapy to glucagon alone for cardiovascular depression associated with propranolol toxicity in a canine model. Am J Emerg Med 1993;11(4):360–3.
70. Love JN, Leasure JA, Mundt DJ, et al. A comparison of amrinone and glucagon therapy for cardiovascular depression associated with propranolol toxicity in a canine model. J Toxicol Clin Toxicol 1992;30(3):399–412.
71. Sato S, Tsuji MH, Okubo N, et al. Milrinone versus glucagon: comparative hemodynamic effects in canine propranolol poisoning. J Toxicol Clin Toxicol 1994; 32(3):277–89.
72. Sato S, Tsuji MH, Okubo N, et al. Combined use of glucagon and milrinone may not be preferable for severe propranolol poisoning in the canine model. J Toxicol Clin Toxicol 1995;33(4):337–42.
73. Toet AE, te Biesebeek JD, Vleeming W, et al. Reduced survival after isoprenaline/dopamine in d,l-propranolol intoxicated rats. Hum Exp Toxicol 1996;15(2): 120–8.
74. Toet AE, Wemer J, Vleeming W, et al. Experimental study of the detrimental effect of dopamine/glucagon combination in d,l-propranolol intoxication. Hum Exp Toxicol 1996;15(5):411–21.
75. Holger JS, Engebretsen KM, Obetz CL, et al. A comparison of vasopressin and glucagon in beta-blocker induced toxicity. Clin Toxicol 2006;44(1):45–51.
76. Kerns W 2nd, Schroeder D, Williams C, et al. Insulin improves survival in a canine model of acute beta-blocker toxicity. Ann Emerg Med 1997;29(6): 748–57.
77. Levine M, Curry SC, Padilla-Jones A, et al. Critical care management ofverapamil and diltiazem overdose with a focus on vasopressors: a 25-year experience at a single center. Ann Emerg Med 2013;62(3):252–8.
78. Cole JB, Arens AM, Laes JR, et al. High dose insulin for beta-blocker and calcium channel-blocker poisoning. Am J Emerg Med 2018;36(10):1817–24.
79. Engebretsen KM, Kaczmarek KM, Morgan J, et al. High-dose insulin therapy in beta-blocker and calcium channel-blocker poisoning. Clin Toxicol 2011;49(4): 277–83.
80. Cole JB, Stellpflug SJ, Ellsworth H, et al. A blinded, randomized, controlled trial of three doses of high-dose insulin in poison-induced cardiogenic shock. Clin Toxicol 2013;51(4):201–7.
81. Cole JB, Corcoran JN, Engebretsen KM, et al. Use of a porcine model to evaluate the risks and benefits of vasopressors in propranolol poisoning. J Med Toxicol 2020;16(2):212–21.
82. Engebretsen KM, Morgan MW, Stellpflug SJ, et al. Addition of phenylephrine to high-dose insulin in dihydropyridine overdose does not improve outcome. Clin Toxicol 2010;48(8):806–12.
83. Skoog CA, Engebretsen KM. Are vasopressors useful in toxin-induced cardiogenic shock? Clin Toxicol 2017;55(4):285–304.
84. Holger JS, Engebretsen KM, Fritzlar SJ, et al. Insulin versus vasopressin and epinephrine to treat beta-blocker toxicity. Clin Toxicol 2007;45(4):396–401.
85. Kline JA, Tomaszewski CA, Schroeder JD, et al. Insulin is a superior antidote for cardiovascular toxicity induced by verapamil in the anesthetized canine. J Pharmacol Exp Ther 1993;267(2):744–50.
86. Katzung KG, Leroy JM, Boley SP, et al. A randomized controlled study comparing high-dose insulin to vasopressors or combination therapy in a porcine model of refractory propranolol-induced cardiogenic shock. Clin Toxicol 2019;57(11):1073–9.

87. De Backer D, Biston P, Devriendt J, et al. Comparison of dopamine and norepinephrine in the treatment of shock. N Engl J Med 2010;362(9):779–89.
88. Page CB, Ryan NM, Isbister GK. The safety of high-dose insulin euglycaemia therapy in toxin-induced cardiac toxicity. Clin Toxicol 2018;56(6):389–96.
89. Schimmel J, Monte AA. Risk of fluid overload from failure to concentrate high-dose insulin as an intravenous antidote. Ann Pharmacother 2019;53(3):325.
90. Corcoran JN, Jacoby KJ, Olives TD, et al. Persistent Hyperinsulinemia Following High-Dose Insulin Therapy: A Case Report. J Med Toxicol 2020. https://doi.org/10.1007/s13181-020-00796-2.
91. Carpenter JE, Murray BP, Saghafi R, et al. Successful treatment of antihypertensive overdose using intravenous angiotensin II. J Emerg Med 2019;57(3):339–44.
92. Jang DH, Donovan S, Nelson LS, et al. Efficacy of methylene blue in an experimental model of calcium channel blocker-induced shock. Ann Emerg Med 2015;65(4):410–5.
93. Laes JR, Williams DM, Cole JB. Improvement in hemodynamics after methylene blue administration in drug-induced vasodilatory shock: a case report. J Med Toxicol 2015;11(4):460–3.
94. LeRoy JM, Boley SP, Corcoran JN, et al. Effect of Methylene Blue on a Porcine Model of Amlodipine Toxicity. J Med Toxicol 2020;16(4):398–404.
95. Sirianni AJ, Osterhoudt KC, Calello DP, et al. Use of lipid emulsion in the resuscitation of a patient with prolonged cardiovascular collapse after overdose of bupropion and lamotrigine. Ann Emerg Med 2008;51(4):412–5, 415.e1.
96. Cole JB, Stellpflug SJ, Smith SW. Refractory hypotension and "ventricular fibrillation" with large U waves after overdose. JAMA Intern Med 2016;176(7):1007–9.
97. Stellpflug SJ, Fritzlar SJ, Cole JB, et al. Cardiotoxic overdose treated with intravenous fat emulsion and high-dose insulin in the setting of hypertrophic cardiomyopathy. J Med Toxicol 2011;7(2):151–3.
98. Stellpflug SJ, Harris CR, Engebretsen KM, et al. Intentional overdose with cardiac arrest treated with intravenous fat emulsion and high-dose insulin. Clin Toxicol 2010;48(3):227–9.
99. Weinberg GL. Lipid emulsion infusion: resuscitation for local anesthetic and other drug overdose. Anesthesiology 2012;117(1):180–7.
100. Mullins ME, Seger DL. Antidotal use of lipid emulsion - the pendulum swings. Clin Toxicol 2020;58(12):1281–3.
101. American College of Medical Toxicology. ACMT position statement: guidance for the use of intravenous lipid emulsion. J Med Toxicol 2017;13(1):124–5.
102. Gosselin S, Hoegberg LCG, Hoffman RS, et al. Evidence-based recommendations on the use of intravenous lipid emulsion therapy in poisoning. Clin Toxicol 2016;54(10):899–923.
103. Hayes BD, Gosselin S, Calello DP, et al. Systematic review of clinical adverse events reported after acute intravenous lipid emulsion administration. Clin Toxicol 2016;54(5):365–404.
104. Cole JB, Stellpflug SJ, Engebretsen KM. Asystole immediately following intravenous fat emulsion for overdose. J Med Toxicol 2014;10(3):307–10.
105. Fettiplace MR, Akpa BS, Rubinstein I, et al. Confusion about infusion: rational volume limits for intravenous lipid emulsion during treatment of oral overdoses. Ann Emerg Med 2015;66(2):185–8.
106. Laes JR, Olinger C, Cole JB. Use of percutaneous left ventricular assist device (Impella) in vasodilatory poison-induced shock. Clin Toxicol 2017;55(9):1014–5.

107. Dalia AA, Lu SY, Villavicencio M, et al. Extracorporeal cardiopulmonary resuscitation: outcomes and complications at a quaternary referral center. J Cardiothorac Vasc Anesth 2020;34(5):1191–4.
108. Ramanathan K, Tan CS, Rycus P, et al. Extracorporeal membrane oxygenation for poisoning in adult patients: outcomes and predictors of mortality. Intensive Care Med 2017;43(10):1538–9.
109. Weiner L, Mazzeffi MA, Hines EQ, et al. Clinical utility of venoarterial-extracorporeal membrane oxygenation (VA-ECMO) in patients with drug-induced cardiogenic shock: a retrospective study of the Extracorporeal Life Support Organizations' ECMO case registry. Clin Toxicol 2020;58(7):705–10.
110. Wang GS, Levitan R, Wiegand TJ, et al. Extracorporeal membrane oxygenation (ECMO) for severe toxicological exposures: review of the toxicology investigators consortium (ToxIC). J Med Toxicol 2016;12(1):95–9.
111. Lewis J, Zarate M, Tran S, et al. The recommendation and use of extracorporeal membrane oxygenation (ECMO) in cases reported to the california poison control system. J Med Toxicol 2019;15(3):169–77.
112. Bowman AJ, Chen CP, Ford GA. Nitric oxide mediated venodilator effects of nebivolol. Br J Clin Pharmacol 1994;38(3):199–204.

Toxin-Induced Seizures *Adapted from "Toxin-Induced Seizures" in Neurologic Clinics, November 2020

Haley N. Phillips, MD[a,*], Laura Tormoehlen, MD[b,c]

KEYWORDS

• Toxin • Seizure • Mechanism • Clinical management

KEY POINTS

- Many toxins can cause seizure in overdose and are changing over time, with new toxins always emerging; we outline common toxins resulting in seizure.
- Mechanisms for toxins are outlined to assist in the identification of future toxins with similar mechanisms of action that may result in seizure.
- Toxidromes of selected toxins are outlined, along with treatment approaches unique to each toxin.
- Treatment should be unique to underlying toxin mechanisms; in general GABA-A agonist treatments are preferred in toxin-induced seizures with adjunctive therapies depending on the mechanism of toxins.

INTRODUCTION

An important distinction in seizure management is the identification of a provoked versus an unprovoked seizure. This distinction allows for proper treatment of seizures and avoidance of unnecessary side effects of treatments that would not reduce the risk of seizure recurrence. Toxicity and withdrawal of medications, chemicals, and environmental toxins can result in seizure with some substances' effects more widely known than others[1,2] It is unclear the national incidence of toxin-induced seizures, but select population studies indicate the most common toxins that result in seizure have

[a] Department of Neurology, Emory University, Emory University Brain Health Center, 12 Executive Park Dr. 2 nd Floor, Suite 250, Atlanta, GA 30329, USA; [b] Department of Neurology, Department of Emergency Medicine, Indiana University, Indiana University Neuroscience Center, 355 W. 16 th Street, Suite 4700, Indianapolis, IN 46202, USA; [c] Department of Emergency Medicine, Indiana University, Indiana University Neuroscience Center, 355 W. 16 th Street, Suite 4700, Indianapolis, IN 46202, USA
* Corresponding author.
E-mail address: haleykathol@gmail.com

Emerg Med Clin N Am 40 (2022) 417–430
https://doi.org/10.1016/j.emc.2022.01.010

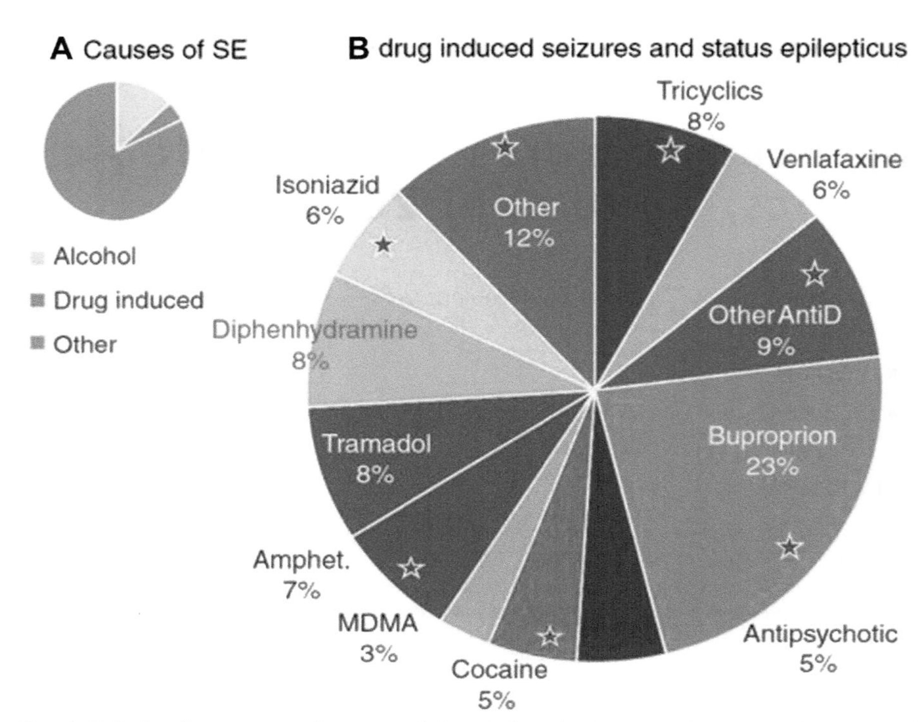

Fig. 1. Relative frequency and causes of drug-induced seizures and status epilepticus. (*A*) Data from a prospective population-based study of status epilepticus (SE, Status Epilepticus, n = 204 cases).[5] (*B*) Data from a retrospective review of cases (n = 386) whereby seizures were reported as an outcome reported as an outcome reported to the California State Poisons Registry in 2003; proportion (%) by drug/drug class. 3.6% of cases overall had status epilepticus (indicated by a star); and 27.7%, 2 or more seizures.[3] amphet, amphetamine; AntiD, Antidepressants; MDMA, 3,4-methylenedioxy-methamphetamine; SE, Status Epilepticus. (*From* "Cock, HR. Drug-induced status epilepticus. *Epilepsy & Behavior.* 2015;49:76-82"[4] with permission.)

evolved over time as prescribing practices evolve and new illicit substances become more widely available, see **Fig. 1**.[3–5] The basic mechanism of seizure activity resulting from chemicals, medications, or toxins (referred to as toxins throughout this article) involves the stimulation of central nervous system (CNS) excitatory pathways, or inhibition of inhibitory pathways within the CNS, or withdrawal of long-term CNS depressants. It is important to distinguish and identify toxin-induced seizure from epilepsy as the long- and short-term treatments differ.[4,6,7] We have identified and will outline the mechanisms and specific examples of toxins that result in seizure in 6 main categories. These categories are stimulants, cholinergics, gamma-aminobutyric acid (GABA) antagonists including GABA agonist withdrawal, glutamate agonists, histamine antagonists, and adenosine antagonists. There are many other drugs and toxins that cause seizures that are outside the scope of this article, see **Table 1** (PLASTICs Mnemonic).[8] Also outside the scope of this article are drug-induced metabolic derangements that cause seizures (eg, insulin and hypoglycemia or carbon monoxide and hypoxia).

The basic mechanism by which toxins cause seizure activity involves (1) increased excitation, (2) decreased inhibition, or (3) withdrawal of depressants. Excitatory

Table 1
PLASTIC mnemonic[a] for the partial listing of drugs and chemicals that may cause acute seizures

P	Phencyclidine, pesticides, phenol, propoxyphene
L	Lead, lithium, lindane, local anesthetics
A	Antidepressants, antipsychotics, anticonvulsants, antihistamines, abstinence syndromes
S	Salicylate, sympathomimetics, strychnine, solvents, shellfish (domoic acid)
T	Theophylline, tricyclic antidepressants, thallium, tobacco (nicotine)
I	Isoniazid, insulin (and other causes of hypoglycemia), insecticides
C	Camphor, cocaine, cyanide/carbon monoxide, chloroquine, cyclonite (C4 plastic explosive), cicutoxin

[a] The authors would like to acknowledge Dr James R. roberts for being the first to develop and teach this mnemonic at the poison control center, Phila.
From "Osterhoudt KC, Henretig FM. A 16-Year-Old With Recalcitrant Seizures. *Pediatric Emergency Care*. 2012;28 (3):304 - 306"[8] with permission.

neuronal activity can be caused by glutamate agonists, stimulants/sympathomimetics, and cholinergic agonists.[9] Excitation is the result of increased cellular sodium influx and decreases in chloride influx and potassium efflux. CNS depression results from GABA, adenosine, and histamine action; antagonizing the activity of these neurotransmitters results in decreased CNS inhibitory activity, thus shifting the balance toward CNS activation with seizure as a potential result.[10,11]

STIMULANTS

Stimulants are substances that shift the excitation-inhibition balance in the brain toward excitation, resulting in an agitated delirium. Many stimulants are sympathomimetic substances that increase the release of dopamine (DA), serotonin (5-HT), norepinephrine (NE), and epinephrine while also blocking their reuptake from the synaptic space, resulting in increased extracellular concentrations of these neurotransmitters. Sympathomimetic syndrome is characterized by anxiety, delusions, diaphoresis, hypertension, tachycardia, hyperreflexia, mydriasis, paranoia, piloerection, and seizures. Complications of severe poisoning include status epilepticus and uncoupling of oxidative phosphorylation.

Cocaine is a sympathomimetic that blocks the DA transporter, thereby increasing synaptic levels of biogenic amines (DA, 5-HT, and NE), and is also a sodium channel blocker. The result is a toxidrome that includes hypertension, but can also result in hypotension, QRS prolongation, and malignant cardiac dysrhythmia from sodium channel blockade.[12] Acute cocaine intoxication can be complicated by seizure, acidosis, hyperthermia, and uncoupling. Cocaine-induced hypertension generally should not be treated with beta-blockers, which could result in unopposed alpha-adrenergic action. The benzodiazepines used for agitated delirium and seizures will be useful in lowering heart rate and blood pressure.

Amphetamines and phenethylamines are sympathomimetics that diffuse into presynaptic vesicles, causing monoamine release. Additionally, they block monoamine oxidase (MAO) and the dopamine re-uptake transporter, which results in DA excess. At higher doses, receptors and synaptic clefts are flooded after increased vesicle release and blockade of 5-HT re-uptake. Amphetamine and methamphetamine block metabolism by inhibiting MAO, increasing the concentration of monoamines in the presynaptic nerve terminal, thereby promoting their release and directly activating postsynaptic receptors. Psychotic symptoms occur in overdose from excess 5-HT and DA activity; designer phenethylamines have variable psychoactive properties including hallucinations from 5-HT receptor agonism.[13] Serotonin syndrome is also possible and clinical features are hyperthermia, mydriasis, clonus, rigidity, and agitated delirium.

Synthetic cathinones, initially sold as “bath salts,” represent an abused class of substances that emerged over the past decade that can result in seizure, with notable prevalence in both pediatric and adult populations.[14,15] Seizure likely results from sympathomimetic toxicity with increased NE, 5-HT, and DA activity. Hyperthermia and seizure activity have been found to be associated in some studies.[14,15] Hyponatremia can also result, and the mechanism is unclear but may be similar to that of 3,4-methylenedioxy-methamphetamine (MDMA), resulting from SIADH, outlined later in discussion.[16]

Other psychostimulant designer drugs which are reported to result in seizure include benzylpiperazine (BZP), trifluoromethylphenylpiperazine (TFMPP), and MDMA. BZP and TFMPP enhance release of DA, NE, and 5-HT at the nerve terminals. BZP primarily increases DA and NE while TFMPP has more 5-HT agonist activity which increases activity at postsynaptic cell receptors.[17] MDMA acts to increase 5-HT activity by promoting its release into the synaptic cleft, inhibiting reuptake. This promotes prolonged 5-HT concentration in the synaptic cleft, resulting in increased binding to postsynaptic 5-HT2a receptors. MDMA also has been shown to reduce glutamic acid decarboxylase in the hippocampus, resulting in the increase of extracellular glutamate within the hippocampus which can lead to seizure, as well as resulting in GABAergic neuronal cell death.[18] The toxidrome for MDMA includes hypertension, hyperthermia, tachycardia, and hepatotoxicity. Serotonergic toxicity can cause serotonin syndrome. SIADH may also be seen, with serum sodium monitoring warranted in addition to seizure treatment with benzodiazepines and correction of hyponatremia if present.

Atypical antidepressants bupropion and venlafaxine are responsible for toxin-related seizures in 23% and 6% of a toxin-induced seizure cohort, respectively.[3] Bupropion, a monocyclic antidepressant and only synthetic cathinone approved by the U.S. Food and Drug Administration for pharmacologic use, inhibits presynaptic DA and NE reuptake transporters as well as increases DA, NE, and 5-HT vesicular transport into presynaptic vesicles and promotes their release to the synaptic space.[19–21] This results in a toxidrome including tremors, agitation, or tachycardia, but seizure can occur without other signs of CNS toxicity and may be delayed up to 24 hours. QRS prolongation caused by bupropion is due to blockade of cardiac gap junctions.[22] QTc interval prolongation may also result from cardiac potassium channel blockade, especially if taken with other agents that can prolong QT intervals, and this should be monitored as Torsade de Pointes can occur. Venlafaxine inhibits 5-HT and NE reuptake. It is associated with both QT and QRS prolongation with the risk of dysrhythmia in high doses. Venlafaxine associated seizure occurs at a reported higher rate than in SSRI or TCA overdose.[23]

Synthetic cannabinoids (eg, “K2” and “Spice”) (SCs) cause psychoactive effects by complete cannabinoid receptor-1 (CB_1R) agonism in the CNS. While not directly sympathomimetic, these drugs do produce a stimulant syndrome. A higher binding affinity for CBRs has been noted in most SCs compared to Δ9-tetrahydrobannabinol (Δ9-THC); it is also known that SCs have full agonist activity compared with the partial agonist activity of Δ9-THC.[24] The toxidrome other than seizures for SCs include anxiety, psychosis, agitation, and tachycardia and are felt to be secondary to the high affinity of SC metabolites for CB_1R and CB_2R, increased direct activity on the receptors, as well as possible upregulation of 5HT-2 receptors from CB_2R activation.[24,25] A potentially additive mechanism for seizure is prolonged or exaggerated effect, as the metabolites of SC parent compounds bind with much higher affinity to CBRs than Δ9-THC does.[26]

Phencyclidine (PCP) is an N-methyl-0064-aspartate (NMDA) receptor antagonist with high affinity for receptors in the limbic system, as well as a DA, NE, and 5-HT reuptake inhibitor. It has a stimulant toxidrome that is often marked by significant agitation, seizure, psychosis, and alteration in awareness.[27] Overall, the initial clinical treatment of stimulant toxicity is benzodiazepines which increase GABA activity to combat the sympathomimetic toxidrome and cease seizures. Frequent monitoring of serum electrolytes (particularly sodium, potassium, and glucose) and cardiac monitoring for QRS and QTc prolongation, arrhythmias, and cardiac ischemia are important in the supportive care for patients with stimulant/sympathomimetic toxidromes. Primary treatment of cardiac dysrhythmias is sodium bicarbonate for QRS prolongation, and potassium repletion (to keep >4.0 mEq/L) and magnesium supplementation for QTc prolongation. Avoidance of beta-blockers in some settings may be warranted depending on the toxins involved. In general, no methods of enhanced elimination or antidotes are indicated. Cyproheptadine has been considered as second-line treatment of serotonin syndrome, but evidence of efficacy is poor and its use remains controversial.[1,16]

CHOLINERGIC AGENTS

Acetylcholine (Ach) agonists stimulate directly by binding nicotinic or muscarinic receptors to promote their activity. Alternatively, some agents inhibit acetylcholinesterase, resulting in an increased amount of acetylcholine at the nerve terminal by preventing its intrasynaptic breakdown. The increased acetylcholine binds to nicotinic and muscarinic receptors. Different studies have shown muscarinic or nicotinic receptors may both be responsible for seizures depending on the region of the brain (basal forebrain by nicotinic receptors or zona incerta by muscarinic).[28,29]

Nerve agents have been observed in vivo to result in seizures and status epilepticus by increasing muscarinic receptor action in the entorhinal cortex–hippocampus complex.[30] In nerve agent poisoning, animal models have also shown an initial response to atropine, an antimuscarinic agent, stopping seizures in the acute setting, but prolonged seizure activity results in neuropathology that causes recurrent seizure activity. This seems to be due to prolonged cholinergic action resulting in NMDA receptor stimulation and glutamatergic excitation and resultant cellular damage.[6,31] Nerve agents bind to serine residues at the active site of the acetylcholinesterase enzyme, resulting in seizure from excessive Ach activity in the CNS.[32] Associated symptoms from neuromuscular junction nicotinic ACh activity include weakness, fasciculations, respiratory depression, and eventual paralysis. The muscarinic symptoms of cholinergic toxicity can be represented by the mnemonic DUMBBELS: defecation, urination, miosis, bradycardia, bronchospasm, emesis, lacrimation, and salivation. Treatment with pralidoxime may be warranted to treat and/or prevent nicotinic symptoms, specifically weakness. Atropine is the treatment of muscarinic symptoms and is dosed to the resolution of bronchorrhea and bronchoconstriction.[33] Seizures should be treated with benzodiazepines.

Organophosphate pesticides have the same mechanism as nerve agents, and can result in convulsions as well, with early seizure resulting from nicotinic ACh receptor hyperstimulation, followed by a mixed cholinergic and noncholinergic phase, then finally into a noncholinergic phase with associated glutamatergic excitotoxicity resulting in permanent damage to neurons.[33] Organophosphates can induce a DUMBBELS toxidrome from the hyperstimulation of muscarinic Ach receptors.[34] Benzodiazepines have primarily been used to treat seizure in these cases. It has been proposed that cholinergic stimulation may cause increased central glutamatergic activity, and thus treatment with glutamate receptor antagonists, adenosine receptor agonists, or antimuscarinics with antiglutamatergic action could hypothetically play a role in future treatment.[34,35] Otherwise, treatment recommendations mirror those for the nerve agents.

Nicotine acts on the central and peripheral nervous systems to result in gastrointestinal, respiratory, cardiovascular, and neurologic effects. One proposed mnemonic is the days-of-the-week "MTWTFSS," for Mydriasis, Tachycardia, Weakness, Tremors, Fasciculations, Seizures and Somnolence, to recall the nicotinic toxidrome.[36] Seizure is hypothesized to result from nicotine by the activation of central nicotinic acetylcholine receptor. Several hypotheses of the mechanism include Excitatory Amino Acid Transporter 3 (EATT3) activity reduction by nicotine, resulting in glutamate accumulation. Other hypotheses include: enhancing NO production through glutamate release and NMDA receptor activation, reducing GABAergic signal to the hippocampus, oxidative stress from nicotine causing glutathione depletion, and oxidative stress causing increased reactive oxygen and nitrogen species leading to epileptogenesis.[37]

Treatment of seizures resulting from excess cholinergic activity relies on benzodiazepines and support for additional associated symptoms with antimuscarinics and/or oximes as described. There are no indicated methods of enhanced elimination other than activated charcoal in pesticide ingestion.

GAMMA-AMINOBUTYRIC ACID ANTAGONISTS

The GABA-A receptor is a chloride ion (Cl-) channel. GABA-ergic neurons have postsynaptic GABA-A receptors and presynaptic GABA-B receptors. When bound to the GABA-A receptor, GABA results in chloride ion influx into the cell resulting in hyperpolarization and thus inhibits action potentials. GABA-A agonists (ie, benzodiazepines and barbiturates) reduce cerebral activity, and toxicity from these drugs results in coma. Withdrawal states can precipitate seizures as well as status epilepticus.[4] GABA-B receptors are metabotropic and have second messenger systems; binding of presynaptic GABA-B results in the prevention of release of GABA. Postsynaptic GABA-B receptor activation induces a slower and longer inhibition than GABA-A.[38] GABA-B activity results in muscle relaxation, decreased cognitive function, pain relief, bronchiolar relaxation, nausea, reduced intestinal peristalsis, and dizziness.[39]

A commonly-used analgesic that is known to cause seizure is the partial *mu*-opioid agonist tramadol.[3] It is notable that therapeutic levels of tramadol have been known to result in seizure, with single exposure overdose ingestion in up to 52.5% of patients in one population. Another state reported 13.7% of toxin-induced seizures were from tramadol over 2.5 years.[40,41] The exact mechanism for seizure is unknown, but likely results from the excessive synaptic accumulation of 5-HT and NE by reuptake inhibition, and inhibition of GABA-A receptors.[42–44]

Baclofen is a known GABA-B receptor agonist that results in seizure from abrupt withdrawal as well as intoxication.[3] Baclofen binds to the GABA-B receptor and promotes presynaptic GABA release by potassium efflux as well as decreased calcium conductance. This hyperpolarizes neurons, resulting in the diminished release of neurotransmitters, but can result in a paradoxic seizure in high doses.[45] The exact mechanism of seizure is unknown, but it has been proposed that in toxic doses baclofen becomes a GABA-A and -B receptor agonist and may decrease GABA release via presynaptic auto receptor activation.[46] Abrupt withdrawal of the GABA-B agonist can also precipitate seizure (see section on withdrawal).[47]

Antimicrobials

A key mechanism in toxin-induced seizures is that GABA synthesis requires glutamate to be converted to GABA via glutamic acid decarboxylase, a reaction that requires pyridoxine as a coenzyme. Depletion of pyridoxine (vitamin B6) can result in excess glutamate activity and GABA depletion. The resulting GABA deficiency will prevent the GABA-A channel from opening, that is GABA itself is required for receptor function. Thus, benzodiazepines alone will not be successful in treating seizure in the setting of pyridoxine deficiency, the deficiency must be treated.

Isoniazid (INH) is an inhibitor of pyridoxine phosphokinase by the hydratization of pyridoxal-5-phosphate, which results in the depletion of active B6 so GABA synthesis from glutamate is unable to proceed. This results in excessive glutamatergic action and absence of GABA tone; pyridoxine and benzodiazepines are both needed to treat seizures resulting from INH.[38,48]

Penicillin, cephalosporins (particularly cefepime), carbapenems, and fluoroquinolones all bind to and inhibit the GABA-A receptor, which results in a reduction of Cl- influx, allowing for convulsive activity to be promoted and not inhibited. Penicillin and aztreonam can also bind the channel to block the influx of chloride resulting in decreased GABA tone. Penicillin has also been postulated to directly bind to the benzodiazepine site on the GABA-A receptor to produce convulsions.[21,49]

Withdrawal of Gamma-Aminobutyric Acid Agonists

Acute or abrupt withdrawal from various sedatives can precipitate seizures via mechanisms of the GABA pathways, which were outlined above. Acute withdrawal from GABA agonists has been shown to result in seizure in the literature and sedative withdrawal has increased as a cause for toxin-induced seizure.[3] Chronic use of GABA agonists such as benzodiazepines, ethanol, GHB, barbiturates, and baclofen result in decreased GABA receptor density in the brain. Then, the abrupt discontinuation of the medication results in seizure from relative unopposed excitatory action with less GABA tone to promote inhibitory action. The medication flumazenil is a partial agonist at the GABA receptor. It is a medication sometimes used as a reversal agent in overdose, but is known to precipitate an acute GABA withdrawal by competitively binding to the receptors, decreasing overall GABA tone, and thus resulting in seizure.[3,50]

Baclofen is a GABA-B receptor agonist that in withdrawal can precipitate seizures and status epilepticus. Seizure has been documented to occur with baclofen toxicity, outlined previously, and withdrawal precipitates seizure from lack of GABA tone that was previously maintained with chronic baclofen administration.[51,52]

Antidepressants and Antipsychotics

Tricyclic antidepressants (TCAs) are medications often prescribed and have been noted in one study to represent nearly 8% of drug-induced seizures. This is less than previously reported, but still the third leading cause of seizure reported to a poison control center.[3] The primary mechanism of inducing seizure is from GABA-A antagonism. TCAs possess antimuscarinic and antihistaminergic properties, as well as cause sodium channel blockade. Hyperthermia, flushing, mydriasis, ileus, and urinary retention occur as a result of antimuscarinic toxicity, QRS prolongation from sodium channel blockade, as well as QTc prolongation from potassium efflux blockade. Physostigmine is contraindicated in TCA toxicity as it has been associated with cardiac arrest in TCA overdose, regardless of the prominent anticholinergic toxidrome.[53]

Other antidepressants including selective serotonin reuptake inhibitors (SSRIs) and selective serotonin and norepinephrine reuptake inhibitors (SNRIs) have been shown to result in seizure.

Venlafaxine increases 5-HT and NE to result in seizure activity alone or with the combination of other serotonergic agents. Citalopram has been cited to more likely cause seizure than escitalopram given its racemic mixture of R and S-enantiomers. SSRIs in overdose can lead to serotonin syndrome as well as hyponatremia, with paroxetine use at therapeutic doses also leading to seizure from hyponatremia.[54–56] Glutamate release increase, AMPA receptor expression increase, and NMDA receptor interaction postsynaptically may also play a role in antidepressant overdose resulting in seizure.[54,57,58]

Antipsychotics, in particular, have been reported to have a 2-fold increase in seizure when used in combination with other antipsychotic drugs, tricyclic antidepressants, or lithium in an inpatient psychiatric population.[3,57] Phenothiazine antipsychotics are also known to result in seizure in toxicity or overdose, common examples include chlorpromazine, prochlorperazine, thioridazine, and perphenazine, though true incidence of these rates is unclear. Clozapine particularly has been reported to cause seizures, often in concomitant use with other antidepressants or antipsychotics as well as in high therapeutic doses. Potassium and sodium channel blockade can result in cardiac dysrhythmia, DA and muscarinic receptor imbalance can result in dystonic reactions, and antidopaminergic effect can result in neuroleptic malignant syndrome.[20,54,58]

Treatment of GABA agonist withdrawal or GABA antagonists involves maintaining or improving GABA tone with benzodiazepines. Pyridoxine should be given in cases of pyridoxine deficiency as benzodiazepines will not be effective without the presence of GABA. Barbiturates may be required for treatment as well if the benzodiazepine site is blocked by an antagonist, or as adjunctive therapy in severe cases.[6]

GLUTAMATE AGONIST

Glutamate agonists bind 3 subgroups of receptors to induce seizure activity: (1) NMDA, (2) α-amino-3-hydroxy-5-methyl-4-isoxazolepropionic acid (AMPA), and (3) kainite. They promote Na + influx and K+ efflux from neurons to further perpetuate action potentials and promote hyperactivity. Glutamate transporter inhibition also results in excess glutamate in the synaptic cleft and promotes neuroexcitability resulting in seizure.[2,9,11] Domoic acid is produced by algae consumed by shellfish, bioaccumulated in the shellfish, and is ingested by humans who consume the shellfish. Seizures result from glutaminergic AMPA receptor activation. This can result in mesial temporal sclerosis; thus patients may develop recurrent complex partial seizures even after acute toxicity has resolved.[59] Amanita muscaria mushrooms, with large red caps and white spots, are ingested for hallucinogenic effects or by accidental ingestion. Ibotenic acid and muscimol are the toxins concentrated in the caps of the mushroom. Ibotenic acid results in CNS excitation while muscimol promotes CNS depression. Ibotenic acid results in excitatory effects at glutamic acid receptors in the CNS, which is responsible for causing seizure. Toxidrome of ingestion of *A. muscaria* includes somnolence or coma (from the action of muscimol to promote GABA action), hallucinations, seizure, nausea and vomiting, diarrhea, and salivation. Treatment of delirium, agitation, or seizures is primarily with benzodiazepines and toxicity generally resolves after 24 hours.[60,61] Treatment of glutamate agonist toxicity includes counteraction with benzodiazepines to promote GABA activity.

HISTAMINE ANTAGONISTS

Histamine can inhibit seizure by binding to its G protein-coupled receptors to promote several intracellular pathways which play a role in GABA, glutamate, DA, 5-HT, and ACh pathways. Seizures result from excitotoxicity from antagonism at histamine receptor 1 (HR1). Dysregulation of the sodium/hydrogen pump has been shown to be caused by HRs. How the loss of HR function lowers seizure threshold is not fully understood. One theory is the sodium/hydrogen pump loss of function causes neuronal cells to have an inability to regulate pH changes and reduce the threshold for cellular signaling resulting in the propagation of epileptic discharges.[62,63]

Diphenhydramine is perhaps the most common antihistamine to result in seizure, the causative agent in 8% of a cohort study population of drug-induced seizures.[3,64] Other examples of antihistamines than can cause seizures to include doxylamine, hydroxyzine, and chlorpheniramine. Sodium channel blockade also contributes to the toxidrome, leading to QRS prolongation and wide complex tachycardia. Status epilepticus is less common.[4,65] Anticholinergic syndrome is characterized by confusion, ataxia, disorientation, hallucinations, agitated delirium, psychosis, dry mucous membranes, and mydriasis. Treatment for seizures includes benzodiazepines, but overall, seizures are usually self-limited and avoidance of further anti-histamines is encouraged.[4]

ADENOSINE ANTAGONISTS

Intracellular adenosine is used in the adenosine-diphosphate (ADP) conversion to adenosine triphosphate (ATP) for cellular energy, the base compound being mediated by adenosine kinase to help formulate adenosine monophosphate from adenosine. It is helpful to understand this as it outlines the relationship of adenosine to seizure activity from a cellular level. The uptake of adenosine by the over activity of adenosine kinase leads to low synaptic adenosine levels, which results in an increased risk of seizure activity. The high likelihood of recurrent seizures or status epilepticus is likely due to adenosine's role in endogenous anti-seizure effects.[3,66,67] Historically, theophylline is a common example of adenosine antagonism resulting in seizure, though its prevalence may be decreasing.[3] It's adenosine receptor antagonism that causes relative increases in cGMP while preventing cAMP increases. Seizure activity results from theophylline's action to block the brain's natural anticonvulsant adenosine; theophylline toxicity typically presents as focal and generalized seizures clinically which do not respond to anticonvulsant drugs. Often, patients with theophylline-induced seizure have elevated serum levels of theophylline, but a therapeutic dose may also result in seizure. The physiology of chronic obstructive pulmonary disease (COPD) results in increased sympathetic response. This, combined with the adenosine antagonism of theophylline puts patients with COPD taking this medication at a higher risk for seizure and toxicity as there is a dual mechanism for CNS excitation.[66] Bronchodilation from phosphodiesterase antagonism is also seen with theophylline toxicity but seizure may be the only presenting symptom. Mortality from theophylline toxicity is as high as 10%, especially if seizures or cardiac dysrhythmia occur.[68]

Other methylxanthines, including caffeine, act via adenosine pathways to result in seizure in toxicity in a similar mechanism. Compared with other stimulants or theophylline, caffeine-induced seizure is less commonly cited in the literature among human studies but has been described in animal models.[69–71] It should be noted though, that some report a lowered seizure threshold in patients with underlying epilepsy during caffeine use.[72] Treatment of adenosine antagonist mediated seizures in toxicity primarily involves discontinuing the offending agent and supportive treatment with benzodiazepines for seizure cessation. Barbiturates or propofol after the initiation of mechanical ventilation may be required for prolonged seizures or status epilepticus.[68] Hemodialysis may be indicated for enhanced elimination.[73]

CLINICS CARE POINTS

- First-line management: Benzodiazepines.
- Second-line treatment should include other GABA agonists, such as propofol or barbiturates rather than traditional anticonvulsants (eg, phenytoin)
- Limited data on the benefit of newer anticonvulsants (eg, levetiracetam) for toxin-induced seizure treatment, but the paucity of data prevents change in practice recommendations at this time.[7]
- Phenytoin has been considered as a second-line agent, but it is often not effective, and may actually worsen toxin-induced seizures and contribute to cardiac toxicity.
- In general, GABA-A agonist treatments (benzodiazepines, barbiturates, and propofol) are preferred in toxin-induced seizures to increase the rate and duration of GABA channel opening.[74]
- Given the variety or multitude of toxidromes that may be present, adjunctive therapy will vary more than first-line treatments for toxin-induced seizures. As an example, given the mechanism of INH causing seizures, pyridoxine will be an important treatment adjunct. Certain toxidromes, such as theophylline may require hemodialysis in addition to benzodiazepines.
- Poison centers are an excellent resource for the most up-to-date recommendations on toxin-induced seizure treatment.

SUMMARY

Many toxins cause seizure in therapeutic use or overdose, as well as in withdrawal states, although the most common culprits change over time.[3] Though not a complete and exhaustive list, the above reviews commonly reported toxins and mechanisms of seizure. Understanding the mechanism, characteristic toxidromes, and treatments of commonly reported toxins is essential to correctly identify and appropriately treat patients who present after a toxin-induced seizure. Physician familiarity with the commonly known toxins that result in seizure is pivotal in the comprehensive evaluation of seizure (see **Fig. 1**).[8] Physician awareness also helps in the ongoing reporting efforts to identify the evolution of toxin trends as new toxins are continually emerging. The mechanisms understood to cause seizure in existing toxins can be helpful in predicting if new toxins will likely result in seizure in the setting of overdose, abuse, or poisoning, as well as therapeutic use.

DISCLOSURE

The authors have nothing to disclose.

REFERENCES

1. Barry JD, Wills BK. Neurotoxic emergencies. Neurol Clin 2011;29(3):539–63.
2. Alldredge BK, Lowenstein DH, Simon RP. Seizures associated with recreational drug abuse. Neurology 1989;39(8):1037–9.

3. Thundiyil JG, Kearney TE, Olson KR. Evolving epidemiology of drug-induced seizures reported to a Poison Control Center System. J Med Toxicol 2007;3(1):15–9.
4. Cock HR. Drug-induced status epilepticus. Epilepsy Behav 2015;49:76–82.
5. DeLorenzo RJ, Hauser WA, Towne AR, et al. A prospective, population-based epidemiologic study of status epilepticus in Richmond, Virginia. Neurology 1996;46(4):1029.
6. Chen H-Y, Albertson TE, Olson KR. Treatment of drug-induced seizures. Br J Clin Pharmacol 2016;81(3):412–9.
7. Lee T, Warrick BJ, Sarangarm P, et al. Levetiracetam in toxic seizures. Clin Toxicol 2018;56(3):175–81.
8. Osterhoudt KC, Henretig FM. A 16-Year-old with recalcitrant seizures. Pediatr Emerg Care 2012;28(3):304–6.
9. Chapman AG. Glutamate receptors in epilepsy. Prog Brain Res 1998;116: 371–83.
10. Schlicker E, Kathmann M. Role of the Histamine H3 Receptor in the Central Nervous System. Handb Exp Pharmacol 2017;241:277–99.
11. Barker-Haliski MW HS. Glutamatergic mechanisms in seizures and epilepsy. Cold Spring Harb Perspect Med 2015;5:a022863.
12. Sanchez-Ramos J. Neurologic complications of psychomotor stimulant abuse. Int Rev Neurobiol 2015;120:131–60.
13. Dean BV, Stellpflug SJ, Burnett AM, et al. 2C or not 2C: phenethylamine designer drug review. J Med Toxicol 2013;9(2):172–8.
14. Riley AL, Nelson KH, To P, et al. Abuse potential and toxicity of the synthetic cathinones (i.e., "Bath salts"). Neurosci Biobehav Rev 2019;110:150–73.
15. Tekulve K, Alexander A, Tormoehlen L. Seizures associated with synthetic cathinone exposures in the pediatric population. Pediatr Neurol 2014;51(1):67–70.
16. Prosser JM, Nelson LS. The toxicology of bath salts: a review of synthetic cathinones. J Med Toxicol 2012;8(1):33–42.
17. Schep LJ, Slaughter RJ, Vale JA, et al. The clinical toxicology of the designer "party pills" benzylpiperazine and trifluoromethylphenylpiperazine. Clin Toxicol 2011;49(3):131–41.
18. Huff CL, Morano RL, Herman JP, et al. MDMA decreases glutamic acid decarboxylase (GAD) 67-immunoreactive neurons in the hippocampus and increases seizure susceptibility: Role for glutamate. Neurotoxicology 2016;57:282–90.
19. Foley KF, DeSanty KP, Kast RE. Bupropion: pharmacology and therapeutic applications. Expert Rev Neurother 2006;6(9):1249–65.
20. Grosset KA, Grosset DG. Prescribed drugs and neurological complications. J Neurol Neurosurg Psychiatry 2004;75(Suppl 3):iii2–8.
21. Wallace KL. Antibiotic-induced convulsions. Crit Care Clin 1997;13(4):741–62.
22. Caillier B, Pilote S, Castonguay A, et al. QRS widening and QT prolongation under bupropion: a unique cardiac electrophysiological profile. Fundam Clin Pharmacol 2012;26(5):599–608.
23. Buckley NA, Faunce TA. 'Atypical' antidepressants in overdose: clinical considerations with respect to safety. Drug Saf 2003;26(8):539–51.
24. Malyshevskaya O, Aritake K, Kaushik MK, et al. Natural ((9)-THC) and synthetic (JWH-018) cannabinoids induce seizures by acting through the cannabinoid CB1 receptor. Sci Rep 2017;7(1):10516.
25. Adamowicz P, Gieroń J, Gil D, et al. The effects of synthetic cannabinoid UR-144 on the human body—A review of 39 cases. Forensic Sci Int 2017;273:e18–21.
26. Tai S, Fantegrossi WE. Pharmacological and toxicological effects of synthetic cannabinoids and their metabolites. Curr Top Behav Neurosci 2017;32:249–62.

27. Bailey DN. Phencyclidine abuse: clinical findings and concentrations in biological fluids after nonfatal intoxication. Am J Clin Pathol 1979;72(5):795–9.
28. Browning R, Maggio R, Sahibzada N, et al. Role of brainstem structures in seizures initiated from the deep prepiriform cortex of rats. Epilepsia 1993;34(3): 393–407.
29. Brudzynski SM, Cruickshank JW, McLachlan RS. Cholinergic Mechanisms in Generalized Seizures: Importance of the Zona Incerta. Can J Neurol Sci 1995; 22:116–20.
30. Friedman A, Behrens CJ, Heinemann U. Cholinergic dysfunction in temporal lobe epilepsy. Epilepsia 2007;48(s5):126–30.
31. McDonough JH Jr, Shih TM. Neuropharmacological mechanisms of nerve agent-induced seizure and neuropathology. Neurosci Biobehav Rev 1997;21(5): 559–79.
32. Albaret C, Lacoutière S, Ashman WP, et al. Molecular mechanic study of nerve agent O-ethyl S-[2-(diisopropylamino)ethyl]methylphosphonothioate (VX) bound to the active site of Torpedo californica acetylcholinesterase. Proteins 1997; 28(4):543–55.
33. King AM, Aaron CK. Organophosphate and carbamate poisoning. Emerg Med Clin North Am 2015;33(1):133–51.
34. Kozhemyakin M, Rajasekaran K, Kapur J. Central cholinesterase inhibition enhances glutamatergic synaptic transmission. J Neurophysiol 2010;103(4): 1748–57.
35. Tattersall J. Seizure activity post organophosphate exposure. Front Biosci (Landmark Ed) 2009;14:3688–711.
36. Walls R, Meehan TJ. Approach to the Poisoned Patient. In Rosen's emergency medicine: Concepts and clinical practice 2nd ed., Ch 139, (1813-1822). (2018).Elsevier.
37. Yoon HJ, Lim YJ, Zuo Z, et al. Nicotine decreases the activity of glutamate transporter type 3. Toxicol Lett 2014;225(1):147–52.
38. DeLorey TMOR. Gamma-aminobutyric acidA receptor structure and function. J Biol Chem 1992;267(24):16747–50.
39. Bowery NG. GABAB receptor: a site of therapeutic benefit. Curr Opin Pharmacol 2006;6(1):37–43.
40. Murray BP, Carpenter JE, Dunkley CA, et al. Seizures in tramadol overdoses reported in the ToxIC registry: predisposing factors and the role of naloxone. Clin Toxicol (Phila) 2019;57(8):692–6.
41. Marquardt KA, Alsop JA, Albertson TE. Tramadol exposures reported to statewide poison control system. Ann Pharmacother 2005;39(6):1039–44.
42. Samadi M, Shaki F, Bameri B, et al. Caffeine attenuates seizure and brain mitochondrial disruption induced by Tramadol: the role of adenosinergic pathway. Drug Chem Toxicol 2019;44:1–7.
43. Shadnia S, Brent J, Mousavi-Fatemi K, et al. Recurrent seizures in tramadol intoxication: implications for therapy based on 100 patients. Basic Clin Pharmacol Toxicol 2012;111(2):133–6.
44. Rehni AK, Singh I, Kumar M. Tramadol-induced seizurogenic effect: a possible role of opioid-dependent γ-aminobutyric acid inhibitory pathway. Basic Clin Pharmacol Toxicol 2008;103(3):262–6.
45. Rush JM, Gibberd FB. Baclofen-induced epilepsy. J R Soc Med 1990;83(2): 115–6.

46. Fakhoury T, Abou-Khalil B, Blumenkopf B. EEG changes in intrathecal baclofen overdose: a case report and review of the literature. Electroencephalogr Clin Neurophysiol 1998;107(5):339–42.
47. Perry HE, Wright RO, Shannon MW, et al. Baclofen overdose: drug experimentation in a group of adolescents. Pediatrics 1998;101(6):1045–8.
48. Sutter R, Ruegg S, Tschudin-Sutter S. Seizures as adverse events of antibiotic drugs: a systematic review. Neurology 2015;85(15):1332–41.
49. Naeije G, Lorent S, Vincent JL, et al. Continuous epileptiform discharges in patients treated with cefepime or meropenem. Arch Neurol 2011;68(10):1303–7.
50. Borowski TB, Kirkby RD, Kokkinidis L. Amphetamine and antidepressant drug effects on GABA- and NMDA-related seizures. Brain Res Bull 1993;30(5–6):607–10.
51. Hyser CL, Drake ME Jr. Status epilepticus after baclofen withdrawal. J Natl Med Assoc 1984;76(5):533–8.
52. Triplett JD, Lawn ND, Dunne JW. Baclofen neurotoxicity: a metabolic encephalopathy susceptible to exacerbation by benzodiazepine therapy. J Clin Neurophysiol 2019;36(3):209–12.
53. Kerr GW, McGuffie AC, Wilkie S. Tricyclic antidepressant overdose: a review. Emerg Med J 2001;18(4):236–41.
54. Judge BS, Rentmeester LL. Antidepressant overdose–induced seizures. Psychiatr Clin North Am 2011;36(2):245–60.
55. Corrington KA, Gatlin CC, Fields KB. A case of SSRI-induced hyponatremia. J Am Board Fam Pract 2002;15(1):63–5.
56. Kirchner V, Silver LE, Kelly CA. Selective serotonin reuptake inhibitors and hyponatraemia: review and proposed mechanisms in the elderly. J Psychopharmacol 1998;12(4):396–400.
57. Druschky K, Bleich S, Grohmann R, et al. Seizure rates under treatment with antipsychotic drugs: Data from the AMSP project. World J Biol Psychiatry 2019 Nov;20(9):732–41.
58. Jobe PC, Browning RA. The serotonergic and noradrenergic effects of antidepressant drugs are anticonvulsant, not proconvulsant. Epilepsy Behav 2005;7(4):602–19.
59. Ramsdell JS, Gulland FM. Domoic acid epileptic disease. Mar Drugs 2014;12(3):1185–207.
60. Benjamin DR. Muschroom poisoning in infants and children: the Amanita pantherina/muscaria group. J Toxicol Clin Toxicol 1992;30(1):13–22.
61. Kondeva-Burdina M, Voynova M, Shkondrov A, et al. Effects of Amanita muscaria extract on different in vitro neurotoxicity models at sub-cellular and cellular levels. Food Chem Toxicol 2019;132:110687.
62. Cox GA, Lutz CM, Yang C-L, et al. Sodium/hydrogen exchanger gene defect in slow-wave epilepsy mutant mice. Cell 1997;91(1):139–48.
63. Bhowmik M, Khanam R, Vohora D. Histamine H3 receptor antagonists in relation to epilepsy and neurodegeneration: a systemic consideration of recent progress and perspectives. Br J Pharmacol 2012;167(7):1398–414.
64. Yokoyama H, Onodera K, Iinuma K, et al. Proconvulsive effects of histamine H1-antagonists on electrically-induced seizure in developing mice. Psychopharmacology (Berl) 1993;112(2–3):199–203.
65. Jang DH, Manini AF, Trueger NS, et al. Status epilepticus and wide-complex tachycardia secondary to diphenhydramine overdose. Clin Toxicol (Phila) 2010;48(9):945–8.

66. Nakada T, Kwee IL, Lerner AM, et al. Theophylline-induced seizures: clinical and pathophysiologic aspects. West J Med 1983;138(3):371–4.
67. Weltha L, Reemmer J, Boison D. The role of adenosine in epilepsy. Brain Res Bull 2019 Sep;151:46–54.
68. Boison D. Methylxanthines, seizures, and excitotoxicity. Handb Exp Pharmacol 2011;200:251–66.
69. Morgan PF, Durcan MJ. Caffeine-induced seizures: apparent proconvulsant action of n-ethyl carboxamidoadenosine (NECA). Life Sci 1990;47(1):1–8.
70. Chu N-S. Caffeine- and aminophylline-induced seizures. Epilepsia 1981;22(1): 85–94.
71. Czuczwar SJ, Gasior M, Janusz W, et al. Influence of different methylxanthines on the anticonvulsant action of common antiepileptic drugs in mice. Epilepsia 1990; 31(3):318–23.
72. Kaufman KR, Sachdeo RC. Caffeinated beverages and decreased seizure control. Seizure 2003;12(7):519–21.
73. Ghannoum M, Wiegand TJ, Liu KD, et al. Extracorporeal treatment for theophylline poisoning: systematic review and recommendations from the EXTRIP workgroup. Clin Toxicol (Phila) 2015;53(4):215–29.
74. Sharma AN, Hoffman RJ. Toxin-related seizures. Emerg Med Clin North Am 2011; 29(1):125–39.

Utilizing the Toxicology Laboratory in the Poisoned Patient

Laura Bechtel, PhD, DABCC[a,*], Christopher P. Holstege, MD[b]

KEY WORDS

• Toxicology • Laboratory • Emergency medicine • Drug testing • Analyte

KEY POINTS

- Urine drug immunoassay screens for the management of intoxicated patients have limited utility in the emergency department, and clinicians using such testing should be aware of the test's potential for both false positive and false negatvie results.
- Ethylene glycol metabolites glycolate and glyoxylic acid can falsely elevate L-lactate results with some blood gas analyzers owing to their interference with specific lactate oxidase enzymes used; depending on the clinical scenario, elevated lactate concentrations should be confirmed by a central chemistry laboratory analyzer with poisoned patients.
- Testing for acetaminophen by automated spectrophotometric methods may be subject to interferences with bilirubin or bilirubin byproducts absorbing at similar wavelengths and causing falsely detectable acetaminophen levels.
- Laboratories may report substance concentrations in terms of milligrams per deciliter and milligrams per liter (eg, salicylate, methanol, ethylene glycol). This important distinction, which involves a 10-fold reporting difference, can cause confusion and unnecessary transfers and treatment (eg, dialysis) of patients.
- Emergency medicine clinicians should communicate closely with their laboratory teams, especially if values reported do not correspond with the clinical scenario.

Emergency medicine clinicians commonly encounter critically poisoned patients. Exposure to potential toxins can occur either unintentionally (eg, occupational or environmental exposures, medication interactions, medication error) or intentionally (eg, substance abuse, intentional overdose, malicious poisoning). A competent clinician needs to determine which diagnostic tests are appropriate for managing each presenting poisoned patient by assimilation of numerous factors, especially focusing on obtaning a thorough history and physical examination. This includes obtaining

[a] Kaiser Permanente Colorado Health System, 11000 45th Avenue, Denver, CO 80239, USA; [b] Division of Medical Toxicology, Department of Emergency Medicine, University of Virginia School of Medicine, Blue Ridge Poison Center, University of Virginia Health System, PO Box 800699, Charlottesville, VA 22908-0699, USA
* Corresponding author.
E-mail addresses: Laura.K.Bechtel@kp.org (L.B.); ch2xf@virginia.edu (C.P.H.)

Emerg Med Clin N Am 40 (2022) 431–441
https://doi.org/10.1016/j.emc.2022.01.003
0733-8627/22/

the time and date of the suspected exposure, a complete medication list, and the pre-existing health status of the patient. The clinician should also perform a thorough assessment of the physical state of the patient at the time of presentation and be able to recognize toxic syndromes (toxidromes).[1]

Stabilization of the poisoned patient is essential until the causative agent or agents can be identified. Useful and timely clinical laboratory results are required to support medical treatment decisions. Design of laboratory test menus used by the emergency department should consider published guidelines from the National Academy of Clinical Biochemistry (NACB).[2] These guidelines recommend specific tests and appropriate sample matrices that have the greatest impact for care of a poisoned patient. Collaboration between the laboratory and the health care team directly managing the poisoned patient is essential for ordering appropriate tests at the right time and ensuring accurate interpretation of the results. Clinical laboratory test menus must provide rapid turnaround times (TATs) and accurate results supporting initial management of the intoxicated patient for short turnaround testing (STAT) testing. STAT testing should include specific quantitative tests in blood (serum or plasma) to determine whether antidotes and/or specific supportive care are necessary for optimal recovery.[3] At a minimum, testing of intentional poisoned patients (eg, suicidal) should include a basic metabolic panel as well as acetaminophen and salicylate levels. Use of qualitative urine drug screens (UDS) for tier-one testing remains controversial. Utilization of UDS typically does not change the acute management of a poisoned patient, and these tests have unique limitations. UDS have reasonable TATs, but the results can be misleading because of false positive or false negative results and lack of correlation with the clinical presentation. Clinical laboratory test menus should also include access to more specific analytes for patients who remain intoxicated, obtunded, or comatose and require long-term care. If these more complex tests are not available at the emergency care facility, specific tests should be accessible at a hospital or reference laboratory that provides reasonable result times for patient management. This article examines the role of diagnostic tests in the evaluation of a poisoned patient presenting to the emergency department.

AUTOMATED LABORATORY TESTING

Chemistry and immunoassay methods are readily available in clinical laboratory laboratories on automated instruments to perform most STAT testing necessary for managing the poisoned patient. Chemistry and ion-selective electrode methods are used for basic and complete metabolic panels, ethanol, lithium, and iron. These methods are highly specific and minimally affected by interferences. Immunoassay methods use antibodies that bind short sequences within proteins or unique functional groups within a chemical compound or drug. The antibodies in homogeneous immunoassay reagents used in automated clinical analyzers are formulated by manufacturers to minimize false positive results and maximize sensitivity to the target compound. Many methodologies for capturing and measuring a compound are available across different manufactured reagents. Each have advantages and disadvantages that are vetted by the laboratory when choosing a specific reagent to maximize what is desired to be measured and minimizes unwanted interferences. These nuances should be communicated to medical personnel managing the intoxicated patient.

Automated Chemistry Tests

Anion gap

Clinicians should obtain a basic metabolic panel from poisoned patients as an important initial screening test. When low serum bicarbonate results on a basic metabolic panel, the clinician should determine whether an elevated anion gap (AG) exists. The formula most commonly used for the AG calculation is as follows:

$$AG = [Na^+] - [Cl^- + HCO_3^-]$$

The AG arose from the "Gamblegram" law of electroneutrality.[4] The number of net positive charges contributed by serum cations must equal the number of net negative charges contributed by serum anions.[5] The primary cation (sodium, 92%) and anions (chloride, 67%, and bicarbonate, 17%) are represented in this equation.[6] Other compounds (potassium, calcium, magnesium, phosphate, sulfate, organic acids, and protein) are relatively low and do not significantly affect the gap. Different clinical analytical instruments produce different AG reference ranges in a population.[7] An increase in the AG beyond an accepted reference limit and accompanied by a metabolic acidosis represents an increase in unmeasured endogenous (eg, lactate) or exogenous (eg, salicylates) anions. Clinically useful mnemonics for causes of high AG metabolic acidosis are the classic MUDPILES (classically representing Methanol; Uremia; Diabetic/alcoholic/starvation ketoacidosis; Propylene glycol; Iron, isoniazid, inhalants; Lactate; Ethylene glycol; Salicylate and stimulants) and the more recently proposed GOLD MARK (Glycols [ethylene and propylene]; Oxoproline; L-lactate; D-lactate; Methanol; Aspirin; Renal failure; Ketoacidosis).[8]

It is imperative that clinicians who admit poisoned patients initially presenting with an increased AG metabolic acidosis investigate the cause of that acidosis. Many symptomatic poisoned patients may have an initial mild metabolic acidosis upon presentation caused by processes resulting in elevated serum lactate (eg, transient hypoxia or hypovolemia). However, with adequate supportive care (eg, oxygenation and hydration), the AG acidosis should steadily improve. If, despite adequate supportive care, an AG metabolic acidosis worsens in a poisoned patient, the clinician should consider continued absorption of exogenous acids (eg, salicylate), formation of acidic metabolites (eg, metabolites of ethylene glycol, methanol, or toluene), and cellular ischemia with worsening lactic acidosis (eg, cyanide) as potential causes.[9,10]

Lactate

Lactic acidosis is the most common cause of metabolic acidosis in hospitalized patients. Lactic acidosis occurs when lactic acid production (>4 mmol/L) exceeds lactic acid clearance. Lactic acidosis is often associated with an elevated AG and reduced arterial pH (depending on the respiratory rate and subsequent CO_2 level), yet moderately increased lactate levels can be observed with a normal AG (eg, in the context of hypoalbuminemia).

STAT lactate levels are commonly performed on point-of-care instruments (POC) for emergency departments.[11] The correlation between lactate on POC versus the laboratory's clinical analyzers is clinically acceptable; however, emergency medicine providers should be aware of the potential of falsely elevated serum lactate concentrations in the setting of poisoned patients. Ethylene glycol metabolites glycolate and glyoxylic acid can falsely elevate L-lactate results with some POC blood gas analyzers owing to their interference with specific lactate oxidase enzymes.[12–14] In specific clinical settings, POC elevated lactate concentrations should be confirmed by a central chemistry laboratory analyzer. An elevated POC lactate level compared with a central chemistry laboratory lactate level has been referred to in literature as the "lactate gap" and should be used with caution for diagnosis of ethylene glycol poisoning using blood gas analyzers.[15]

Osmolal gap

The main osmotically active constituents of serum include Na^+, Cl^-, HCO_3^-, glucose, and urea. The osmol gap is the difference between measured (OSMm) and calculated osmolality (OSMc) in serum. Basic metabolic panel and serum osmol laboratory tests are required for this calculation. The osmol gap is used to screen for the possible presence of exogenous toxic substances. Several empirical formulas based on measurement of these substances have been used to estimate the serum osmolality. In practice, one has not shown itself to be superior to the others, yet each equation demonstrates significant differences in the osmol gap reference interval.[16] Therefore, reference intervals must be validated on appropriate patient populations. A commonly used formula (in conventional units) is as follows:

$$\text{OSMc (mOsm/kg)} = 2\ \text{Na (mmol/L)} + \text{glucose (mg/dL)}/18 + \text{urea (mg/dL)}/2.8.$$

The difference between the actual osmolality (OSMm), measured by freezing-point depression, and the OSMc is referred to as delta-osmolality, or the osmolar gap (OSMg).

$$\text{OSMg} = \text{OSMm} - \text{OSMc}$$

Elevated OSMg implies the presence of unmeasured osmotically active substances. Volatile alcohols (acetone, ethanol, isopropanol, and methanol) and ethylene glycol, when present at significant concentrations, increase serum osmolality, thus resulting in an increased OSMg. The calculation of OSMg is commonly used as a clinical screening test. However, it is important to remember that volatile alcohols are not detected when osmolality is measured with a vapor pressure osmometer. Therefore, for the purpose of determining the OSMg, only osmolality measurements based on freezing-point depression are acceptable.

What constitutes a normal osmol gap is widely debated. Traditionally, a normal osmol gap has been defined as less than 10 mOsm/kg.[17] Further clinical studies have not shown this assumption to be accurate, and large variability is seen in the normal population.[18–21] By considering the effect of ethanol on the serum osmolality, it is possible to determine what portion of an increased OSMg is due to ethanol. The contribution of ethanol to the OSMm can be calculated (ethanol, mg/dL/4.6 $\times$ 0.83). However, it has been observed that ethanol and methanol do not follow a completely predictable relationship with OSMg. In severe ethanol and methanol intoxication, OSMg increases with increasing concentration, making it appear that another agent is present and impacting serum osmolality besides the ethanol.

A significant residual OSMg (>10 mOsm/kg) would suggest the possible presence of acetone, ethanol, ethylene glycol, isopropanol, and methanol, or another osmotically active substance. This information, in conjunction with the presence or absence of metabolic acidosis or serum acetone, is helpful to the clinician when specific measurements of alcohols, other than ethanol, are not available on an emergency basis. It must be realized that ketones and substances administered to patients, such as polyethylene glycol (burn cream), mannitol (osmotic diuretic), and propylene glycol (diluent used with intravenous diazepam, lorazepam, and phenytoin), may increase serum osmolality.[22]

For the diagnosis of ethanol intoxication, OSMg has lost its usefulness because ethanol can be measured quickly on most chemistry analyzers. However, because other toxic alcohols can be measured only by chromatographic techniques, OSMg is still useful. Unfortunately, OSMg as a screening method is insensitive to low, yet clinically significant, concentrations of ethylene glycol (<50 mg/dL) and methanol

(<30 mg/dL). Tier-two toxic alcohol panels may be required for confirmation of late presenting ethylene and methanol exposures to detect metabolites.

Automated Immunoassays Tests

STAT immunoassay methods for intoxicated patients require specific, sensitive, and quantitative measurement of drug concentrations in serum or plasma. These tests may use monoclonal or polyclonal antibodies covalently attached to particles permitting the binding domain of the antibody to attach to a drug present in the blood specimen. Particles used and detection technology of the antibody-drug complex is dependent on the manufacturer formulation. For example, the complex may be washed to remove unwanted nonspecific compounds in the specimen and then a second labeled antibody specific for the bound complex may be detected. Labeled detection reagents are used by the manufacturer based on the level of sensitivity required for detecting specific analytes (high-sensitivity pg/mL to ng/mL, to low-sensitivity μg/mL). Chromophore, chemiluminescence, electrochemiluminescence, and fluorometry are common detection technologies (low sensitivity to high sensitivity, respectively).[23] Alternatively, the method may use an antibody-drug complex that results in the formation of insoluble aggregates causing light scatter and is detected at a specific wavelength. Immunoassays methods typically run 15 to 30 minutes to result once received in the central laboratory, supporting required TATs to support emergency care of poisoned patients. Typical automated immunoassays include such drugs as acetaminophen, salicylate, carbamazepine, digoxin, phenobarbital, and valproic acid.

Acetaminophen

The initial clinical findings in acetaminophen toxicity can be absent and are relatively mild or nonspecific (nausea, vomiting, and abdominal discomfort) and thus are not predictive of impending hepatic necrosis, which typically begins 12 to 36 hours after toxic ingestion. Although uncommon, with severe overdose, both coma and metabolic acidosis may occur before development of hepatic necrosis.[24]

Specific therapy for acetaminophen overdose is the administration of N-acetyl cysteine (NAC). The time of administration of NAC is critical. Maximum efficacy is observed when NAC is administered within 8 hours, and efficacy declines with time; therefore, it is most effective when administered before hepatic injury occurs, as signified initially by elevations of AST and ALT. However, NAC treatment provides beneficial effects even after liver injury has occurred.

The measurement of serum acetaminophen concentrations becomes paramount for proper assessment of the severity of overdose and for appropriate decision making for antidotal therapy. If serum acetaminophen results are not available locally within 8 hours of suspected ingestion, treatment with NAC should begin until levels are available. The Rumack-Matthew nomogram relates serum acetaminophen concentration and time following acute ingestion to the probability of hepatic necrosis.

Many spectrophotometric and immunoassay methods are available for the determination of acetaminophen. Automated spectrophotometric methods may be subject to interferences, such as bilirubin or bilirubin byproducts, absorbing at similar wavelengths. Some methods measure the nontoxic metabolites and parent acetaminophen and thus may produce especially misleading results. Therefore, only methods specific for parent acetaminophen should be used. A different spectrophotometric approach uses aryl-acylamide amidohydrolase to hydrolyze acetaminophen (but not conjugates) to *p*-aminophenol and acetate. Subsequent formation of the absorbing species depends on the reaction of generated *p*-aminophenol with 8-hydroxyquinoline or *o*-

cresol. Aryl-acylamide amidohydrolase methods are susceptible to interference by NAC, bilirubin, and immunoglobulin M monoclonal immunoglobulins. Most chromatographic methods are very accurate and are considered reference procedures. A qualitative, one-step lateral flow immunoassay (cutoff of 25 μg/mL) may be suitable for POC application, yet it has a low positive predictive value.[25]

Salicylate

Acetylsalicylic acid (aspirin) has analgesic, antipyretic, and anti-inflammatory properties. These therapeutic benefits derive from acetylsalicylic acid and its metabolite, salicylate, and their ability to inhibit biosynthesis of prostaglandins. Aspirin also interferes with platelet aggregation and thus prolongs bleeding time. The platelet inhibitory effect is a consequence of the ability of aspirin to acetylate and irreversibly inhibit platelet cyclooxygenase, thereby reducing the formation of thromboxane A_2, a potent mediator of platelet aggregation. Platelets have little or no capacity for protein synthesis; therefore, the duration of this enzyme inhibition is the normal lifespan of the platelets (8–11 days).

Interpretation of salicylate concentrations as a guide for clinical management decisions can be difficult. Treatment for salicylate intoxication is directed toward decreasing further absorption, increasing elimination, and correcting acid-base and electrolyte disturbances. Toxic concentrations alone are of poor prognostic value; however, certain clinical findings predict a poor prognosis, including pulmonary edema, fever, coma, and acidosis. Initial serial concentrations should be performed every 2 hours while the patient is monitored clinically. When the concentrations begin to decline and the patient's clinical status is improved, concentrations can be measured less frequently.

Automated serum salicylate methods are chemistry or immunoassay based. The units reported with each concentration should be documented before management decisions are made. Laboratories may alternatively report concentrations in terms of milligrams per deciliter and milligrams per liter.[26] This important distinction, which involves a 10-fold difference in reporting, can cause confusion and unnecessary transfers to tertiary referral centers. In extreme cases of these miscommunications, hemodialysis has been ordered for patients thought to have astronomically high salicylate concentrations that were later proven to be nontoxic.

Methemoglobin

An acquired (toxic) methemoglobinemia may be caused by various drugs and chemicals. In addition, oxides of nitrogen and other oxidant combustion products make smoke inhalation a potential cause of methemoglobinemia. The normal percentage of methemoglobin is less than 1.5% of total hemoglobin. The severity of symptoms usually correlates with measured methemoglobin levels; methemoglobin percentages up to 20% may cause slate-gray cutaneous discoloration, cyanosis, and chocolate-brown blood. Percentages between 20% and 50% may cause dyspnea, exercise intolerance, fatigue, weakness, and syncope. More severe symptoms of dysrhythmias, seizures, and metabolic acidosis have been reported with methemoglobin percentages greater than 50%.[23] A normal pO_2 in a cyanotic patient with low cutaneous measured oxygen saturations is a significant indication for the possible presence of methemoglobinemia.

Specific therapy for toxic methemoglobinemia involves the administration of methylene blue, which acts as an electron transfer agent in the NADPH-methemoglobin reductase reaction, thereby increasing the activity of this system several-fold. Methylene blue and sulfhemoglobin cause spectral interference in the measurement of methemoglobin with some co-oximeters but not with the Evelyn-Malloy method. Ascorbic acid can also reverse methemoglobin by an alternate metabolic pathway but is of minimal benefit acutely because of its slow action.

Methemoglobin is commonly determined using automated multiwavelength measurements with a co-oximeter or manual spectrophotometric method of Evelyn and Malloy. Because methemoglobin is not stable at room temperature, specimens should be kept on ice or refrigerated, but not frozen. Freezing results in an increase in methemoglobin concentration. Abnormal noninvasive pulse oximetry results have occurred because of methemoglobin interference, when measuring the absorbance of light at 660 nm (oxyhemoglobin) and 940 nm (deoxyhemoglobin).

Urine drug screens

Urine drug immunoassay screens (UDS) for the acute management of intoxicated patients have limited clinical utility in emergency medicine.[27,28] UDS may continue to be used in small or rural hospitals that may not have access to clinical toxicology specialists that understand the analytical limitations of UDS.[2] NACB guidelines support emergency physicians and clinical laboratories by encouraging the in vitro diagnostic industry to take steps to improve analytical methodologies to improve UDS results.

UDS use antibody-drug binding complexes like those described for tier-one analyses. However, to minimize the number of toxicology tests required to screen for possible agents causing intoxication, some tests were developed to capture or bind to a drug class (eg, benzodiazepines, opiates, amphetamines) rather than a specific substance (eg, fentanyl, heroin metabolite, hydrocodone, oxycodone, tramadol). Modest improvements over the last decade by in vitro diagnostic manufacturers have emerged with improved specificity for opioid and benzodiazepine drug classes. These improvements have been driven by patient medical needs in the emergency department as well as pain management, chemical dependency, and behavioral health. Opioid drug class tests have improved sensitivity to a wider range of natural opium alkaloids (eg, morphine and codeine) and semisynthetic opiates (eg, heroin, hydrocodone, hydromorphone, oxycodone). Immunoassay screens with improved selectivity for specific compounds within the opioid drug class have emerged (eg, tramadol, fentanyl, oxycodone). Utilization of glucuronidase enzyme within the benzodiazepine immunoassay reagent to cleave phase II conjugates, glucuronides, from compounds improves sensitivity for more benzodiazepine compounds, but does not improve specificity. This improvement permits more readily detectable clonazepam, alprazolam, and lorazepam compounds.

Proper identification of a particular toxidrome may be used to exclude some drug classes as the cause of the symptoms without urine drug testing. Polypharmacy exposure and delayed presentation may misguide the clinician and can cause analytical interferences. Emergency medicine clinicians have been trained to treat the syndrome encountered at the time of presentation and not rely on results of urine drug testing for emergent management decisions. This is in part because immunoassays, although rapid, have limitations in sensitivity and specificity, and chromatographic assays, which are more definitive, are more labor-intensive. The US Centers for Medicare and Medicaid Services–covered indications for presumptive UDS are determined by local coverage determinations (eg, L36037).[29] Presumptive urine drug tests may be medically necessary as part of the evaluation and management of a patient (termed "group A") who presents in an urgent care setting with any one of the following: coma, altered mental status in the absence of a clinically defined toxic syndrome or toxidrome, severe or unexplained cardiovascular instability (cardiotoxicity), unexplained metabolic or respiratory acidosis in the absence of a clinically defined toxic syndrome or toxidrome, seizures with an undetermined history, or to provide an antagonist to a specific drug. The presumptive findings, definitive drug tests ordered, and reasons for the testing must be documented in the patient's medical record.

NONAUTOMATED LABORATORY TESTING

Not all testing can be supported with rapid TATs to support poisoned patients, especially in remote or rural areas. These tests require specialized instrumentation and personnel to perform the analyses and interpret the results. Therefore, clinical laboratories supporting intoxicated patients must establish mechanisms to coordinate testing with centralized hospital or commercial reference laboratories to provide specific quantitative tests in blood (serum or plasma) where antidotes and specific supportive care are necessary.

Ethylene Glycol

Ethylene glycol itself has initial central nervous system effects resembling those of ethanol. Metabolism of ethylene glycol by alcohol dehydrogenase to glycoaldehyde, which is then metabolized to glycolic, glyoxylic, and oxalic acids, is a cause for toxicity. Oxalate readily precipitates with calcium to form insoluble calcium oxalate crystals in kidneys and other tissues. Ethylene glycol has a short elimination half-life and serum, and the concentration may be low or undetectable at a time when glycolic acid remains elevated. Therefore, serum glycolic acid concentration correlates more closely with clinical symptoms and mortality. The mainstay of therapy for ethylene glycol toxicity includes the administration of ethanol or fomepizole, as competitive alcohol dehydrogenase inhibitors, and dialysis.

The presence of AG, osmol gap, and urine oxalate crystals suggests ethylene glycol poisoning. Oxalate crystals may be visible under a microscope after centrifugation of the urine specimen, but only present in half of ethylene glycol–toxic patients.[30] Confirmatory testing of both ethylene glycol and glycolic acid by gas chromatography with flame ionization detection (GC-FID) methodology is the gold standard and provides crucial clinical and confirmatory information for ethylene glycol–poisoning cases.

Volatile Alcohols

Methanol poisoning can be lethal if not recognized early. Unfortunately, in some instances, a latent period can be as long as 12 to 24 hours before toxicity is recognized, making laboratory identification of this poisoning critical. GC-FID remains the most common method for the detection and quantitation of volatile alcohols in biological samples. Not only does it distinguish between ethanol, methanol (and its toxic metabolite, formic acid), isopropanol, and acetone, but also it has the capability to measure concentrations as low as 10 mg/dL (0.01%). The volatility of the alcohols is used to separate them from the matrix. Specifically, the "Gas Law" states that at a given temperature, the amount of volatile substance in the air space, "headspace," above the liquid is proportional to the concentration of the volatile alcohol in the solution. Therefore, the sample in the headspace allows calculation of the concentration in urine or blood specimens.

Comprehensive Urine Drug Screens

Larger hospitals or health systems with readily available central reference laboratory or commercial laboratories have developed comprehensive gas or liquid chromatography mass spectrometry screens to improve specificity and sensitivity to analytes encountered in intoxicated patients. These facilities can maintain instrumentation and staff to run highly specialized testing and have higher volumes to justify the increased cost. Typical instrumentation includes either gas chromatography mass spectrometry (GC-MS), liquid chromatography tandem mass spectrometry (LC-MS/MS), or liquid chromatography high-resolution mass spectrometry (HRMS). These methods use specific cutoffs important for detecting analytes with minimal method run times to improve time to result. Preliminary results can be sent to the ordering physician while a more specific mass spectrometry method is used to confirm the analyzed drug. Although these comprehensive mass spectrometry screening tests expand the number of drugs analyzed, they also may be subject to interferences owing to coelutions of drugs with the same mass from the chromatography column, matrix interferences, or poor extraction recovery. Interference can be overcome with optimized chromatography, longer run times, or HRMS detectors. These types of targeted screening methods are laboratory-developed tests and require communication between the emergency medicine physician and the laboratory personnel to accurately interpret results. Rapid comprehensive UDS lack supportive evidence that the results change clinical management.[31,32]

Urine Drug Confirmations

Urine drug confirmations use targeted analytical methodologies performed on GC-MS, LC-MS/MS, or liquid chromatography HRMS. All methodologies incorporate preanalytical sample preparation steps, such as dilution, concentration, precipitation, derivatization, hydrolysis, liquid-liquid extraction, or sold phase extraction.[33] These preanalytical steps "clean up the specimen" and optimize detection of specific drugs and their metabolites (analytes). Utilization of gas or liquid chromatography of a mass spectrometer for detection provides high sensitivity and specificity. Ultimately, the sample must be introduced into the mass spectrometer as a gas phase ion. Once the ions enter into the mass spectrometer, they are sorted and filtered based on their mass-to-charge (*m/z*) ratio. Targeted ions of specific mass are selected and detected. Other contaminant ions are filtered out because their *m/z* is not specifically selected. The resolution of the mass spectrometer is important to identifying the correct target ion. When a mass spectrometer can reliably distinguish between 1 mass unit, this means it can distinguish between a drug that is 299 and 300. It cannot distinguish between a drug that is 299.364 *m/z* (codeine) and 299.368 *m/z* (hydrocodone). The 2 analytes must be separated by an analytical column (gas or liquid chromatography) or detected within a high-resolution mass spectrometer that can distinguish between 299.364 *m/z* and 299.368 *m/z*.

Clinical mass spectrometry drug confirmation methods must be validated in a clinical laboratory meeting high regulatory standards (eg, Clinical Laboratory Improvement Amendments or College of American Pathologists). These methods must produce reproducible results, and the clinician must be aware of not only what the test detects but also what it does not detect. A negative confirmatory test may be due to a parent drug resulting under the cutoff, the parent drug is metabolized and metabolite is not included in the test, or the drug or metabolite was not present. Invalid test results for a particular analyte means the anticipated ion ratio (targeted masses anticipated for detection) do not meet validated method criteria or an interference is present. Reanalysis of an invalid result typically does not overcome an invalid result. If the methodology has robust validation and reproducibility, the same interference will continue to be extracted from the same specimen. Sometimes alternative methodologies (GC vs LC, or alternate method run time) can overcome invalid results (eg, interferences). Selection or implementation of a robust test methodology for urine drug confirmations is important. The fastest or least-expensive test method is not necessarily the best choice for monitoring the poisoned patient.

SUMMARY

Clinical laboratory tests used to support the poisoned patient are essential. Emergency medicine clinicians should continue their quest to eliminate indiscriminate broad-range test orders for poisoned patients. They are encouraged to work with laboratorians to permit test utilization that optimizes the care of their patients. Test results should always be reviewed in the context of the clinical scenario. Feedback from clinicians concerning inconsistent results is welcomed by laboratorians and typically leads to improved testing and results.

DISCLOSURE

The authors have nothing to disclose.

REFERENCES

1. Holstege CP, Borek HA. Toxidromes. Crit Care Clin 2012;28(4):479–98.
2. Wu AH, McKay C, Broussard LA, et al. National Academy of Clinical Biochemistry Laboratory Medicine practice guidelines: recommendations for the use of laboratory tests to support poisoned patients who present to the emergency department. Clin Chem 2003;49(3):357–79.
3. Thompson JP, Watson ID, Thanacoody HK, et al. Guidelines for laboratory analyses for poisoned patients in the United Kingdom. Ann Clin Biochem 2014; 51(Pt 3):312–25.
4. Kraut JA, Madias NE. Serum anion gap: its uses and limitations in clinical medicine. Clin J Am Soc Nephrol 2007;2(1):162–74.
5. Gabow PA. Disorders associated with an altered anion gap. Kidney Int 1985; 27(2):472–83.
6. Ishihara K, Szerlip HM. Anion gap acidosis. Semin Nephrol 1998;18(1):83–97.
7. Pratumvinit B, Lam L, Kongruttanachok N, et al. Anion gap reference intervals show instrument dependence and weak correlation with albumin levels. Clin Chim Acta 2020;500:172–9.
8. Mehta AN, Emmett JB, Emmett M. GOLD MARK: an anion gap mnemonic for the 21st century. Lancet 2008;372(9642):892.
9. Ross JA, Borek HA, Holstege CP. Toxic alcohols. Crit Care Clin 2021;37(3): 643–56.
10. Parker-Cote JL, Rizer J, Vakkalanka JP, et al. Challenges in the diagnosis of acute cyanide poisoning. Clin Toxicol (Phila) 2018;56(7):609–17.
11. Bhalla A. Bedside point of care toxicology screens in the ED: utility and pitfalls. Int J Crit Illn Inj Sci 2014;4(3):257–60.
12. Meng QH, Adeli K, Zello GA, et al. Elevated lactate in ethylene glycol poisoning: true or false? Clin Chim Acta 2010;411(7–8):601–4.
13. Manini AF, Hoffman RS, McMartin KE, et al. Relationship between serum glycolate and falsely elevated lactate in severe ethylene glycol poisoning. J Anal Toxicol 2009;33(3):174–6.
14. Brindley PG, Butler MS, Cembrowski G, et al. Falsely elevated point-of-care lactate measurement after ingestion of ethylene glycol. CMAJ 2007;176(8): 1097–9.

15. Hauvik LE, Varghese M, Nielsen EW. Lactate gap: a diagnostic support in severe metabolic acidosis of unknown origin. Case Rep Med 2018;2018:5238240.
16. Choy KW, Wijeratne N, Lu ZX, et al. Harmonisation of osmolal gap - can we use a common formula? Clin Biochem Rev 2016;37(3):113–9.
17. Smithline N, Gardner KD Jr. Gaps–anionic and osmolal. JAMA 1976;236(14): 1594–7.
18. Chabali R. Diagnostic use of anion and osmolal gaps in pediatric emergency medicine. Pediatr Emerg Care 1997;13(3):204–10.
19. Glasser L, Sternglanz PD, Combie J, et al. Serum osmolality and its applicability to drug overdose. Am J Clin Pathol 1973;60(5):695–9.
20. McQuillen KK, Anderson AC. Osmol gaps in the pediatric population. Acad Emerg Med 1999;6(1):27–30.
21. Aabakken L, Johansen KS, Rydningen EB, et al. Osmolal and anion gaps in patients admitted to an emergency medical department. Hum Exp Toxicol 1994; 13(2):131–4.
22. Bruns DE, Herold DA, Rodeheaver GT, et al. Polyethylene glycol intoxication in burn patients. Burns Incl Therm Inj 1982;9(1):49–52.
23. Rifai N, Horvath A, Wittwer C, editors. Clinical chemistry & molecular diagnostics. 6th edition. Elsevier, Inc.; 2018.
24. Flanagan RJ, Mant TG. Coma and metabolic acidosis early in severe acute paracetamol poisoning. Hum Toxicol 1986;5(3):179–82.
25. Dale C, Aulaqi AA, Baker J, et al. Assessment of a point-of-care test for paracetamol and salicylate in blood. QJM 2005;98(2):113–8.
26. Simpson D. Units for reporting the results of toxicological measurements. Ann Clin Biochem 1980;17(6):328–31.
27. Stellpflug SJ, Cole JB, Greller HA. Urine drug screens in the emergency department: the best test may be no test at all. J Emerg Nurs 2020;46(6):923–31.
28. Moeller KE, Lee KC, Kissack JC. Urine drug screening: practical guide for clinicians. Mayo Clin Proc 2008;83(1):66–76.
29. Medicare Coverage Database (MCD) - Local coverage determination (LCD): urine drug testing (L36037). CMS.gov. Available at: https://www.cms.gov/medicare-coverage-database/search.aspx. Accessed November 26, 2021.
30. Jialal I, Devaraj S. Laboratory diagnosis of ethylene glycol poisoning: the cup is half full? Am J Clin Pathol 2011;136(2):165–6.
31. Metushi I. Performing drug screening through high resolution mass spectrometry in the clinical laboratory: to implement or not? AACC Scientific shorts. American Association for Clinical Chemistry; 2017. Available at: https://www.aacc.org/science-and-research/scientific-shorts/2017/validation-of-a-broad-spectrum-drug-screening-method.
32. Christian MR, Lowry JA, Algren DA, et al. Do rapid comprehensive urine drug screens change clinical management in children? Clin Toxicol (Phila) 2017; 55(9):977–80.
33. McMillin GA, Slawson MH, Marin SJ, et al. Demystifying analytical approaches for urine drug testing to evaluate medication adherence in chronic pain management. J Pain Palliat Care Pharmacother 2013;27(4):322–39.

9780323848862